CARDIOVASCULAR
FLUID DYNAMICS

VOLUME 2

CARDIOVASCULAR
FLUID DYNAMICS

Edited by

D. H. BERGEL

Fellow of St. Catherine's College,
University Laboratory of Physiology, Oxford, England

VOLUME 2

1972

ACADEMIC PRESS

LONDON AND NEW YORK

ACADEMIC PRESS INC. (LONDON) LTD.
24/28 Oval Road,
London NW1

United States Edition published by
ACADEMIC PRESS INC.
111 Fifth Avenue
New York, New York 10003

Library of Congress Catalog Card Number: 79–185200
ISBN: 0–12–089902–7

PRINTED IN GREAT BRITAIN BY
THE WHITEFRIARS PRESS LIMITED
LONDON AND TONBRIDGE

List of Contributors

B. J. BELLHOUSE, *Magdalen College and Department of Engineering Science, Oxford, England.*

JAN E. W. BENEKEN, *Research Group on Cardiovascular Physics, Institute of Medical Physics TNO, Da Costakade, Utrecht, The Netherlands.*

D. H. BERGEL, *St. Catherine's College and University Laboratory of Physiology, Oxford, England.*

J. R. BLINKS, *Department of Physiology, Mayo Medical School, Rochester, Minnesota, U.S.A.*

*STANLEY E. CHARM, *Department of Physiology, Tufts University Medical School, Boston, Massachusetts, U.S.A.*

*GARY G. FERGUSON, *Department of Biophysics, Faculty of Medicine, University of Western Ontario, London, Ontario, Canada.*

*J. M. FITZ-GERALD, *Department of Mathematics, University of Queensland, St. Lucia, Brisbane, Australia.*

IVOR T. GABE, *M.R.C. Cardiovascular Research Unit and Department of Medicine, Hammersmith Hospital, London, England.*

U. GESSNER, *Department of Biomedical Engineering, Hoffmann-La Roche & Co., A.G., Basel, Switzerland.*

*B. S. GOW, *Department of Physiology, University of Sydney, Sydney, Australia.*

B. R. JEWELL, *Department of Physiology, University College, London, England.*

*G. S. KURLAND, *Department of Medicine, Beth Israel Hospital and Harvard Medical School, Boston, Massachusetts, U.S.A.*

*C. C. MICHEL, *The Queen's College and University Laboratory of Physiology, Oxford, England.*

CHRISTOPHER J. MILLS, *Cardiovascular Research Unit, Royal Postgraduate Medical School, London, England.*

*W. R. MILNOR, *Department of Physiology, Johns Hopkins University School of Medicine, Baltimore, Maryland, U.S.A.*

*DALI J. PATEL, *Section on Experimental Atherosclerosis, National Heart and Lung Institute, National Institutes of Health, Bethesda, Maryland, U.S.A.*

*MARGOT R. ROACH, *Departments of Biophysics and Medicine, University of Western Ontario, London, Ontario, Canada.*

K. SAGAWA, *Department of Biomedical Engineering, Johns Hopkins University School of Medicine, Baltimore, Maryland, U.S.A.*

D. L. SCHULTZ, *St. Catherine's College and Department of Engineering Science, Oxford, England.*

*R. SKALAK, *Department of Civil Engineering and Engineering Mechanics, Columbia University, New York, U.S.A.*

*RAMESH N. VAISHNAV, *Department of Civil and Mechanical Engineering, The Catholic University of America, Washington, D.C., U.S.A.*

.* Contributors to Volume 2.

Preface

The purpose of this book is to make available, in as concise and manageable a form as possible, the results of the intensive study of the fluid dynamics of the mammalian cardiovascular system undertaken in the previous decade. In the ten years that have elapsed since the publication of McDonald's monograph on "Blood Flow in Arteries", so much has been achieved that a new assessment is needed.

I hope that the various chapters will show what is the present situation in this field, and how this point has been reached through experimentation based on a proper understanding of the physical background. The methods and concepts used in this work will be only partly familiar to biologists, physicians and fluid dynamicists. It has been my intention to produce a book which will serve these specialists in introducing them to a very active field of experimental research and will allow them to enter it with a good understanding of the established physical and biological features of the fascinating cardiovascular system.

At this point it is customary for the editor to thank all those who have contributed to the work. I hope it will be clear that my expressions of thanks are a great deal more than conventional. My own contribution here has been quite modest, for although I have myself worked in many of the areas discussed, I have been aware that others are much better qualified now to deal with these subjects. It has been a great privilege to work with so large and varied a team and I can only hope that our friendship will survive the strain. I wish especially to thank all the Oxford authors, and also Dr. Colin Clark, whose continuing criticisms and suggestions have helped me greatly. Finally, the publishers, who have transformed a great heap of paper into what I hope is now a coherent whole; may they never regret the effort.

D. H. BERGEL

Oxford
October, 1972

Acknowledgements

Grateful acknowledgement is made to the following Journals and Publishers, and to the Authors, for permission to use the following figures and tables: Circulation Research and the American Heart Association Inc. for Figs. 21 and 26 in Chapter 5, Fig. 9 in Chapter 7, Figs. 2, 3, 4, 5, 11, 12 and Tables 1, 2, 3, 4 in Chapter 11, and Figs. 11, 13 and 14 in Chapter 12; *Acta Physiologica Scandinavica* for Fig. 7 in Chapter 7; *The American Journal of Physiology* for Figs. 10, 27, 28a and 28b in Chapter 5, Fig. 8 in Chapter 7, Figs. 8 and 9 in Chapter 12; *Pflügers Archiv* for Fig. 31 in Chapter 5; W. B. Saunders Company for Figs. 12, 24 and 25 in Chapter 5, and Figs. 9 and 10 in Chapter 6; Pergamon Press for Fig. 29 in Chapter 5; *The Journal of Applied Physiology* for Fig. 21 in Chapter 6; *Archives Internationales de Physiologie et Biochemie* for Fig. 29 in Chapter 5; The Federation of American Societies for Experimental Biology for Fig. 2 in Chapter 6; *The Journal of Physiology* for Fig. 1, and the Cambridge University Press for Fig. 4 in Chapter 7.

CONTENTS

Chapter 11

The Rheology of Large Blood Vessels

DALI J. PATEL and RAMESH N. VAISHNAV

Chapter 12

The Influence of Vascular Muscle on the Viscoelastic Properties of Blood Vessels

B. S. GOW

Chapter 13
Poststenotic Dilatation in Arteries
MARGOT R. ROACH

Chapter 14
Flow Conditions at Bifurcations as Determined in Glass Models, with Reference to the Focal Distribution of Vascular Lesions
GARY G. FERGUSON and MARGOT R. ROACH

Chapter 15
Blood Rheology
STANLEY E. CHARM and GEORGE S. KURLAND

Chapter 16
The Mechanics of Capillary Blood Flow
J. M. FITZ-GERALD

Chapter 17
Flows across the Capillary Wall
C. C. MICHEL

Chapter 18

Pulmonary Hemodynamics

WILLIAM R. MILNOR

Chapter 19

Synthesis of a Complete Circulation

RICHARD SKALAK

Glossary

Adventitia | The outermost coat of a blood vessel.

Aneurysm | A localized dilatation of an artery.

Angiogram | An X-ray picture in which the contents of the blood vessels have been rendered radio-opaque by the injection of a contrast medium.

Arteriole | The finest subdivision of the arterial tree, typically vessels of 100–200 μm in diameter. The walls are relatively muscular and variations in the activity of this muscle play a major part in the control of the circulation.

Arteries | The vessels carrying the blood from the left or right ventricles to the tissues.

Atherosclerosis, arteriosclerosis | Varieties of degenerative disease of the arteries. Atheroma is a fatty degeneration of the inner layers of an artery; in the early stages intimal plaques of atheromatous material may be visible.

Attenuation | See Decibel, Neper.

Baroreceptors | Areas of the vascular system which function as pressure receptors. Nerve endings in the vessel wall respond to its deformation. The most important systemic arterial baroreceptors are found in the arch of the aorta (near its origin) and near the point at which the carotid artery in the neck divides into two branches, at about the level of the angle of the jaw.

Blood | Blood is a suspension of cells in the fluid plasma. The cells comprise the red cells (erythrocytes), white cells (leucocytes) and the platelets (thrombocytes), the average numbers of each per mm^3 of blood being about 5×10^6, 10^4, and 3×10^5, respectively.

Bode plot | A diagram which presents the frequency response of a system as an amplitude ratio (gain) and the phase shift as functions of frequency, on a logarithmic scale. The unit of gain is the decibel where gain in dB = 20 log (output amplitude/input amplitude).
For a first-order system (q.v.) the gain is zero up to the corner frequency (q.v.) and falls thereafter with a slope of −20 dB/decade. The phase shift tends towards −90° (90° lag) at high frequencies and has a value of −45° at the corner frequency. For a second-order system the attenuation is −40 dB/decade and the maximal phase shift is −180°.

Boundary conditions | Known conditions at one or several of the boundaries of the physical process considered; they are in general required in order to obtain full solutions to the equations governing the process.

Boundary layer (viscous)   Usually a rather thin layer of fluid adjacent to a solid surface in which shear forces due to viscosity predominate and give rise to steep velocity gradients.

Capillary   The finest blood vessels, normally about 5–6 μm in diameter, and about 0·5 mm long in the systemic circulation.

Cavitation   The formation of cavities filled with vapour or gas within a moving liquid due to the local pressure being reduced to below the vapour pressure for the liquid.

Cervical rib   An abnormal small rib in the lower neck.

Coarctation   An isolated narrowing of an artery; generally refers to a congenital defect of the aorta.

Complex number   A complex number is an expression of the form $X = a + ib$, where a and b are real numbers, and i is the imaginary unit $\sqrt{(-1)}$. Such numbers are used to describe time varying quantities which are characterized by an amplitude or modulus ($M = (a^2 + b^2)^{\frac{1}{2}}$), together with a phase relationship with some time reference. They may be visualized as vectors in a Cartesian coordinate system. The projection on one axis has the value a and is termed the real part ($Re\ X$), the projection on the other axis is ib, the imaginary part (Im X). A real number, A, can be considered as a vector lying along the real axis, rotation by 90° will result in an imaginary number, iA, with no real part. A further rotation by 90° returns the vector to the real axis but it is reversed, i.e. $-A$. Thus if one rotation is indicated by multiplication by the imaginary operator i, two such rotations are equivalent to multiplying by -1; i can then be seen to be equal to $\sqrt{(-1)}$.

Compliance (distensibility)   A measure of the ability of a hollow structure to change its volume, generally the ratio of volume change to internal pressure change (dV/dP). The inverse of compliance is elastance.

Corner frequency (break frequency)   A frequency analogous to the resonant frequency of a mechanical system. For a first-order system the relation of the corner frequency to the time constant, τ, is $\tau = 1/\omega_0$. where ω_0 is the corner frequency in radians/second. In the electrical analog of a first-order system the product RC has the value $\omega_0/2\pi$.

Decibel (dB)   A logarithmic measure of the ratio between two quantities. The gain of a system may be expressed in dB, where gain = 20 log (output amplitude/input amplitude).

Diastole (atrial or ventricular)   The resting phase of the cardiac cycle.

Drag   A force induced on a solid surface by fluid moving past it, and in the direction of the fluid motion. Drag may be due to viscous shear forces alone, for example, on the

	wall of a pipe, or may also have a component due to relatively low pressures in the wake region behind an immersed body.
Elasticity	A measure of a material's resistance to deformation. See Modulus.
Electrocardiogram (E.C.G.)	A record of the electrical activity of the heart, normally obtained with electrodes on the skin.
Endothelium.	The layer of cells lining the blood vessels.
Energy (ML^2T^{-2})	Unit energy or work is that exchanged when unit force acts through unit displacement in the direction of the force. One joule is the work done when one newton acts through one metre. $(J = 10^7$ ergs.)
First-order delay (or lag) system	A system whose input-output relationships are those of a parallel resistance-capacitance unit (time constant $= RC$). As such a system is excited with an input of increasing frequency the output becomes reduced and lags progressively with a maximal lag of 90°. The performance of a first-order system depends both on the input function and its first time-differential.
Force (MLT^{-2})	Unit force is that which gives unit acceleration to unit mass. One newton gives an acceleration of 1 m s^{-2} to 1 kg, one dyne gives an acceleration of 1 cm s^{-2} to 1 g. Unit force (gravitational) is the force of gravitation on unit mass in the locality in question and is therefore expressed in mass units. Thus a mass of M grams is attracted to the earth with a force of M grams weight which is equal to Mg dynes, where g is the local acceleration due to gravity in cm s^{-2}. The accepted value for g is $9 \cdot 80665$ m s^{-2}.
Haematocrit	The relative volume of the cells in blood, normally about 45 per cent.
Heart	The mammalian heart consists of four chambers, right and left atria, right and left ventricles. The atria are thin walled chambers into which blood flows at low pressure from the veins. Between atria and ventricles are the tricuspid (right) and mitral (left) valves. Blood at high pressure leaves the ventricles by the pulmonary artery (right) and aorta (left); there are valves at the origin of each of these. The blood supply to the heart itself comes from the coronary arteries which spring from the aorta at its origin. Normally both atria beat together a short time before the synchronous beat of the ventricles.
Histology	The microscopic study of tissue structure.
Hookean material	An ideally elastic material for which tensile stress is proportional to strain, i.e. the Young's modulus, E, is constant.
Hypertension, pulmonary or systemic	A condition in which the arterial blood pressure is abnormally high (cf. hypotension, which is low pressure).

Intima	The innermost coat of a blood vessel, comprises the endothelium and a thin connective tissue layer.
Isometric contraction	One in which no change of muscle length is allowed to occur.
Isotonic contraction	One in which the load on the muscle is constant.
Impedance (Z, electrical, acoustic, mechanical, hydraulic)	The resistance to disturbance of a system or material. It is measured as the complex ratio of a force (voltage, pressure, stress) to the resulting change (current, fluid flow, strain) at a specified frequency. An impedance plot shows the impedance as a function of frequency. The hydraulic input impedance is the complex ratio of pressure to flow at the input to a hydraulic system, e.g. the root of the aorta or pulmonary artery, and is both a function of frequency and of position.
Inertia	In fluid flows inertia is represented by the property density and is the force required to accelerate fluid particles, provided by a pressure gradient.
Inlet length (entrance length)	The region of a pipe or channel near the inflow point, in which the thickness of the boundary layer progressively increases. At the end of this region, where the final velocity profile is established, the flow is said to be fully developed.
Karman trail (or vortex steet)	A regular series of fluid vortices in a wake region, in which alternate eddies rotate with opposite sense.
Kinetic energy	The energy associated with the velocity of a material particle or system, and is given by: $\frac{1}{2}$ (speed)^2 per unit mass.
Laminar flow	In laminar pipe flow the fluid velocity remains constant on cylindrical surfaces within the fluid which are concentric with the axis. The flow is well ordered and stable and can be considered as individual cylindrical laminae of fluid sliding over each other.
Laplace transform	The Laplace transform of a function is expressed by an integral formula. This enables the algebraic solution of linear differential equations in terms of initial conditions. For fuller details the reader is referred to the textbooks listed in the references to Chapter 5.
Media	The middle coat of a blood vessel, generally the thickest. It contains the fibrous proteins elastin and collagen, and smooth muscle.
Modulus	The real part of a complex number. Such a number can be visualized as a vector whose length is the modulus and whose angle with the real axis is its phase.
Modulus, of elasticity	A measure of the resistance to deformation of a material, the stress (force/unit area, $ML^{-1}T^{-2}$) required to cause unit strain. The three moduli are the tensile modulus (Young's modulus, E), the shear modulus (G) and the bulk modulus (modulus of compressibility, K).
Murmur (bruit)	An abnormal sound heard over a blood vessel or the heart.

Muscle	Three broad types of muscle are distinguished. Skeletal or striated muscle is normally used for conscious movement and is that commonly referred to as "muscle". Cardiac muscle is the muscle forming the walls of the cardiac chambers. Smooth muscle is a broad term describing the muscle, normally not under voluntary control, which is contained in the walls of the alimentary canal, blood vessels, and other structures. Papillary muscles are strands of cardiac muscle which support the mitral and tricuspid valves and are convenient for studies on the properties of cardiac muscle.
Myocardium	The muscle of the heart.
Neper	A measure of attenuation. If a wave attenuates with distance travelled (L) as $\exp(-\alpha L)$, the attenuation is α nepers/unit length.
Nerva vasorum	The nerves that supply the wall of a blood vessel.
Newtonian fluid	One in which the ratio of shear stress to shear strain is constant.
Nyquist diagram	An alternative to the Bode plot (q.v.) for plotting the frequency response of a system. The transfer function is plotted as a vector with its amplitude representing the gain and the angle with the real axis as the phase shift. The locus of the vector tips at different frequencies is the Nyquist plot. By convention, for a negative feedback system the phase delay at zero frequency is plotted as zero degrees rather than as $-180°$. Thus a delay on this diagram of 180° represents a difference of 360° between input and output. If the plot shows a gain >1 at a phase shift of 180° then the system is likely to be unstable and go into feedback oscillations at the frequency at which the 180° phase shift line is crossed.
Peripheral resistance	The ratio of the mean pressure drop across a circulatory bed to the mean flow through it.
Phonocatheter	A catheter bearing a small microphone for the recording of intravascular sounds.
Plethysmograph	A device for measuring the volume changes of an organ or part of the body.
Polycythaemia	An abnormal increase in the number of red cells in blood.
Potential energy	The energy associated with position in a gravitational field relative to some datum level at which the potential energy may arbitrarily be set equal to zero.
Power $(M\,L^2\,T^{-3})$	Unit power is that rate of doing work in which unit energy is exchanged in unit time. 1 watt (W) is 1 J s^{-1}.
Power, hydraulic	The energy flux associated with a given flow and having, in general, "pressure", kinetic and potential components.
Pressure $(M\,L^{-1}\,T^{-2})$	A measure of the force per unit area exerted by a fluid. The SI unit of pressure is one newton/sq. metre $(N\,m^{-2})$ or one pascal (pa). This is equal to 10 dynes cm^{-2}. The

	conventional millimetre of mercury (mmHg) is equal to $13 \cdot 5951 \times 980 \cdot 665 \times 10^{-2}$ N m^{-2}. One Torr is equal to 1 mmHg to within 2×10^{-7} Torr. One bar is 10^5 N m^{-2}.
Pressure gradient	The pressure drop per unit length along a flow channel.
Pressure, static	The pressure measured in still fluid; ideally that also measured in flowing fluid with a device sensitive only to the force perpendicular to the direction of flow. The dynamic pressure is that measured with a device sensitive to force parallel to the direction of flow, and is different from the static pressure by the quantity $\frac{1}{2}\rho V^2$ where ρ is the fluid density and V the local velocity vector.
Pressure, transmural	The difference in pressure between the inside and outside of a hollow structure.
Radian (r or rad)	A measure of angle. An angle of $360°$ is equal to 2π radians, thus 1 r $= 57 \cdot 34°$, $1° = 0 \cdot 017453$ r.
Reynolds number (Re)	An important dimensionless group in fluid mechanics defined as the product of a characteristic length and flow speed divided by the kinematic viscosity of the fluid. The magnitude of the number represents the relative importance of inertia forces compared with viscous forces.
Sarcomere	The functional unit of a fibre of striated muscle.
Sarcoplasm	The material in which the contractile apparatus of a muscle cell is embedded.
Second-order system	A system whose transfer function depends on terms up to the second time-differential of the input. Such properties are shown, for example, by a mechanical system containing elements with frictional, elastic and inertial properties.
Stenosis	A narrowing of a blood vessel or of a valve.
Strain	A measure of the deformation of a material relative to some reference dimension. Tensile and volumetric strains are changes in length (along some defined axis) and in volume, respectively. Shear strain refers to a relative displacement of material elements in two parallel planes in a direction within the planes.
Stream function	A measure of the flux of fluid volume; it remains constant along streamlines. Velocity components may be computed as appropriate derivatives of the stream function.
Stress ($M L^{-1} T^{-2}$)	A measure of the deforming force applied to a material, the units are force/unit area.
Surfactant, pulmonary	A material lining the finest air spaces of the lungs, the alveoli, which is normally present and which lowers the surface tension at the air–fluid interface.
Sympathomimetic drug	A drug whose action is similar to that produced by stimulation of the sympathetic nervous system, this being generally an increase in the rate and force of cardiac contraction and an increase in the peripheral

vascular resistance. Catecholamines are a chemically defined group of sympathomimetic agents including adrenalin and noradrenalin.

Systemic circulation	The circulation to the body, the term excludes the pulmonary circulation which contains the gas-exchanging pulmonary capillaries.
Systole (atrial or ventricular)	The active part of the cardiac cycle.
Transportation lag (dead time, latency)	If there is a time lag, L, between an input signal change and the alteration in the output the system is said to have a transportation lag. This is often represented in control system engineering by the transfer function $\exp(-sL)$ where s is the Laplace operator.
Transfer function	The transfer function of a control system (or subsystem) is the ratio of the Laplace transforms of its output and input, and so characterizes the response of the system.
Turbulence	Turbulent flows are characterized by random fluctuations of the fluid motions which cannot be predicted in detail. These fluctuations may be superimposed upon a particular average direction of flow as occurs, for example, in pipe flow. This feature is due to the inherent instability of the flow, i.e. induced disturbances will grow with time whereas, in laminar flow, such disturbances would be damped out.
Vasa vasorum	The blood vessels that supply the walls of the larger blood vessels.
Vasomotor control system	A term describing the physiological mechanisms, both nervous and endocrine, which alter the hydraulic resistance of the vascular bed. This is brought about by changes in the activity of the muscle in the vessel walls, thereby altering the size of the vascular lumen.
Veins	The vessels carrying blood from the tissues to the atria of the heart.
Venomotor control system	The physiological control system whereby the compliance of the veins, and hence the volume of contained blood, may be altered by changes in the activity of the muscles in their walls.
Viscoelasticity	A viscoelastic material is one in which both the strain (elastic response) and the rate of strain (viscous response) are functions of the imposed stress.
Viscosity ($M L^{-1}T^{-1}$)	The property of resisting deformation in a fluid, it gives rise to tangential or shear stresses. Kinematic viscosity is the dynamic viscosity divided by density and can be considered as the diffusion coefficient governing the transport of molecular momentum within a fluid. The units of viscosity are the poise (P) and the centipoise (cP), one poise is the viscosity of that material which requires unit shear stress (1 dyne cm^{-2}) to maintain a shear velocity gradient of 1 (cm s^{-1} cm^{-1}) or

Windkessel $1\,s^{-1}$. The SI unit of viscosity is the newton second per sq. metre ($N\,s\,m^{-2}$) and is equal to 10 poise. The unit of kinematic viscosity is the Stoke (St). ($1\,St = 10^{-4}$ $m^2\,s^{-1}$.)

Windkessel · A term used by Otto Frank in 1899 to describe the elastic reservoir function of the aorta. In the simple windkessel theory the systemic bed was modelled as an elastic reservoir connected to a peripheral hydraulic resistance.

Zero-order system (zero-memory system) · A system in which the output follows the input with no lag. The electrical analogue is an ohmic resistance.

Contents of Volume 1

To Nicolette, Timothy, Stephen, Oliver
and Matthew; with great love

Chapter 11

The Rheology of Large Blood Vessels†

DALI J. PATEL

Section on Experimental Atherosclerosis,
National Heart and Lung Institute, National Institutes of Health,
Bethesda, Maryland 20014, U.S.A.

and

RAMESH N. VAISHNAV

Department of Civil and Mechanical Engineering,
The Catholic University of America,
Washington, D.C. 20017, U.S.A.

† Part of this material was presented by Dr. Patel at the 91st Winter Annual Meeting of the American Society of Mechanical Engineers, December 1970.

1

1. INTRODUCTION

Knowledge of mechanical properties of the blood vessels has long been recognized as an important aspect of the understanding of the behavior of the cardiovascular system. For instance, in 1808 Thomas Young described a relation between vessel elasticity and circulatory hemodynamics. Most of the subsequent work done in this area prior to 1960 has been summarized by Bergel (1960), McDonald (1960), Burton (1962) and Hardung (1962); it still represents a useful approximation to the true state of affairs. However, during the last decade systematic approaches have been made to progressively more complicated and realistic characterization of the mechanical properties of blood vessels. Typical examples of these are: Patel *et al.* (1960); Peterson *et al.* (1960); Bergel (1961a,b); Fry *et al.* (1962); Patel *et al.* (1962); Remington (1963); Patel *et al.* (1964); Patel and Fry (1964); Wiener *et al.* (1966); Apter (1967); Iberall (1967); Lee *et al.* (1967); Tickner and Sacks (1967); Apter and Marquez (1968); Anliker *et al.* (1968); Atabek (1968); Attinger (1968); Attinger *et al.* (1968); Cox (1968); Gow and Taylor (1968); Blatz *et al.* (1969); Patel (1969); Patel *et al.* (1969); Apter *et al.* (1970); Azuma *et al.* (1970); Dobrin and Doyle (1970).

This recent upsurge in research activity was motivated by a need to answer questions that have arisen in a number of areas which require a more detailed and realistic picture of vascular rheology. For example: (1) An intelligent design of vascular prostheses or artificial organs should include detailed consideration of vascular architecture and rheology. (2) Any meaningful approach to the analysis of pulse contours or other circulatory variables for diagnostic or therapeutic purposes requires accurate knowledge of the principal rheologic parameters of the blood vessel. (3) Vascular 'rheology may be intimately related to degenerative vascular diseases. It is well recognized that the elastic properties of the arterial tree change significantly with the aging process; the artery becomes dilated, non-uniform, less compliant, and elongated, occasionally to the extent that it may assume a kinked and tortuous course. (4) Finally, recent evidence (Fry, 1969) indicates that the permeability and the integrity of the endothelial surface are sensitive to adjacent hydrodynamic events, such as existence of high shearing stress and high frequency components of turbulence and that the underlying cause of vessel damage in these cases is an increase in the strain energy density at the intimal layer of the vessel wall. The magnitude of the strain energy density is determined among other things by the geometry and rheology of the vessel wall. It thus becomes necessary to re-examine the older data and concepts of vascular rheology in light of these modern needs.

In this chapter, we plan to review some of the more recent concepts that have been developed in our laboratory in the past decade. The theoretical concepts together with experimental data supporting these will be presented. Pertinent results from various other laboratories will also be discussed; however, it is important to point out that no attempt will be made to cover systematically all the literature in the field. Limiting the discussion to large blood vessels such as the aorta, we may say that the relevant work done in this area can be classified into four basic types:

A. EXPERIMENTAL VERIFICATION OF BASIC ASSUMPTIONS CONCERNING GENERAL MATERIAL PROPERTIES

The first type includes works concentrating on the general properties of the aortic wall material. These include the work of Carew et al. (1968) establishing that the arterial wall is incompressible, and of Patel and Fry (1969) establishing the curvilinearly orthotropic nature of the aorta. These general properties considerably simplify the subsequent theoretical treatment of material properties in a realistic manner.

B. LONGITUDINAL TETHERING OF THE AORTA

The second type of work considers the role of vascular tethering in aortic mechanics. Blood vessels in situ are attached (tethered) to the surrounding tissues. Vascular tethering plays such an important role in influencing the mechanical behavior of the blood vessel that no rheological study would be complete without taking tethering into account (Womersley, 1957a, b). Although tethering restrains the motion of the blood vessel wall in all directions, it is relatively stronger in the longitudinal direction. Therefore we have included a discussion on longitudinal vascular tethering as examined by Patel and Fry (1966).

C. INCREMENTAL VISCOELASTIC PROPERTIES

The third type of work deals with the mechanical properties of the aorta from the incremental point of view. In this approach one recognizes the non-linear character of the aortic material response but attempts to characterize the material properties in the linear regime sufficiently close to a chosen state of deformation. Such work is typified by the work of Patel *et al.* (1969) which considers the anisotropic nature of the incremental response of the aortic wall.

D. NON-LINEAR ELASTIC PROPERTIES

Finally, the fourth type of work attacks head on the problem of characterizing the non-linear behavior of the blood vessel wall (Vaishnav *et al.*, 1972; Young, 1970). In such an approach, the incremental properties result from a postulated constitutive relation which may then be experimentally validated.

2. EXPERIMENTAL VERIFICATION OF BASIC ASSUMPTIONS CONCERNING GENERAL MATERIAL PROPERTIES

It is essential here as elsewhere to make definite simplifying assumptions in developing a theory so that the mathematics and physics remain tractable. However, it is very important to keep these assumptions constantly in sight and whenever possible to verify them experimentally since the theory applies to the real situation only to the extent that the various assumptions are valid. The theoretical structure can be improved progressively as newer, more refined experimental procedures become available. The assumptions made in developing the theory of mechanical behavior of large arteries will be discussed in detail in this section and whenever possible their experimental basis will be presented.

A. HOMOGENEITY

Throughout this article the analysis is based on the assumption of homogeneity, i.e. that the observed mechanical properties of a small volume of the arterial wall at one place can be considered to have mechanical properties identical with those of one taken from another place. Histologically, an arterial segment can be considered to have reasonably uniform structure in the longitudinal and circumferential directions, but not in the radial direction (Wolinsky and Glagov, 1964, 1967). Therefore, the wall properties may be considered uniform at least in the longitudinal and the circumferential directions. Since in most experiments on an artery, measurements are based on uniform states of stress and strain, the results will be relatively more accurate for the longitudinal and the circumferential directions in the local sense also, but not for the radial direction; in the radial direction they will reflect only the average properties. However for many practical applications, such as the study of pressure-volume relationships, or the propagation of pressure waves, only the average properties of the blood vessel wall are relevant, and the results obtained using the homogeneity assumption are valid.

Another implication of the assumption of homogeneity is that no distinction is made between the contributions made by the different constituents of the wall such as elastin and collagen. When the overall mechanical behavior is the property of interest this implication is unimportant. However, a more detailed understanding of the deformational response would require knowledge of the separate contributions of elastin and collagen fibers to the total response. In this connection we mention the work of Roach and Burton (1957), who studied the effects of differential digestion of collagen and elastin on the elastic properties of human iliac arteries. They concluded that the resistance to stretch at low pressures was almost entirely due to elastin fibers, that at physiological pressures it was due to both collagen and elastin fibers, and that at high pressures it was almost entirely due to collagen fibers.

B. CYLINDRICALITY AND THINNESS OF ARTERIAL SEGMENT

Here we shall be concerned with a segment of the canine middle descending thoracic aorta, approximately 8 cm long, having a small longitudinal taper (the difference in end diameters being 1 to 2 mm). We shall treat the segment as a thin circular cylindrical tube of constant thickness. Although at a very low intravascular pressure the cross section of the segment may not be circular, it assumes an essentially circular shape with more or less uniform thickness as the intravascular pressure is raised. Moreover, the ratio of the midwall radius R and the wall thickness h is essentially constant along the length of the segment (Bergel, 1960). It will be seen later that the circumferential and longitudinal stresses due to the intraluminal pressure depend essentially on the R/h ratio only.

The consequences of the assumption of thinness can be analyzed as follows. Let us refer a cylindrical arterial segment of length L, midwall radius R and wall thickness h, to a cylindrical coordinate system (see Fig. 1) such that the z axis coincides with the center line of the lumen. We shall frequently use the term "physiologic loading" to mean an axially symmetric loading consisting of an intraluminal pressure p, a pair of equal and opposite longitudinal forces F applied axially on opposite ends, and distributed inertial forces proportional to local accelerations. Frequently, we shall talk about the static case wherein the inertial forces will not appear. Such a loading will cause in the segment a state of stress consisting of only the three normal stresses, S_r (radial), S_θ (circumferential) and S_z (longitudinal). In the absence of inertial forces, non-uniformity of material properties and end-effects, these stresses will be uniform along the θ and z directions but will vary along the r direction due to the circular geometry of the cross section;

the exact variation will depend upon the stress-strain relation for the material. If the segment is considered thin-walled, then the stresses can be taken to be uniform through the thickness of the segment and can be obtained using the following formulae:

$$S_\theta = p \left(\frac{R}{h} - \tfrac{1}{2} \right) \tag{2.1}$$

$$S_z = \frac{p}{2} \left(\frac{R}{h} - 1 \right) + F/2\pi R h \tag{2.2}$$

$$S_r = -p/2 \tag{2.3}$$

Equation 2.1 for S_θ can be obtained by imagining a longitudinal bisecting cut in the arterial segment and equating the force due to the intraluminal pressure p acting over the area $2(R-h/2)L$ of the interior surface projected on the diametral plane and dividing by the area $2hL$ opened up by the cut and over which S_θ is acting. Equation (2.2) for S_z can be derived in a similar manner by imagining a transverse cut in the segment. The total longitudinal force acting on the cross section is $p\pi(R-h/2)^2 + F$, the first term being due to the intraluminal pressure when the segment is capped at the ends and the second being the additional force due to longitudinal tethering, instrument restraint, or other such source. Division by the wall cross-sectional area $2\pi R h$, after neglecting a very small quantity $ph/8R$, yields the desired formula (2.2). The value of the radial stress from (2.3) is simply the average of the pressures on the inner and outer surfaces.

In engineering practice it is customary to consider a tube to be thin-walled if the ratio R/h is approximately 10 or larger (McDonald, 1960). For the segments of the descending thoracic aorta that we are concerned with, R/h is between 8 and 10 in physiologic range of strain (Patel et al., 1969). Similar values for other arteries are also obtained, e.g. Bergel (1961a) has reported R/h values of 9·9, 8·2 and 7·1 for the thoracic aorta, and the femoral and the carotid arteries, respectively at a pressure of 136 cm H_2O. Thus, (2.1) to (2.3) obtained using the assumption of a thin vessel wall can be applied to an aortic segment with reasonable confidence. The degree of error incurred by assuming its wall to be thin cannot be simply evaluated as it depends on the constitutive relation of the material. However, some insight can be gained by a systematic reduction of the well-known Lamé formulas (Timoshenko and Goodier, 1970) for a pressurized thick-walled cylinder of an isotropic, linearly elastic material. We shall dispense with the details of calculations and point out that, in this case, the assumption of uniform distribution through the thickness causes a maximum error of $50h/R$ per cent in the circumferential stress. For $R/h = 8$, this is an error of about 6 per cent.

Equations (2.1) and (2.2) can be further simplified by neglecting, in the parentheses, the terms $\frac{1}{2}$ and 1, respectively, since $R/h \gg 1$. This leads to the formulae

$$S_\theta = pR/h \tag{2.4}$$

$$S_z = pR/2h + F/2\pi Rh \tag{2.5}$$

$$S_r = -p/2 \tag{2.6}$$

Equations (2.4) and (2.5) are not as accurate as (2.1) and (2.2), but are very frequently used in view of their simplicity.

C. INCOMPRESSIBILITY

(1) General remarks

Rubber-like materials, i.e. solids capable of undergoing large deformations, show, in general, a very low degree of compressibility. In other words, they resist volume changes to a much higher degree than they do shape changes. Thus, for a majority of practical applications, their resistance to change in volume can be considered infinite, i.e. these materials are incompressible, and if this is true for arteries it would simplify both the theoretical considerations and the experimental work.

Several investigators have reported experimental findings on the compressibility of the arterial wall. For example, Lawton (1954) found excised aortic strips to remain isovolumic under varying degrees of stretch. Dobrin and Rovick (1969) reported similar conclusions from experiments on canine carotid arteries. As will be seen later, this information *per se* is not enough to establish the validity of the incompressibility assumption. Moreover, Tickner and Sacks (1967) came to the opposite conclusion. Their findings were based on the measurement of wall thickness from X-ray photographs, a method of questionable accuracy. Carew *et al.* (1968) considered the problem in greater depth and reported definitive findings on the degree of compressibility of the arterial tissue, and concluded that under physiologic states of stress, the assumption of incompressibility can safely be made.

(2) The notion of incompressibility

An ideally incompressible material, by definition, preserves its volume under all states of stress.† Whereas all materials can undergo isochoric (volume-preserving) deformations, an ideally incompressible material can undergo only isochoric deformations. From a molecular standpoint it is easy to see that no real material can be ideally incompressible; however, the

---

† We exclude here volume changes associated with thermal and other non-mechanical phenomena.

notion of such a material is very useful in the study of materials whose mechanical behavior can be approximated by that of an ideally in-compressible material under certain circumstances.

This will be clarified if we use the concepts of hydrostatic (or isotropic) and deviatoric stress and strain, e.g. see Attinger (1964). An arbitrary state of stress can be represented as a sum of two states of stress: hydrostatic and deviatoric. As the name implies, the hydrostatic state of stress is like the state of stress in a body submerged in a fluid at rest. In a body in a hydrostatic state of stress, the stress on all planes is simply tensile or compressive, and is the same on all planes. The part of the state of stress that remains after subtracting the hydrostatic part is called the deviatoric stress. When the state of strain in an infinitesimally strained continuum is decomposed in a similar manner into a hydrostatic (or volumetric) and a deviatoric part, the former is a measure of change in volume per unit volume and the latter is a measure of the change of shape in a certain sense. In an isotropic, linearly elastic body, the ratios of the hydrostatic and the deviatoric parts of the states of stress to the corres-ponding parts of the strain are independent of the amount of strain and define two independent material constants. Specifically, the ratio of the hydrostatic part of the stress to the volumetric strain (which is three times the hydro-static part of the strain) is called the bulk modulus of elasticity and the ratio of one half of the deviatoric part of the stress to the deviatoric part of the strain is called the modulus of rigidity or the shear modulus. The bulk modulus and the shear modulus form a pair of elastic moduli which can be used to characterize a material instead of the familiar pair of constants, namely, Young's modulus and Poisson's ratio. For an ideally incompressible isotropic, linearly elastic material the bulk modulus is infinitely large and Poisson's ratio equals $\frac{1}{2}$. For such a material, all the strain is deviatoric and thus the deviatoric stress alone is determined by the strain. The hydrostatic stress is determined from the knowledge of the boundary values of the stress. The degree to which a given isotropic, linearly elastic material approaches to incompressibility can be quantified by the ratio of the bulk modulus to the shear modulus or even the ratio of the bulk modulus to Young's modulus. The value of the bulk modulus, *per se*, is no indication of the compressibility of a given material. For example, the bulk modulus of water is $2 \cdot 18 \times 10^{10}$ dynes cm^{-2} and that of steel is $12 \cdot 8 \times 10^{11}$ dynes cm^{-2} but as the correspond-ing shear moduli are approximately zero and $8 \cdot 11 \times 10^{11}$ dynes cm^{-2}, respectively, water can be considered incompressible in most applications but steel cannot. On the other hand, when responses to a purely hydrostatic stress of a given magnitude are compared, both the materials are compressible, steel being less so. Whereas this discussion relates to isotropic, linearly elastic bodies, the basic ideas apply to the study of incompressibility of the arterial tissue.

Thus, whether an arterial tissue can be considered as incompressible or not is determined by subjecting it to a known state of stress which is neither predominantly hydrostatic nor deviatoric, and comparing the relative magnitudes of the hydrostatic and deviatoric parts of the associated strain. We outline below study by Carew *et al.* (1968), which was carried out with this in mind.

(3) *Methods and results*

Studies were carried out on 11 segments from the descending thoracic aorta of eight dogs. First, the *in vivo* length of the segment and the arterial pressure were measured and then segments from the upper and lower descending thoracic aorta were excised. Finally, after completion of the experiment, the unstretched midwall radius, R_o, length, L_o, and tissue volume, V_o, were determined.

A typical experiment was carried out in two steps: (1) The segment was filled with saline and submerged in a saline-filled flask designed specifically for the measurement of the changes in the volume of the vessel wall associated with straining of the vessel. The segment was stretched to a length above that of the *in vivo* length and pressurized to above the *in vivo* pressure. The change in wall volume, ΔV, was then measured as the segment returned to the unstressed state. (2) Another experiment was carried out, outside the flask, to determine the value of hydrostatic stress, S_h, for the amount of stretch applied in step 1. The vessel was stretched and held between two legs of a force gauge (Janicki and Patel, 1968) at the same length and pressure as before. Thus the longitudinal force, F, needed in addition to that due to intraluminal pressure, p, was determined. From these measurements the various stresses were calculated using (2.4) to (2.6). The hydrostatic stress S_h, was calculated as

$$S_h = \tfrac{1}{3}(S_r + S_\theta + S_z). \tag{2.7}$$

From the values obtained for S_h, ΔV and V_o, the bulk modulus, k, of the arterial wall was computed as

$$k = \frac{S_h}{\Delta V / V_o}. \tag{2.8}$$

The bulk modulus is thus the hydrostatic stress required to cause unit volumetric strain.

The results are summarized in Table 1. S_d is the magnitude of the deviatoric stress and is computed as the square root of the sum of the squares of the three differences between the principal stresses S_θ, S_z and S_r, namely, $S_\theta - S_z$, $S_z - S_r$, and $S_\theta - S_r$. Note that the hydrostatic stress, S_h, is of the same order of magnitude as the deviatoric stress, S_d, and that the bulk modulus, k, has

TABLE 1

Summary of data to demonstrate incompressibility of the arterial tissue

$(\Delta L/L_o) \times 100$	40
$(\Delta R/R_o) \times 100$	70
p (cm H_2O)	246
S_θ (dynes $cm^{-2} \times 10^6$)	2·72
S_z (dynes $cm^{-2} \times 10^6$)	2·70
S_r (dynes $cm^{-2} \times 10^6$)	−0·12
S_h (dynes $cm^{-2} \times 10^6$)	1·76
S_d (dynes $cm^{-2} \times 10^6$)	4·00
k (dynes $cm^{-2} \times 10^9$)	4·35

Average values for 11 segments from the descending aorta are shown. $\Delta L/L_o$ and $\Delta R/R_o$ are the longitudinal and circumferential strains; S_θ, S_z and S_r are the circumferential, longitudinal and radial stresses; S_h and S_d are the hydrostatic and deviatoric stresses; k is the bulk modulus; and p is intravascular pressure. (Adapted from Carew *et al.*, 1968.)

the high value $4·35 \times 10^9$ dynes cm^{-2}. Before assigning a proper meaning to this value of k one needs to consider two questions: (1) How much is ΔV affected by the possibility of influx or outflux of water as the arterial wall is deformed during an experiment? Carew *et al.* (1968), conducted supplementary experiments to provide semiquantitative evidence that this factor did not invalidate their results. (2) Do the results justify assuming the arterial tissue to be incompressible? To answer this one needs to compare the value $4·35 \times 10^9$ dynes cm^{-2} obtained for k with a representative value of shear modulus for the tissue. Taking a value of Young's modulus from Bergel's (1961a) data as $4·3 \times 10^6$ dynes cm^{-2}, one then finds the approximate value of the shear modulus, G, as one-third of Young's modulus or $1·4 \times 10^6$ dynes cm^{-2}. Thus the k/G ratio is approximately 3000, indeed large compared to unity. Thus for most applications, where the state of stress is not predominantly hydrostatic, the arterial wall can be considered to be incompressible. It can be shown (Carew *et al.*, 1968) that in physiologic states of stress the hydrostatic and deviatoric parts are of the same order of magnitude, and thus the assumption of incompressibility in the study of an arterial segment under physiologic loading is justified.

D. CURVILINEAR ORTHOTROPY

(1) *General remarks*

To determine the constitutive relation of a material, one has to hypothesize the nature of symmetry of the material response. The higher the degree of symmetry of material response, the smaller the number of independent constitutive parameters necessary to describe it; the lower the degree of symmetry, the larger the number of independent constitutive parameters required to characterize the material. If a material does not have a certain kind of symmetry but the experimentor erroneously assumes that it has, then the predictions based on the theory could be erroneous. On the other hand, if the material symmetry is overlooked, a part of the experimental effort is redundant and the true constitutive parameters get disguised in a larger set of interdependent parameters. It is thus important, if possible, to define by means of preliminary experiments, the exact degree of material symmetry exhibited by a material before launching a more involved program to determine the constitutive parameters.

The preceding remarks will be explained in more specific terms by considering the material symmetry of the arterial tissue. For simplicity, in this section, the arterial wall will be considered to be linearly elastic. Consider

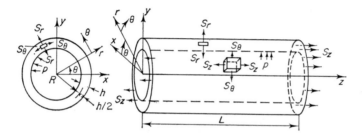

FIG. 1. A thin cylindrical arterial segment referred to a cylindrical coordinate system (r, θ, z); $p =$ intraluminal pressure; $S_\theta, S_z, S_r =$ circumferential, longitudinal and radial stresses; $R, L, h =$ midwall radius, length and wall thickness of the segment, respectively.

an arterial segment in the form of a thin-walled circular cylinder referred to a polar cylindrical co-ordinate system (r, θ, z) as shown in Fig. 1. Let us isolate, for purposes of discussion, an infinitesimal element bounded by the co-ordinate surfaces, i.e. two radial planes, two transverse planes and two concentric cylinders. The state of stress on this element will, in general, consist of six components: three normal stresses S_r, S_θ, S_z perpendicular to the faces of the element and three shear stresses $S_{\theta z} = S_{z\theta}$, $S_{zr} = S_{rz}$ and $S_{r\theta} = S_{\theta r}$. (For a shear stress, e.g. $S_{z\theta}$, the first subscript, z, indicates that the shear stress is acting on a plane perpendicular to the z axis and the second subscript, θ, indicates the direction in which it is acting.) The state of strain for this element will in general consist of three elongating (or contracting) strains γ_r, γ_θ and γ_z and three shearing strains $\gamma_{z\theta}$, γ_{rz} and $\gamma_{r\theta}$. (The shearing strain $\gamma_{z\theta}$ denotes the change, due to deformation, in the angle between the line elements initially in the θ and z directions; physically, this represents twisting of the tube. Similarly, the shearing strain $\gamma_{r\theta}$ is due to the circumferential movement of the outer cylindrical surface relative to the inner cylindrical surface, and γ_{rz} represents the axial movement of the outer cylindrical surface relative to the inner one. These shearing strains are illustrated in Fig. 2.)

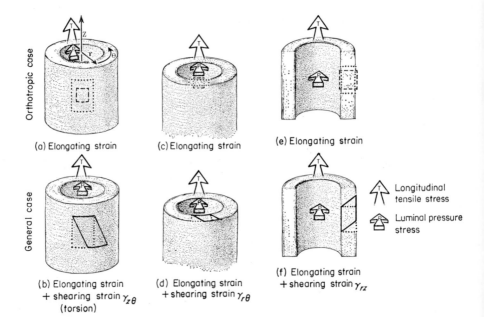

(a) Elongating strain

(c) Elongating strain

(e) Elongating strain

Orthotropic case

General case

(b) Elongating strain
+ shearing strain $\gamma_{z\theta}$
(torsion)

(d) Elongating strain
+ shearing strain $\gamma_{r\theta}$

(f) Elongating strain
+ shearing strain γ_{rz}

Longitudinal tensile stress

Luminal pressure stress

FIG. 2. Schematic drawing of an arterial segment under physiologic loading. Under such loading only normal stresses exist on the planes perpendicular to the r, θ and z axes, i.e. shearing stresses on these planes are zero. The broken lines indicate the position of the particles in the unstressed state, and the dotted lines indicate the position of the same particles in the stressed state. For the orthotropic case, only elongating (or contracting) strains develop as shown in (a), (c) and (e). In the general anisotropic case, superimposed shearing strains develop as indicated by the solid lines in (b), (d) and (f). The subscripts for the shearing strains are used in the following sense: $\gamma_{r\theta}$ implies change in the angle between two line elements initially in the r and θ directions. (From Patel and Fry, 1969.)

If the arterial segment has no elastic symmetry then a state of stress with only one non-zero component would produce all six types of strains. Conversely, any attempt to produce a single type of elongating or shearing strain will call for a state of stress in which all six components are non-zero. Thus, all the stresses depend on all the strains and vice versa. Assuming linear relationships between stresses and strains, we may write down the following equivalent forms of the symmetrized generalized Hooke's law (e.g. see Sokolnikoff, 1956):

$$\left.\begin{aligned}
\gamma_r &= B_{11}S_r + B_{12}S_\theta + B_{13}S_z + B_{14}S_{r\theta} + B_{15}S_{rz} + B_{16}S_{z\theta} \\
\gamma_\theta &= B_{12}S_r + B_{22}S_\theta + B_{23}S_z + B_{24}S_{r\theta} + B_{25}S_{rz} + B_{26}S_{z\theta} \\
\gamma_z &= B_{13}S_r + B_{23}S_\theta + B_{33}S_z + B_{34}S_{r\theta} + B_{35}S_{rz} + B_{36}S_{z\theta} \\
\gamma_{r\theta} &= B_{14}S_r + B_{24}S_\theta + B_{34}S_z + B_{44}S_{r\theta} + B_{45}S_{rz} + B_{46}S_{z\theta} \\
\gamma_{rz} &= B_{15}S_r + B_{25}S_\theta + B_{35}S_z + B_{45}S_{r\theta} + B_{55}S_{rz} + B_{56}S_{z\theta} \\
\gamma_{z\theta} &= B_{16}S_r + B_{26}S_\theta + B_{36}S_z + B_{46}S_{r\theta} + B_{56}S_{rz} + B_{66}S_{z\theta}
\end{aligned}\right\} \quad (2.9)$$

and

$$\left.\begin{aligned}
S_r &= A_{11}\gamma_r + A_{12}\gamma_\theta + A_{13}\gamma_z + A_{14}\gamma_{r\theta} + A_{15}\gamma_{rz} + A_{16}\gamma_{z\theta} \\
S_\theta &= A_{12}\gamma_r + A_{22}\gamma_\theta + A_{23}\gamma_z + A_{24}\gamma_{r\theta} + A_{25}\gamma_{rz} + A_{26}\gamma_{z\theta} \\
S_z &= A_{13}\gamma_r + A_{23}\gamma_\theta + A_{33}\gamma_z + A_{34}\gamma_{r\theta} + A_{35}\gamma_{rz} + A_{36}\gamma_{z\theta} \\
S_{r\theta} &= A_{14}\gamma_r + A_{24}\gamma_\theta + A_{34}\gamma_z + A_{44}\gamma_{r\theta} + A_{45}\gamma_{rz} + A_{46}\gamma_{z\theta} \\
S_{rz} &= A_{15}\gamma_r + A_{25}\gamma_\theta + A_{35}\gamma_z + A_{45}\gamma_{r\theta} + A_{55}\gamma_{rz} + A_{56}\gamma_{z\theta} \\
S_{z\theta} &= A_{16}\gamma_r + A_{26}\gamma_\theta + A_{36}\gamma_z + A_{46}\gamma_{r\theta} + A_{56}\gamma_{rz} + A_{66}\gamma_{z\theta}
\end{aligned}\right\} \quad (2.10)$$

The symmetry of the mutually reciprocal matrices A_{ij} and B_{ij} follows from the assumption of the existence of a strain energy density function. Each of the two arrays thus has 21 independent constants, but they are, however, interdependent through reciprocity and one can be calculated from the other. A complete lack of symmetry in an arterial segment would thus imply that 21 constitutive constants would be required for a complete characterization of its elastic response. As mentioned before, physiologic loading of an artery consists mainly of an intravascular pressure and a longitudinal force due to tethering. This type of loading would correspond to three non-zero stresses only, S_r, S_θ and S_z, and the shearing stresses would vanish. Thus only the 15 constants B_{ij} appearing in the left half of the right-hand side of (2.9) would be necessary to determine all the strains due to physiologic loading. Conversely, if the strains are known, only the 15 independent constants A_{ij} appearing in the first three of (2.10) need be known to compute all the non-zero stresses associated with physiologic loading. However, histological considerations suggest the existence of elastic symmetry in the arterial segment. In large arteries extensible fibers of collagen, elastic tissue and smooth muscle are oriented predominantly in the circumferential and longitudinal directions (Wolinsky and Glagov, 1964, 1967). This suggests the possibility of curvilinear orthotropy (Green and Adkins, 1960; Love, 1927) in the elastic response. This means that a typical arterial element described above should show symmetry of material response about the planes perpendicular to the r, θ and z axes. Mathematical analysis shows that this would imply the vanishing of shearing strains $\gamma_{r\theta}$, γ_{rz} and $\gamma_{z\theta}$ when S_r, S_θ and S_z are the only non-zero components. Of the 15 constants B_{ij} in (2.9) relevant to physiologic loading, the nine constants in the lower left quadrant vanish, leaving only six $(B_{11}, B_{22}, B_{33}, B_{12}, B_{13}, B_{23})$ to be determined experimentally. A complete characterization would also involve determining B_{44}, B_{55} and B_{66}, but they are not relevant for physiologic loading. Similarly, in (2.10), A_{11}, A_{22}, A_{33}, A_{12}, A_{13} and A_{23} are the only pertinent non-vanishing constants. Thus considerable saving of experimental effort would result if it can be shown that the arterial segment does indeed have curvilinear orthotropy. To demonstrate this would involve simulating physiologic loading on an excised arterial segment and measuring the resulting shearing strains, if any. Patel and Fry (1969) carried out such experiments which are described below.

(2) *Methods*

Segments from the middle descending thoracic aorta were studied in five dogs. The vessel was exposed and a relatively uniform segment was selected for study. The *in vivo* length and radius and the intravascular pressure were measured. The segment was then excised and mounted for study as shown in Fig. 3. The pressure was controlled by a reservoir containing saline (P.R.) connected to the segment via a hollow metal rod, A, passing through the fixed plug, C. In addition, a glass whisker (shown as an arrow in the figure) was passed perpendicularly through the wall in the middle of the segment.

A typical experiment was carried out in the following manner: The segment was inflated to the control pressure of 130 cm H_2O and its *in situ* length was restored by hanging weights on the lower end. The pressure was then varied, in steps, from 7 to 270 cm H_2O, and the corresponding values of R, L, the angular displacement of the pointer, E, and the angular displacement of the glass whisker were recorded. Finally the unstretched radius, R_o, and length, L_o, were measured.

From these data the shearing strain, $\gamma_{z\theta}$ (associated with the torsion), the shearing strain, $\gamma_{r\theta}$, as well as the circumferential and the longitudinal elongating strains were calculated. The torsional shearing strain, $\gamma_{z\theta}$, for a circular cylinder (Nash, 1957) is given by

$$\gamma_{z\theta} = \Omega R/L \tag{2.11}$$

where R/L is the ratio of radius to length and Ω is the angular rotation in radians of the pointer, E, representing the rotation of the lower end of the cylinder with respect to the upper fixed end. The circumferential strain, γ_θ, is given by $\Delta R/R_o$ and the longitudinal strain, γ_z, by $\Delta L/L_o$; ΔR and ΔL being the changes in radius and length associated with a corresponding

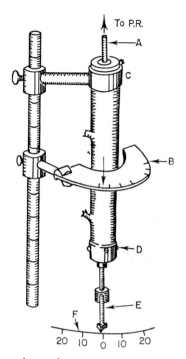

FIG. 3. Diagram of experimental arrangement showing pressurized blood vessel hanging vertically from ring stand support. A, hollow rod; C, proximal plug; D, distal plug and metal end cap; E, pointer; F, protractor scale; P.R., pressure reservoir; B, protractor to measure the change in the angle of the glass whisker indicated by a small arrow. (From Patel and Fry, 1969.)

change in pressure. The value of $\gamma_{r\theta}$ was obtained from the angular displacement of the glass whisker with respect to the vessel surface after making appropriate correction for torsional displacement.

(3) Results and discussion

The results are summarized in Table 2. It can be seen that the shearing strain, $\gamma_{z\theta}$, associated with torsion is at least an order of magnitude smaller than the corresponding circumferential and longitudinal strains. The value of $\gamma_{r\theta}$, although somewhat larger than $\gamma_{z\theta}$, is still much smaller than the corresponding circumferential or longitudinal strains. Moreover, the greatest increase in $\gamma_{r\theta}$ occurs at pressures greater than 179 cm H_2O. These results indicate that under physiologic loading the shearing strain $\gamma_{z\theta}$, is always small compared to the corresponding elongating strains, and that the shearing strain $\gamma_{r\theta}$, is also small for pressures below 180 cm H_2O. It can be shown that if the two shearing strains $\gamma_{z\theta}$ and $\gamma_{r\theta}$ are zero then the third one, γ_{rz}

TABLE 2

Summary of data from middle descending thoracic aorta of five dogs
showing range of averaged values of strains produced by normal stresses

Pressure Range (cm H_2O)	$\gamma_{z\theta} \times 100$	$\gamma_{r\theta} \times 100$	$\dfrac{\Delta R}{R_o} \times 100$	$\dfrac{\Delta L}{L_o} \times 100$
24–136	0–0·5	0–2·2	21–56	30–48
24–179	0–0·6	0–3·7	21–67	30–53
24–270	0–0·9	0–11·5	21–83	30–62

$\gamma_{z\theta}$ = shearing strain associated with torsion.
$\gamma_{r\theta}$ = shearing strain due to the circumferential movement of the outer cylindrical surface relative to the inner cylindrical surface.
$\dfrac{\Delta R}{R_o}$ = circumferential strain.
$\dfrac{\Delta L}{L_o}$ = longitudinal strain.
(Adapted from Patel and Fry, 1969.)

must be zero also (Green and Zerna, 1968). This greatly simplifies the analysis of the elastic properties of these blood vessels since one can consider them to be cylindrically orthotropic tubes, having elastic symmetry about the planes perpendicular to r, θ and z directions.

3. Longitudinal Tethering of the Aorta

The aorta, like all blood vessels *in situ*, is tethered to the surrounding perivascular tissues. As pointed out by Womersley (1957a, b), the mechanical behavior of the aorta is strongly influenced by the tethering, particularly its longitudinal component which enters the equation of dynamic equilibrium in the longitudinal direction. Also, as demonstrated by Patel *et al.* (1969), the longitudinal component of tethering contributes significantly to the difference between the *in vitro* and *in vivo* mechanical properties of a blood vessel segment. Thus it is important to quantify the longitudinal restraint on a blood vessel due to vascular tethering.

By the longitudinal tethering force on a segment we mean the force with which the perivascular tissues resist its longitudinal motion. This force can be measured by isolating an aortic segment with two transverse cuts, approximately 5 cm apart, without disturbing the perivascular tissues, subjecting the segment to a known uniform longitudinal motion and measuring the force required. It is, of course, necessary to ensure that all other longitudinal forces are either known, negligible, or carefully eliminated. Patel and Fry (1966) carried out such experiments which are summarized below.

A. METHODS

Experiments were performed, immediately *post mortem*, on the middle descending thoracic aorta of nine dogs (average weight 26 kg). Following exposure of the blood vessel, a cylindrical plug was inserted into the lumen and the ends of the vessel tied snugly to it. The vessel was then cut cleanly across at either end of the plug. The close coupling of the rigid plug to the inner surface of the vessel prevented development of any longitudinal stress gradients. One end of the segment-plug assembly was attached to a displacement sensing device and the other was attached, through a bar containing a force sensing device to a mechanical driver. The other end of the displacement sensing device (Mallos, 1962) was attached to the skeleton, which, in turn, was tightly coupled to the operating table. The force-gauge was constructed by mounting foil strain gauges to stiff elastic elements, and its internal displacement for the forces used in this instance, was extremely small (always less than 0·1 per cent of the vessel displacements). The mechanical driver imposed step or sinusoidal motion of known amplitude and frequency on the plug. The steady-state response to sinusoidal displacements (0 to 22 Hz) was studied in great detail because of its physiological importance (McDonald, 1960). To isolate the response of the blood vessel from that of the instrument system, each experiment was repeated with the instruments assembled in exactly the same manner but without the vessel segment.

All sinusoidal functions were subjected to harmonic analysis and the impedance functions corresponding to the different harmonics were calculated as complex ratios of force per unit endothelial surface area (dynes cm^{-2}) to the displacement (cm). The data for the plug-instrument system were subjected to further analysis by representing the system as a parallel combination of an elastic element of stiffness K_R and a viscous element of coefficient η_R, this combination, in turn, being in series with an inertial element with mass M_R. The representation was judged extremely faithful in the frequency range (0 to 22 Hz) of interest (see Fig. 3 of Patel and Fry, 1966, for details).

B. RESULTS AND DISCUSSION

Figure 4 shows typical raw experimental data obtained for three types of experiment. Figures 4(a) and 4(b) show that sinusoidal displacements result in sinusoidal force responses, suggesting a linear type of response. This was later verified by comparing system impedances for three different amplitudes of displacement. Figure 4(a) also shows that at low frequencies the force and displacement curves are almost in phase, suggesting that one of the dominant characteristics of the system is its elasticity. Figure 4(c) illustrates that the system exhibits stress relaxation. Finally, Fig. 4(d) shows the transient

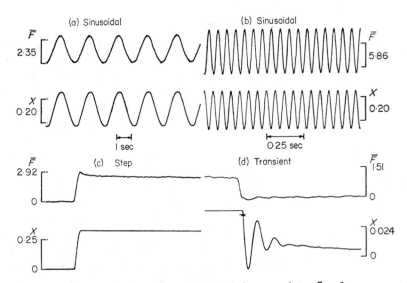

FIG. 4. Typical experimental data obtained from a dog. $F =$ force per unit surface area of the plug (dynes cm^{-2} × 10^3); $X =$ displacement (cm). Note that the time scale for (a) and (c) is different from that for (b) and (d). (From Patel and Fry, 1966.)

response to a sudden removal of impressed force. The displacement curve appears to be composed of a damped oscillatory response superimposed on a quasi-exponential creep recovery curve.

Patel and Fry (1966) suggested a linear mechanical model† consisting of a mass M in series with a parallel combination of an elastic element of stiffness K, a viscous element of viscosity η and a Maxwell element which is a series combination of an elastic element of stiffness K_2 and a viscous element with viscosity η_2. Using a least-squared-error curve fitting procedure they obtained numerical values for the model parameters. It was found that the model with the computed parameter values simulated well the impedance curve of the real system in the experimental frequency range. By subtracting the parameter values M_R, K_R and η_R for the plug-instrument assembly from M, K and η for the vessel-plug-instrument system, they obtained the parameters $M_V + M_A = M - M_R$, $K_1 = K - K_R$, $\eta_1 = \eta - \eta_R$, K_2 and η_2 of the model shown in Fig. 5, which represents the vessel only. Physically, M_V represents the mass of the vessel and M_A the mass of "added" tissue consisting of short stubs of intercostal arteries, immediately adjacent parietal pleura and some retroaortic areolar tissue. The series coupled spring (K_2) and the dashpot (η_2) of the Maxwell element represent

† For a simple discussion of various mechanical models see Patel and Janicki (1966).

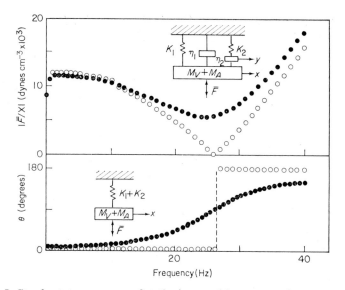

Fig. 5. Steady-state response of tethering models. ●●● 5-parameter model proposed by Patel and Fry; ○○○ 2-parameter model proposed by Womersley. $|\bar{F}/X|$ = magnitude of impedance; θ = angle by which force, $\bar{F}$, leads displacement, X. (Adapted from Patel and Fry, 1966.)

the stress relaxation and added "dynamic" component of the tethering elasticity. The spring (K_1) represents the static elastic coefficient and the dash-pot (η_1) represents the remaining part of the frictional resistance of the system.

The average values ($\pm$ SEM) of K_1, K_2, η_1, η_2, $M_V + M_A$ and M_V from nine dogs are given in Table 3. The value of M_V was obtained by excluding as much as possible of the extra tissue and weighing the vessel segment. From the values in Table 3 one can generate the impedance vs. frequency

TABLE 3

Numerical values of the parameters of the tethering model of
Patel and Fry shown in Fig. 5

	K_1	K_2	η_1	η_2	$M_V + M_A$	M_V
Average	8350	3350	34	1715	0·435	0·130
$\pm$ SEM	1128	382	6	344	0·1	0·011

Average values (per unit endothelial surface area) $\pm$ SEM from the middle descending thoracic aorta of nine dogs are shown. K_1 and K_2 are the spring constants in dynes cm^{-3}; η_1 and η_2 are the dashpot coefficients in dyne s cm^{-3}; M_V and M_A are the vessel mass and the added mass in dyne s^2 cm^{-3}. (Adapted from Patel and Fry, 1966.)

diagram for the vessel segment which is shown in Fig. 5. It represents the dynamic behavior of the blood vessel that should be used with the equation of longitudinal motion for the blood vessel wall, which, in turn, is one of the necessary boundary equations for the solution of the flow equations. At zero frequency the impedance of the complete model consists only of the spring constant K_1. The impedance rises very rapidly below 1 Hz; it then decreases slightly to a minimum at about 25 Hz, and then gradually rises. The complete model representing the actual vessel behavior is also compared to Womersley's frictionless model (1957a, b). If we substitute the values for the mass $(M_V + M_A)$ and dynamic spring constant $(K_1 + K_2)$ from Table 3 into Womersley's model, setting the remaining parameters to zero, and then compute its dynamic response characteristics, we obtain the curve shown by open circles in Fig. 5. It can be seen that the magnitude of the impedance decreases to zero at resonance, around 26 Hz, and then rises monotonically thereafter. The phase angle changes abruptly from 0° to 180° at the resonant frequency. Clearly, this simplified model does not simulate the behavior of the real vessel.

In conclusion the longitudinal tethering of a segment of the middle descending thoracic aorta has been described. Its effect on the general mechanical behavior of the aorta is indicated; its effect on the elastic behavior of the vessel wall will be illustrated in Section 4 in which the wall properties in the tethered and untethered state will be compared.

4. INCREMENTAL VISCOELASTIC PROPERTIES

A. THEORETICAL CONSIDERATIONS

(1) *General remarks*

A constitutive relation relates the state of stress in a continuum to its history of motion. For an elastic body this means a relation between stress and strain; for a visco-elastic body it means a relation between stress and stress rates and strain and strain rates. In developing constitutive relations for blood vessels one observes the following. A blood vessel like the descending thoracic aorta normally operates around an initially stressed state where the average strain in the wall may be as much as 70 per cent. The fluctuations of strain around this value are, however, small, typically only about 3 or 4 per cent in the circumferential direction and 1 per cent in the longitudinal direction (Patel et al., 1961; Patel et al., 1964). This suggests a simplified approach to the problem of large strains which has proved useful, both in engineering and for the mechanical behavior of blood vessels (Patel et al., 1969). In this approach one considers the incremental stress-strain relation at some initially stressed state. This is convenient for *in vivo* measurements and is satisfactory for most applications. The major disadvantage is that in situations where wide ranges of stress and strain must be considered it is necessary to define the mechanical behavior around a number of average strains over the range of interest. Moreover, if one wishes to compare the incremental constitutive constants obtained under different experimental conditions or obtained from different animals, it must be made sure that their values are measured around identical average strains. Thus, we conclude that even if the overall response is non-linear, it is possible to consider a blood vessel to be incrementally linear in mechanical response over restricted ranges of strain. Furthermore, the concept of linear incremental behavior allows the application of certain equations of linear elasticity or visco-elasticity theory to calculate corresponding incremental constitutive constants which describe the response of the blood vessel around selected average values of strain. For a detailed treatment of the incremental approach one is referred to Biot (1965).

(2) Large average stress and strain

As mentioned previously, a segment of a large blood vessel such as the aorta may be assumed to be a thin-walled circular cylinder. Referring the vessel segment to the cylindrical coordinate system shown in Fig. 1, the state of stress due to intraluminal pressure p and an evenly applied additional longitudinal force F can be shown to consist of purely normal (tensile or compressive) stresses S_θ, S_z and S_r along each of the coordinate axes given by (2.1) to (2.3). Thus, it is possible to calculate the average stress acting in the three coordinate directions from measurements of intraluminal pressure, longitudinal force, vessel radius and wall thickness. Under the assumption of homogeneity and neglecting end-effects and effects of intercostal branches, the state of stress is uniform throughout the segment and equals the average state.

The corresponding elongating (or contracting) strains can be computed by comparing the radial, circumferential and longitudinal dimensions of the blood vessel in the unstressed and stressed condition. The average "engineering" or "conventional" strains γ_θ, γ_z and γ_r in the θ, z and r directions, respectively, are given by

$$\gamma_\theta = (R - R_o)/R_o \qquad (4.1)$$

$$\gamma_z = (L - L_o)/L_o \qquad (4.2)$$

$$\gamma_r = (h - h_o)/h_o \qquad (4.3)$$

where h_o, R_o and L_o are the values of thickness, midwall radius and length, respectively, in the unstressed state; and h, R and L are the corresponding values of these quantities at a given intravascular pressure and longitudinal force. Again, under the same assumptions, γ_θ, γ_z and γ_r define the average strain everywhere in the segment. Equivalently, as is often convenient in the theory of large deformations, the state of deformation can also be defined by the extension ratios (or stretches) λ_θ, λ_z and λ_r which are obtained as

$$\lambda_\theta = R/R_o \tag{4.4}$$

$$\lambda_z = L/L_o \tag{4.5}$$

$$\lambda_r = h/h_o. \tag{4.6}$$

Clearly, the stretches exceed the corresponding conventional strains by unity, i.e. $\lambda_\theta = \gamma_\theta + 1$.

Having established orthotropic elastic symmetry we know that no significant shearing strains (in the coordinate surfaces of the chosen cylindrical coordinate system) will develop under physiologic loading. This fact greatly simplifies the problem of strain measurement, since only the three orthogonal elongating strains need to be considered.

(3) Small superposed sinusoidal stresses and strains

If we now connect this blood vessel segment (under initial mean stresses S_θ, S_z and S_r) to a sinusoidal pump which moves a small quantity of blood in and out of it at a given frequency, and impose an additional longitudinal force varying sinusoidally at the same frequency, then sinusoidally varying incremental stresses P_θ, P_z and P_r will develop in the circumferential, longitudinal and radial directions, respectively, along with corresponding incremental strains e_θ, e_z and e_r. As long as the stresses are small, the corresponding steady-state incremental strains will also be small and vary sinusoidally at the same frequency (Patel et al., 1970). The blood vessel will behave incrementally as an orthotropic linearly viscoelastic material and no shearing strains will develop in the coordinate system. The incremental stresses and strains will, in general, not be in phase; however, the phase difference between any two of these will remain constant throughout the cycle. One could calculate these quantities by continuously measuring the pressure, radius, length and longitudinal force.

In the following, we shall make use of the so-called phase diagram on which a sinusoidally varying quantity is represented as the real or imaginary part of a vector rotating at a constant rate in the complex plane. This method of representation is very convenient in showing phase relations among various quantities and is employed in Figs. 6, 7 and 8. As a result of sinusoidal variations of Δp in the equilibrium intraluminal pressure p, and ΔF in the longitudinal force F, the equilibrium midwall radius R undergoes a sinusoidal variation of ΔR (see Fig. 6). If Δp and ΔF have a frequency of $\omega/2\pi$ cycles per unit time, so also will the variation (ΔR) of the midwall radius. Choosing the origin of time ($t = 0$) as the instant when the midwall radius has the maximum value of $R + |\Delta R|$, at any instant t it will be given by

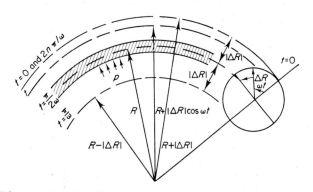

FIG. 6. Diagram showing sinusoidal variation in midwall radius along with its phase diagram. R is the midwall radius at the mean internal pressure, p, at time $t = \pi/2\omega$ where ω is the circular frequency of the sinusoidal variation, ΔR, in R. The midwall radius varies from $R + |\Delta R|$ at $t = 0$ to $R - |\Delta R|$ at $t = \pi/\omega$ and back to $R + |\Delta R|$ at $t = 2\pi/\omega$. The incremental change at any time t is given by $|\Delta R| \cos \omega t$ which is the projection on $t = 0$ axis of ΔR in the phase diagram on the right. The centerline of the wall cross section occupies the same position at $t = 2n\pi/\omega$ as at $t = 0$ where n is any positive integer.

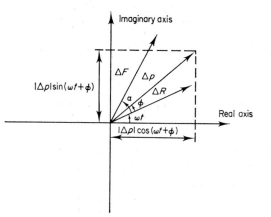

FIG. 7. Phase diagrams for ΔR, Δp and ΔF. ΔR, Δp and ΔF are the complex vectors representing incremental changes in the midwall radius R, internal pressure p and the longitudinal force F. The projections of these vectors on the real axis (or the imaginary axis) vary sinusoidally as the vectors rotate counter-clockwise with a circular frequency ω. Note that at any time t, Δp and ΔF lead ΔR by angles ϕ and α respectively.

$R + |\Delta R| \cos \omega t$. This can be more easily visualized in Fig. 6 where in the circle of radius $|\Delta R|$ a vector ΔR is shown at an angle of ωt with the $t = 0$ direction. With the convention that ΔR rotates counter-clockwise with an angular frequency of ω, the position shown corresponds to the instant t, when the distance of the projection of the tip of the arrow on the $t = 0$ axis from the axis of the blood vessel gives the midwall radius $R + |\Delta R| \cos \omega t$. In this representation, ΔR can be viewed as a representation of a complex number whose modulus is $|\Delta R|$ and phase angle is ωt. The projection $|\Delta R| \cos \omega t$ of ΔR on the $t = 0$ axis (real axis) is called the real part of ΔR and the projection $|\Delta R| \sin \omega t$ on the $t = \pi/2\omega$ axis (imaginary axis) is called the imaginary part of ΔR. Thus we can write

$$\Delta R = |\Delta R| \exp (j\omega t) = |\Delta R| \cos \omega t + j|\Delta R| \sin \omega t \qquad (4.7)$$

where $j = \sqrt{(-1)}$.

Similar representations can be obtained for all the sinusoidally varying quantities involved. For example, in Fig. 7 the incremental complex vectors ΔR, Δp and ΔF are shown as three vectors rotating counter-clockwise as a rigid body at an angular frequency ω. If ΔR is chosen to lie along the real axis at $t = 0$ and if Δp and ΔF lead ΔR by angles ϕ and α, respectively, then at time t the vectors ΔR, Δp and ΔF are given by

$$\Delta R = |\Delta R| \exp (j\omega t) \qquad (4.8)$$

$$\Delta p = |\Delta p| \exp [j(\omega t + \phi)] \qquad (4.9)$$

$$\Delta F = |\Delta F| \exp [j(\omega t + \alpha)] \qquad (4.10)$$

where $|\Delta R|$, $|\Delta p|$, $|\Delta F|$ are the moduli of ΔR, Δp and ΔF, respectively, and thus are positive quantities. Phase differences ϕ and α may be positive or negative. To (4.8) – (4.10) we add the following equation for ΔL (not shown in Fig. 7),

$$\Delta L = |\Delta L| \exp [j(\omega t + \psi)] \qquad (4.11)$$

which describes similarly the complex incremental change in the vessel length.

As neither the moduli of these vectors nor the phase angles relative to ΔR depend on t, we shall use the positions of all vectors at $t = 0$ in all that follow. At $t = 0$, we have

$$\Delta R = \Delta R' = |\Delta R| \qquad (4.12)$$

$$\Delta p = \Delta p' + j\Delta p'' = |\Delta p| \cos \phi + j|\Delta p| \sin \phi \qquad (4.13)$$

$$\Delta F = \Delta F' + j\Delta F'' = |\Delta F| \cos \alpha + j|\Delta F| \sin \alpha \qquad (4.14)$$

$$\Delta L = \Delta L' + j\Delta L'' = |\Delta L| \cos \psi + j|\Delta L| \sin \psi \qquad (4.15)$$

where primes denote the real parts and double primes denote the imaginary parts of the respective quantities.

The phasic relations between the vectors ΔR, and Δp are further clarified

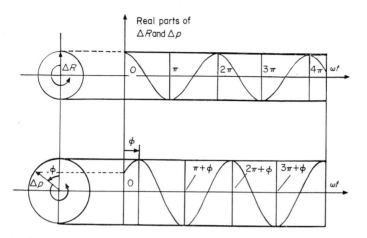

Fig. 8. Sinusoidal variations ΔR and Δp, in midwall radius and intravascular pressure, respectively, vs. ωt where ω is the circular frequency and t is the time. Note that Δp leads ΔR by the angle ϕ; the peaks and nadirs of Δp occur at ϕ, $\pi + \phi$, $2\pi + \phi$, etc.

in Fig. 8 where the real parts of ΔR and Δp are plotted as functions of ωt. On the left of each curve is shown the corresponding phase diagram with the real axis directed upwards and the imaginary axis directed leftward.

Below we show how one can obtain the moduli and phases of the incremental strains and stresses from the moduli and phase angles of ΔR, Δp, ΔF and ΔL and the equilibrium values of R, p, F, L and h.

By definition, incremental strain describes a small (theoretically, infinitesimal) increment which may be positive or negative, in a dimension of a specimen as a fraction of the dimension just prior to the increase. For small increments ΔR, ΔL and Δh we get the following circumferential, longitudinal and radial incremental strains e_θ, e_z and e_r:

$$e_\theta = d\lambda_\theta/\lambda_\theta = \Delta R/R \qquad (4.16)$$

$$e_z = d\lambda_z/\lambda_z = \Delta L/L \qquad (4.17)$$

$$e_r = d\lambda_r/\lambda_r = \Delta h/h \qquad (4.18)$$

where e_θ, e_z, e_r, ΔR, ΔL and Δh are complex and R, L and h are real. By considering infinitesimal change in the volume $2\pi RLh$ of the vessel wall it is easy to show that for constancy of the tissue volume the sum of the incremental strains should vanish, i.e.

$$e_\theta + e_z + e_r = 0. \qquad (4.19)$$

Thus, if the moduli and phase angles of any two of the complex incremental strains are known, those for the third strain can be determined from (4.19).

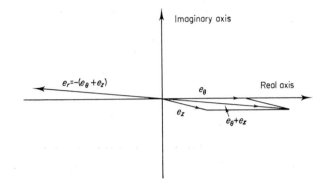

FIG. 9. Complex representation of incremental strains e_r, e_θ and e_z in radial, circumferential and longitudinal directions, respectively, for an incompressible material, which must satisfy the relation $e_r + e_\theta + e_z = 0$ at all times. Note that only two of the incremental strains need be determined experimentally.

This is illustrated in Fig. 9. Algebraically, this can be done by computing the real and imaginary parts of the third strain as negatives of the sums of the corresponding parts of the other two strains and evaluating the modulus and the phase angle therefrom. Using (4.19) we can write (4.18) as

$$e_r = -\left(\frac{\Delta R}{R} + \frac{\Delta L}{L}\right) \tag{4.20}$$

thus obviating independent measurement of Δh. The wall thickness h which is needed in what follows can be obtained from the tissue volume, V, as

$$h = V/2\pi RL \tag{4.21}$$

if the mean radius R is known, or by an equivalent formula if the internal or the external radii are known.

The incremental stresses P_θ, P_z and P_r are the differentials of the mean stresses S_θ, S_z and S_r given by (2.1) to (2.3). Neglecting terms of order higher than one in ΔR, Δp and ΔF in the Taylor series expansions of S_θ, S_z and S_r, we have

$$P_\theta \simeq \Delta S_\theta \simeq \left(\frac{R}{h} - \tfrac{1}{2}\right)\Delta p + \frac{p}{h}\Delta R - \frac{pR}{h^2}\Delta h \tag{4.22}$$

$$P_z \simeq \Delta S_z \simeq \left(\frac{R}{2h} - \tfrac{1}{2}\right)\Delta p + \left(\frac{p}{2h} - \frac{F}{2\pi R^2 h}\right)\Delta R -$$

$$-\left(\frac{pR}{2h^2} + \frac{F}{2\pi Rh^2}\right)\Delta h + \frac{\Delta F}{2\pi Rh} \tag{4.23}$$

$$P_r \simeq \Delta S_r \simeq -\tfrac{1}{2}\Delta p. \tag{4.24}$$

Eliminating Δh in favor of ΔR and ΔL by using (4.20) we obtain

$$P_\theta \simeq \left(\frac{R}{h} - \tfrac{1}{2}\right)\Delta p + \frac{2p\Delta R}{h} + \frac{pR\Delta L}{Lh} \tag{4.25}$$

$$P_z \simeq \left(\frac{R}{2h} - \tfrac{1}{2}\right)\Delta p + \frac{p\Delta R}{h} + \frac{\Delta F}{2\pi Rh} + \left(\frac{pR}{2Lh} + \frac{F}{2\pi RLh}\right)\Delta L \tag{4.26}$$

$$P_r \simeq -\tfrac{1}{2}\Delta p. \tag{4.27}$$

Equations (4.25) to (4.27) determine the complex incremental stresses in terms of the measured or calculated quantities Δp, ΔR, ΔF, ΔL, p, F, R, L and h.

(4) Constitutive relations for the incremental theory

In the following treatment we consider an arterial segment exhibiting incrementally orthotropic linear viscoelastic behavior. Under a set of sinusoidal incremental stresses P_θ, P_z and P_r, the steady state response consists of a set of sinusoidal incremental strains e_θ, e_z and e_r, each strain being a linear combination of all the stresses. Thus we have the relations[†]

$$e_\theta = C_{\theta\theta}P_\theta - C_{\theta z}P_z - C_{\theta r}P_r \tag{4.28}$$

$$e_z = -C_{z\theta}P_\theta + C_{zz}P_z - C_{zr}P_r \tag{4.29}$$

$$e_r = -C_{r\theta}P_\theta - C_{rz}P_z + C_{rr}P_r \tag{4.30}$$

where the coefficients C_{ij} are complex, as are the stresses and strains. Equation (4.28) states that e_θ depends not only on P_θ but also on P_z and P_r. This is the same type of consideration as that giving rise to Poisson's ratio in the linear isotropic elasticity theory,[‡] and similarly with (4.29) and (4.30). The use of negative signs before the coefficients with unidentical suffixes is for convenience only.

[†] Similar equations were used by Hardung (1964) for relating overall stresses and strains in a blood vessel treated as an orthotropic linearly elastic tube. However, it is important to note that (4.28) to (4.30) are more general in that they are valid for evaluating the orthotropic incremental viscoelastic properties of the blood vessel wall.

[‡] It should be pointed out that if the incremental response were isotropic, we would have

$$C_{\theta\theta} = C_{zz} = C_{rr}; \quad C_{\theta z} = C_{z\theta} = C_{zr} = C_{rz} = C_{r\theta} = C_{\theta r}.$$

However, we shall not assume that these equalities hold for a blood vessel segment; for, even if the segment is initially isotropic (i.e. isotropic in the undeformed state), its incremental response will, in general, be orthotropic (Biot, 1965; Fung, 1968) due to the fact that the blood vessel has non-linear mechanical response and the incremental response in a given direction depends greatly on the stretch in that direction. Since, in general, under physiologic loading the state of strain in an artery would involve unequal stretches in the three principal directions, the incremental properties in these directions can not be expected to be identical.

Equations (4.28) to (4.30) can be written equivalently in the following matrix† form:

$$
\begin{bmatrix} e_\theta \\ e_z \\ e_r \end{bmatrix} = \begin{bmatrix} C_{\theta\theta} & -C_{\theta z} & -C_{\theta r} \\ -C_{z\theta} & C_{zz} & -C_{zr} \\ -C_{r\theta} & -C_{rz} & C_{rr} \end{bmatrix} \begin{bmatrix} P_\theta \\ P_z \\ P_r \end{bmatrix} \tag{4.31}
$$

We shall assume that the coefficient matrix C_{ij} in (4.31) is symmetric.‡ Accordingly, we have

$$C_{zr} = C_{rz} \tag{4.32}$$

$$C_{z\theta} = C_{\theta z} \tag{4.33}$$

$$C_{r\theta} = C_{\theta r} \tag{4.34}$$

Because of (4.32) to (4.34), only six of the coefficients C_{ij} are independent. In addition, because of the incompressibility condition, (4.19), the following three relations hold among the remaining six coefficients:

$$C_{\theta\theta} - C_{z\theta} - C_{r\theta} = 0 \tag{4.35}$$

$$C_{zz} - C_{z\theta} - C_{zr} = 0 \tag{4.36}$$

$$C_{rr} - C_{r\theta} - C_{rz} = 0 \tag{4.37}$$

This can be proved by requiring that the sum of the right-hand side of (4.28), (4.29) and (4.30) should vanish for arbitrary choice of P_θ, P_r and P_z.

Equations (4.35), (4.36) and (4.37) further yield the equalities

$$C_{zr} = \tfrac{1}{2}(C_{zz} + C_{rr} - C_{\theta\theta}) \tag{4.38}$$

$$C_{r\theta} = \tfrac{1}{2}(C_{rr} + C_{\theta\theta} - C_{zz}) \tag{4.39}$$

$$C_{\theta z} = \tfrac{1}{2}(C_{\theta\theta} + C_{zz} - C_{rr}) \tag{4.40}$$

Using these relations the matrix C_{ij} can be expressed solely in terms of the three coefficients $C_{\theta\theta}$, C_{zz} and C_{rr} which are now the only unknown constitutive parameters. With this in mind (4.28), (4.29) and (4.30) can be

---

† Readers unfamiliar with matrix notation may consult any good book on Applied Mathematics. For example, see Jeffreys and Jeffreys (1962).

‡ The justification for the assumption of symmetry of C_{ij} is as follows: For incremental deformations of initially unstressed or hydrostatically stressed compressible elastic bodies, such symmetry follows from assuming existence of a strain energy density function that is a quadratic form in strains. For incremental deformations of incompressible elastic bodies it is not necessary for the initial stress to be hydrostatic for such symmetry to obtain. Symmetry of C_{ij} for the incremental deformations of an incompressible visco-elastic body under an arbitrary state of stress depends, in addition, on Onsager's reciprocity relations of irreversible thermodynamics and on the existence of a quadratic dissipation function (Biot, 1965).

expanded and rearranged in the following form:

$$
\begin{bmatrix} e_\theta \\ e_z \\ e_r \end{bmatrix} =
\begin{bmatrix} P_{\theta\theta} & P_{\theta z} & P_{\theta r} \\ P_{z\theta} & P_{zz} & P_{zr} \\ P_{r\theta} & P_{rz} & P_{rr} \end{bmatrix}
\begin{bmatrix} C_{\theta\theta} \\ C_{zz} \\ C_{rr} \end{bmatrix}
\tag{4.41}
$$

where

$$
\begin{aligned}
& P_{\theta\theta} = P_\theta - \tfrac{1}{2}P_z - \tfrac{1}{2}P_r && P_{\theta z} = -\tfrac{1}{2}P_z + \tfrac{1}{2}P_r && P_{\theta r} = \tfrac{1}{2}P_z - \tfrac{1}{2}P_r \\
& P_{z\theta} = -\tfrac{1}{2}P_\theta + \tfrac{1}{2}P_r && P_{zz} = -\tfrac{1}{2}P_\theta + P_z - \tfrac{1}{2}P_r && P_{zr} = \tfrac{1}{2}P_\theta - \tfrac{1}{2}P_r \\
& P_{r\theta} = -\tfrac{1}{2}P_\theta + \tfrac{1}{2}P_z && P_{rz} = \tfrac{1}{2}P_\theta - \tfrac{1}{2}P_z && P_{rr} = -\tfrac{1}{2}P_\theta - \tfrac{1}{2}P_z + P_r
\end{aligned}
\tag{4.42}
$$

At first sight it appears that (4.41) can be solved for $C_{\theta\theta}$, C_{zz} and C_{rr} by inverting the square matrix and premultiplying the strain vector on the left by it. In fact, this is not quite possible as the square matrix is singular (that is, its determinant vanishes) and can not be inverted. However, any two of the equations can be used to solve for two ratios of coefficients and further information on the values of all three coefficients has to come from an independent experiment. This experiment can be of the same type as the first or completely different, but the important thing is that it must involve different relative ratios of incremental strains; of course, for the results to be valid, the second experiment must be carried out around the same overall state of strain as that of the first experiment.

Given that the choice of the second experiment generates one more equation that is linearly independent of the previous set, any three linearly independent equations can be chosen from the available set and solved simultaneously to obtain $C_{\theta\theta}$, C_{zz} and C_{rr}. While maintaining the same overall state of strain several independent experiments may be carried out involving various ratios of the incremental strains and solve the resulting equations by the method of least squares.

For the static, incremental elastic response of a blood vessel, all the quantities in (4.41) are real; however, for the dynamic incremental visco-elastic case they are, in general complex. In this case the three complex equations (4.41) in fact embody six real equations—three for the real parts of $C_{\theta\theta}$, C_{zz} and C_{rr}, and three for their imaginary parts. The real equations can be extracted from (4.41) in a rather straightforward manner. We shall not give their explicit forms here, but merely point out that the real and imaginary parts of the known quantities ΔR, Δp, ΔF, ΔL, e_θ, e_z, e_r, $P_{\theta\theta}$, $P_{\theta z}$, etc. can be easily obtained from (4.12) to (4.15), (4.16), (4.17), (4.20) and (4.42).

(5) Physical meaning of the viscoelastic coefficients

We have discussed the theory for experimental evaluation of the complex constitutive constants $C_{\theta\theta}$, C_{zz} and C_{rr}. Once these are determined, the remaining constants C_{ij} $(i \neq j)$ appearing in (4.28) to (4.30) can be determined from (4.38) to (4.40). Instead of the nine constants C_{ij} (only three of which are independent), we can express the relations among the incremental stresses and strains in terms of nine other complex constants, namely, E_θ, E_z, E_r, $\sigma_{\theta z}$, $\sigma_{z\theta}$, σ_{zr}, σ_{rz}, $\sigma_{r\theta}$ and $\sigma_{\theta r}$. The first three of these are akin to the familiar Young's modulus, E, and the remaining six are akin to the familiar Poisson's ratio, σ, for an isotropic linearly elastic material. We shall develop the relations expressing C_{ij} in terms of the new constants and vice versa.

Let us consider a blood vessel segment stretched in the three orthogonal directions, r, θ and z, so that it acquires a chosen state of initial stress. If we subject the segment to a sinusoidal incremental stress P_θ in the circumferential direction, while keeping stresses in the z and r directions constant, we shall have not only sinusoidally varying incremental strains e_θ, but also sinusoidal strains e_z and e_r. Specifically, for $P_z = P_r = 0$, we have, from (4.28) to (4.30).

$$e_\theta = C_{\theta\theta}P_\theta; \quad e_z = -C_{z\theta}P_\theta; \quad e_r = -C_{r\theta}P_\theta. \tag{4.43}$$

Similarly, for a uniaxial sinusoidal stress in the z direction, we have $P_\theta = P_r = 0$ and

$$e_\theta = -C_{\theta z}P_z; \quad e_z = C_{zz}P_z; \quad e_r = -C_{rz}P_z. \tag{4.44}$$

Finally, for a uniaxial sinusoidal stress in the r direction, we have $P_\theta = P_z = 0$, and hence,

$$e_\theta = -C_{\theta r}P_r; \quad e_z = -C_{zr}P_r; \quad e_r = C_{rr}P_r. \tag{4.45}$$

From the first equations of the sets (4.43), (4.44) and (4.45) we immediately see that, if E_θ denotes the complex incremental Young's modulus in the θ direction (being the ratio of uniaxial incremental stress in the θ direction to the corresponding incremental strain), and E_z and E_r the complex incremental Young's moduli in the z and r directions, respectively, then

$$E_\theta = \frac{1}{C_{\theta\theta}}; \quad E_z = \frac{1}{C_{zz}}; \quad E_r = \frac{1}{C_{rr}}. \tag{4.46}$$

Denoting the real and imaginary parts of E_θ by E_θ' and E_θ'', respectively, and defining† C_{ij}' and C_{ij}'' through the relation $C_{ij} = C_{ij}' - jC_{ij}''$, we get

$$E_\theta' = \frac{C_{\theta\theta}'}{(C_{\theta\theta}')^2 + (C_{\theta\theta}'')^2}; \quad E_\theta'' = \frac{C_{\theta\theta}''}{(C_{\theta\theta}')^2 + (C_{\theta\theta}'')^2}$$
$$C_{\theta\theta}' = \frac{E_\theta'}{(E_\theta')^2 + (E_\theta'')^2}; \quad C_{\theta\theta}'' = \frac{E_\theta''}{(E_\theta')^2 + (E_\theta'')^2} \tag{4.47}$$

† The choice of C_{ij}'' to denote the negative of the imaginary part of C_{ij} is motivated by the fact that C_{ij}'' so defined would be positive for a viscoelastic material.

Similar relations can be written down for E'_z, E''_z, C'_{zz}, C''_{zz}, E'_r, E''_r, C'_{rr} and C''_{rr}.

Now, for isotropic linearly elastic materials, Poisson's ratio, σ, is a real number defined as the ratio of the contraction per unit length in an orthogonal direction to the extension per unit length in the direction of the stress in a uniaxial experiment. This definition may be generalized for the case of incremental deformations of an orthotropic viscoelastic material so that Poisson's ratio σ_{ij} means the ratio of the contractile strain in the i direction to the elongating strain in the j direction in an experiment where only $P_j \neq 0$. We note that σ_{ij} will be a complex number since the strain in the i direction will lag the strain in the j direction. Accordingly, we may evaluate the six Poisson's ratios σ_{ij} from (4.43) through (4.45) as

$$\sigma_{\theta z} = \frac{C_{\theta z}}{C_{zz}}; \quad \sigma_{zr} = \frac{C_{zr}}{C_{rr}}; \quad \sigma_{r\theta} = \frac{C_{r\theta}}{C_{\theta\theta}}$$

$$\sigma_{z\theta} = \frac{C_{z\theta}}{C_{\theta\theta}}; \quad \sigma_{rz} = \frac{C_{rz}}{C_{zz}}; \quad \sigma_{\theta r} = \frac{C_{\theta r}}{C_{rr}}$$

(4.48)

From (4.48) we note that even when $C_{ij} = C_{ji}$, $\sigma_{ij} \neq \sigma_{ji}$.

Let us express

$$\sigma_{ij} = \sigma'_{ij} + j\sigma''_{ij}.$$

(4.49)

Now using relations $C_{ij} = C'_{ij} - jC''_{ij}$ together with (4.48) and (4.49) we get the following relations:

$$\sigma'_{\theta z} = \frac{C'_{\theta z}C'_{zz} + C''_{\theta z}C''_{zz}}{(C'_{zz})^2 + (C''_{zz})^2}$$

$$\sigma''_{\theta z} = \frac{C'_{\theta z}C''_{zz} - C''_{\theta z}C'_{zz}}{(C'_{zz})^2 + (C''_{zz})^2}$$

(4.50)

Similar relations can be obtained for the real and imaginary parts of the remaining Poisson's ratios.

Conversely, we can express the real and imaginary parts of the coefficients C_{ij} ($i \neq j$) in terms of the real and imaginary parts of σ_{ij} and E_θ, E_z and E_r by using (4.46) and (4.48). For $C_{\theta z}$, for example, we have

$$C'_{\theta z} = \frac{\sigma'_{\theta z}E'_z + \sigma''_{\theta z}E''_z}{(E'_z)^2 + (E''_z)^2}$$

$$C''_{\theta z} = \frac{\sigma'_{\theta z}E''_z - \sigma''_{\theta z}E'_z}{(E'_z)^2 + (E''_z)^2}$$

(4.51)

with similar relations for other C_{ij} ($i \neq j$).

Now we demonstrate how the complex coefficients E_θ, E_z, E_r, $C_{\theta\theta}$, C_{zz} and C_{rr} can be interpreted in terms of a model consisting of a combination of springs and dashpots. Although more complicated models might be appropriate, as a first approximation we shall choose a relatively simple model consisting of a parallel combination of a spring and a dashpot (Fig. 10) in each of the three principal directions (θ, z and r), with cross-coupling between different directions.

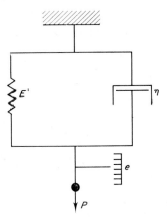

Fig. 10. A linear two-parameter Voigt model for visualizing the physical significance of real and imaginary parts of complex coefficients relating an incremental stress, P, to the corresponding incremental strain, e. E' = spring stiffness constant; η = dashpot viscosity constant.

We assume that the overall mechanical behavior of this model is non-linear (as is the case with an artery); however, for sufficiently small incremental deformations, the behavior of the model will be linear. When such a model is subjected to a small incremental sinusoidal stress denoted by a complex number P it will respond, in the steady state, with a complex sinusoidal strain, e, at the same frequency. The impedance function E, which is given by the ratio P/e is also a complex number. If the spring has an incremental stiffness E' (stress required to cause a unit strain) and the dashpot has an incremental viscosity η (stress required to cause a unit strain rate), then, neglecting inertia, it can be shown that the system has an impedance $E' + jE''$ where $E'' = \omega\eta$. Thus the real part of the impedance (E') can be identified with the incremental elastic properties and the imaginary part (E'') with the incremental viscous properties of the system. We note that $E'' = 0$ when $\omega = 0$.

From (4.47) we see that

$$C'_{\theta\theta} = \frac{E'_{\theta}}{(E')^2 + \omega\eta_{\theta})^2}; \quad C''_{\theta\theta} = \frac{\omega\eta_{\theta}}{(E'_{\theta})^2 + (\omega\eta_{\theta})^2} \tag{4.52}$$

where E'_θ is the incremental modulus similar to Young's modulus denoting stiffness in the circumferential direction; η_θ is the incremental coefficient of viscosity in that direction. Equations (4.52) are valid for all values of ω; however when ω is small the expressions for $C'_{\theta\theta}$ and $C''_{\theta\theta}$ can be simplified. In that case, $\omega\eta_\theta \ll E'_\theta$ and $\omega^2\eta_\theta^2$ can be neglected in comparison with $(E'_\theta)^2$. Thus

$$C'_{\theta\theta} \approx \frac{1}{E'_\theta}; \quad C''_{\theta\theta} \approx \frac{\omega\eta_\theta}{(E'_\theta)^2} \tag{4.53}$$

Similar relations hold for C_{zz} and C_{rr}. The viscous coefficients η_θ, η_z and η_r may be obtained from these relations.

(6) Static incremental elastic theory as a special case

The theory developed so far started with an aortic segment in an initially stressed state with superposition of small additional sinusoidal stresses. The steady state incremental strain response showed a combination of elastic and viscous behavior. All the incremental quantities involved—stresses, strains and constitutive coefficients—were complex numbers. Now, if instead of sinusoidally varying stresses, one suddenly superimposes incremental stresses that remain constant in value, the blood vessel will respond by exhibiting instantaneous incremental strains which will increase with time at a decreasing rate tending toward an equilibrium state. This is the phenomenon of creep exhibited by all viscoelastic materials. Many viscoelastic materials behave as fluids in that they never reach an equilibrium state under a non-hydrostatic stress. Blood vessels, when subjected to small increments of loading, do appear to reach, in approximately one minute, what may be considered to be an equilibrium state for most practical purposes (Patel *et al.*, 1969). Upon removal of the superimposed incremental stresses, the incremental strains disappear at a decreasing rate tending toward the original state. Thus, if sufficient time is allowed to lapse between the application of stress and the measurement of strains, the response of the blood vessel could be considered purely elastic. Similarly, for sinusoidally varying incremental stresses at an extremely low frequency, the dynamic response will tend towards the static elastic case, i.e. $C''_{ij} \to 0$ as $\omega \to 0$. The formulae applicable for very low frequency dynamic experiments, i.e. quasistatic experiments, follow very simply from the formulae for the dynamic viscoelastic case outlined in Section A. The imaginary parts of all complex quantities—stresses, strains and the constitutive constants—vanish. Thus for the static elastic case the symbols e_θ, e_z, e_r, P_θ, P_z, P_r, C_{ij}, etc., are real numbers and can be interpreted as the *time-independent* values of incremental strains, stresses or constitutive constants,

B. EXPERIMENTAL DETERMINATION OF THE INCREMENTAL CONSTITUTIVE
COEFFICIENTS

Although incremental theory applies to the general dynamic viscoelastic case, it has thus far only been used for the static case. The dynamic aspects are currently being studied. Therefore, we shall first describe static experiments and results and then discuss briefly the preliminary results of the dynamic studies.

(1) *The static elastic coefficients*

The static elastic case follows from the general viscoelastic theory as a special case and the fundamental equations (4.28) to (4.30) and (4.41) apply. For the static case all the quantities in these equations become real. As mentioned before, a single experiment wherein the strains e_θ, e_z and e_r, and the associated stresses P_θ, P_z and P_r are measured does not suffice for the evaluation of the three unknown elastic constants $C_{\theta\theta}$, C_{zz} and C_{rr} from (4.41), of which only two are independent; therefore an independent experiment is required. Patel *et al.* (1969) were able to evaluate static *in vivo* C_{ij} by choosing for the first experiment one wherein a blood vessel with a chosen average intravascular pressure was subjected to a variation in pressure at constant length, and for the second experiment, variations of the length with small variations in pressure so as to keep the circumferential and radial stresses constant. We summarize here their experiments and results.

(a) *Experimental details.* Experiments were performed on 14 anesthetized open-chested dogs of average weight 28·6 kg. Ventilation was maintained with a positive pressure respiratory pump. For a typical dog a 7·5 cm long segment of the thoracic aorta was marked out and the mean aortic pressure (p) was noted. The segment was isolated and by-passed from the main systemic circulation. An assembly of two plastic cylindrical plugs connected by a hollow metal rod was fitted into the segment, holding it at the original length L as shown in Fig. 11. The proximal end of the segment was connected to a reservoir (D) of oxygenated blood, which could be raised or lowered to change the intraluminal pressure, this was adjusted to that obtaining when the segment length was marked. A displacement measuring device (R) was then sutured to the segment wall (for details see Mallos, 1962). A gauge (F) for measuring the longitudinal force (see Janicki and Patel, 1968) was attached to the plugs and zeroed. The threaded rod of the plug assembly was unscrewed, withdrawn and re-engaged to the proximal plug (see steps 1 and 2, Fig. 11). The force gauge reading now corresponded to the longitudinal force required to maintain the vessel segment at the chosen length.

To minimize hysteresis effects the vessel was subjected to three inflation-deflation cycles over the physiologic range of pressure (from 110 to 190

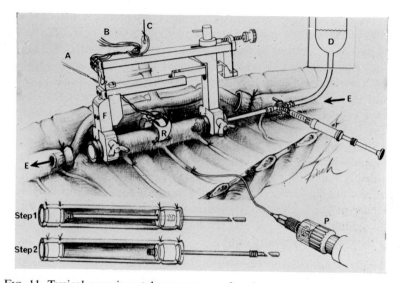

FIG. 11. Typical experimental arrangement for the study of incremental static elastic moduli. A and B = lead wires from the electrical calipers and the force gauge, respectively; C = supporting bracket; D = blood reservoir; E = descending thoracic aorta with by-pass; F = force gauge; P = pressure transducer; R = electrical calipers for sensing displacements. (From Patel *et al.*, 1969.)

cm H_2O). Subsequently, data consisting of pressure, radius and longitudinal force at three segment lengths (L, L^+, L^-) were collected from the ascending limb of the pressure vs. radius curve. The pressure was raised in steps of 20 cm H_2O and data collected at least one minute after the step was imposed.

The oxygen, hydrogen and carbon dioxide concentrations of the blood were carefully controlled. The segment was kept moist during the experiment and the blood temperature was maintained around 26 or 27 °C. The wall volume, V, was determined for each specimen by measuring its loss of weight when excised and suspended in distilled water. The thickness of the vessel wall was computed therefrom for various values of R and L.

(b) *Computation procedures.* For a given dog two experiments were performed around a given state of strain. First, with length L constant the intraluminal pressure was increased from a value p_1, 10 cm H_2O below the pressure (p), to a value p_2, 10 cm H_2O above (p). The associated values of R and F were measured and those for the thickness, h, were calculated assuming constancy of wall volume. The incremental strains and stresses were calculated from these data. As L was unchanged, e_z was zero. e_θ was computed from (4.16). The incremental stresses P_z, P_θ and P_r were obtained from the differences of S_θ, S_z and S_r evaluated with (2.4) to (2.6), using values corresponding to

pressures p_2 and p_1. (Equations (4.22) to (4.24) or (4.25) to (4.27) could
equally well have been used.) Entering these values for e_θ, e_z, P_θ, P_z, P_r in
(4.41) gave two relations in the three unknown quantities $C_{\theta\theta}$, C_{zz} and C_{rr}.
The third relation was obtained through the second experiment mentioned
above. This involved measuring the pressure-radius-longitudinal force relations at three segment lengths L, L^+ and L^-. The experiment was designed
to create an incremental state of stress wherein P_θ was zero and P_r was almost
so. The incremental stresses and strains were calculated as before. For the
second experiment, however, (4.29) or equivalently the second of the set of
(4.41), reduced to a simple ratio between e_z and P_z with C_{zz} as the proportionality constant. The coefficients $C_{\theta\theta}$ and C_{rr} were subsequently
obtained from the data of the first experiment. From these coefficients, the
remainder of the coefficients C_{ij} were obtained using (4.38) to (4.40). The
elastic moduli E_θ, E_z and E_r and the Poisson's ratios $\sigma_{\theta z}$, etc. were obtained
using the elastic equivalents of (4.53).

(c) *Results and discussion.* The results of these *in vivo* studies are summarized
in Table 4 and Fig. 12. Data are grouped according to the range of extension
ratios, λ_θ and λ_z. The following points are noteworthy: (1) The incremental
stresses and strains were small compared to the average stresses and strains.
(2) The values of the incremental Poisson's ratios were positive and always
averaged to 0·5 because of the incompressibility constraint.† (3) The elastic
moduli were higher for group 3 than for group 1 which indicated that the
vessel has non-linear elastic properties. (4) In general, $E_z > E_\theta > E_r$ at
physiologic pressures indicating locally anisotropic behavior of the vessel
wall. (5) The results were repeatable: E_θ and E_r within 2 per cent and E_z
within 16 per cent.

In four dogs the experiment was repeated *in vitro*. The vessel segment was
removed from the thorax with all the instruments in place, stripped of
surrounding tissue up to the adventitia and then studied again. Results
showed a decrease in the values of all the elastic moduli compared to the
in vivo values at corresponding stretches; E_z decreased by 32 per cent
($p < 0·01$), E_r by 20 per cent ($0·2 < p < 0·05$), and E_θ by 9 per cent
($0·05 < p < 0·1$). It was felt that the loss of normal *in situ* tethering of the
aorta could account for the *in vitro* decrease in E_z. To demonstrate this, the
contribution of vascular tethering to the *in vivo* value of E_z was calculated
using the tethering constant K_1 described in Table 3, and was found to be
40 per cent. Thus it was concluded that the 32 per cent decrease in E_z noted
in vitro could easily be explained by the loss of longitudinal tethering.

† The fact that Poisson's ratio is 0·5 for incompressible isotropic linearly elastic
materials is well known. It turns out that the six incremental Poisson's ratios for an incrementally orthotropic elastic material can be grouped in three pairs, each with an average of
0·5, see (5.47).

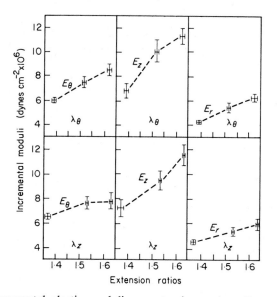

FIG. 12. Incremental elastic moduli vs. extension ratios. E_θ = circumferential modulus; E_z = longitudinal modulus; E_r = radial modulus; λ_θ = circumferential extension ratio; λ_z = longitudinal extension ratio. Horizontal and vertical bars indicate the standard error of the mean for each of the groups. In the upper panels the moduli are plotted vs. the mean λ_θ for each of three groups; the corresponding values of λ_z (from left to right) are $1\cdot45 \pm 0\cdot04$ SE, $1\cdot56 \pm 0\cdot02$ and $1\cdot51 \pm 0\cdot02$. In the lower panels the moduli are plotted vs. λ_z; the corresponding values of λ_θ for each of these groups (left to right) are $1\cdot46 \pm 0\cdot02$, $1\cdot58 \pm 0\cdot02$ and $1\cdot48 \pm 0\cdot02$. (From Patel et al., 1969.)

(2) Dynamic viscoelastic coefficients

There are many ways in which one can attempt to study the dynamic aspects of the problem. We will describe briefly a method currently under study and report the preliminary findings.

As mentioned previously, two independent experimental procedures are required to solve (4.41) for the complex coefficients $C_{\theta\theta}$, C_{zz} and C_{rr}. The experiment was thus carried out in two steps: (1) The middle descending thoracic aorta of a dog was isolated and held at constant in vivo length and pressure in a manner similar to that shown in Fig. 11; however, in this case the force gauge was connected in series with the segment. The blood vessel segment was then connected to a sinusoidal pump via a calibrated syringe, which moved a small quantity of blood in and out of the segment. Data consisting of Δp, ΔF, ΔR, p, F, R and L were collected at frequencies varying from $0\cdot5$ to 5 Hz in steady state. (2) The segment length was now varied by connecting its other end to the sinusoidal pump by a solid metal rod

TABLE 4

Summary of data from static elastic experiments

	Group 1 (λ_θ from 1·29 to 1·45)	Group 2 (λ_θ from 1·46 to 1·55)	Group 3 (λ_θ from 1·56 to 1·72)
No. experimental points	18	18	16
p (cm H_2O)	145	154	162
R (cm)	0·62	0·60	0·63
R/h	8·1	9·8	10·0
$e_\theta \times 100$	4·2	4·5	3·8
$e_z^* \times 100$	2·8	2·7	2·7
P_θ (dynes cm$^{-2} \times 10^6$)	0·255	0·324	0·317
P_z (dynes cm$^{-2} \times 10^6$)	0·068	0·078	0·080
P_z^* (dynes cm$^{-2} \times 10^6$)	0·184	0·276	0·300
S_θ (dynes cm$^{-2} \times 10^6$)	1·150	1·480	1·600
S_z (dynes cm$^{-2} \times 10^6$)	1·040	1·150	1·190
$\sigma_{r\theta}$	0·71	0·80	0·79
$\sigma_{\theta r}$	0·52	0·58	0·59
$\sigma_{\theta z}$	0·29	0·26	0·27
$\sigma_{z\theta}$	0·29	0·20	0·21
σ_{rz}	0·71	0·74	0·72
σ_{zr}	0·48	0·42	0·41

Average values of various parameters are shown. $p =$ intravascular pressure; $R =$ midwall radius; $h =$ wall thickness; $e_\theta =$ circumferential incremental strain; P_θ, $P_z =$ incremental stresses in the circumferential and longitudinal directions; e_z^*, $P_z^* =$ values of incremental longitudinal strain and stress, respectively, for the special case wherein $P_\theta = 0$; S_θ, $S_z =$ stresses in the circumferential and longitudinal directions; $\sigma_{ij} =$ incremental Poisson's ratios. (Adapted from Patel et al., 1969.)

and pulsing sinusoidally at the same frequencies as in step (1). ΔL, ΔF, Δp, ΔR, p, R, L and F were measured. From these data it was possible to calculate various incremental stresses and strains and solve (4.41) for C_{ij}. The complex elastic moduli E_θ, E_z and E_r and Poisson's ratios $\sigma_{\theta z}$ etc. were obtained using (4.53).

Results from six dogs are shown in Table 5. The experiments were carried out in vitro around a mean pressure of 148 cm H_2O and around an initial state of strain given by $\lambda_\theta = 1·53$ and $\lambda_z = 1·51$. The values of static elastic coefficients (0 frequency) from the same dogs are also included in the table for comparison. The following points are noteworthy: (1) The values of E_θ, E_z and E_r tend to increase with frequency. (2) E'_θ, E'_z and E'_r are much greater than E''_θ, E''_z and E''_r. However, it is important to point out that, at this stage, the values of E''_θ, E''_z and E''_r should only be considered approximate but useful for indicating the order of magnitude relative to their primed counterparts.

TABLE 5

Results from the middle descending thoracic aorta of six dogs

Frequency (Hz)	E_θ (dynes cm^{-2} × 10^6)		E_z (dynes cm^{-2} × 10^6)		E_r (dynes cm^{-2} × 10^6)	
	E_θ'	E_θ''	E_z'	E_z''	E_r'	E_r''
0·0	7·38	0·0	6·72	0·0	4·58	0·0
0·5	9·13	0·06	9·96	0·95	6·25	0·59
1·0	9·18	0·10	10·11	0·96	6·31	0·59
2·0	9·30	0·12	10·25	0·95	6·36	0·65
3·0	9·47	0·18	10·19	0·96	6·44	0·69
4·0	9·39	0·32	10·11	1·00	6·28	0·77
5·0	9·50	0·29	10·18	1·04	6·46	0·81

E_θ, E_z and E_r are the complex incremental viscoelastic moduli in the θ, z and r directions; E_θ', E_z' and E_r' are the real parts of the complex moduli representing the elastic coefficients and E_θ'', E_z'' and E_r'' are the imaginary parts related to the viscous coefficients.

C. COMPARISON OF ELASTIC DATA FROM VARIOUS STUDIES IN THE
LITERATURE

As mentioned earlier, various authors have studied the elastic properties of large blood vessels in great detail in the last decade. It will be interesting to compare these studies with the study by Patel *et al.* 1969. described in Section 4B1. Unfortunately no direct comparison is possible because the other studies, (1) assume the blood vessel wall to have isotropic elastic properties, (2) do not include the unstressed dimensions and (3), in some instances do not include the measurement of wall thickness. In spite of these limitations, it was possible to calculate a common parameter, E_{inc}, for all studies using the formula

$$E_{inc} \simeq 0.75 \frac{\Delta p}{\Delta R} \frac{R^2}{h} \qquad (4.54)$$

where E_{inc} is the "isotropic incremental elastic modulus" as defined by Bergel (1960). Although E_{inc} does not describe the material properties of the anisotropic vessel wall, it was used here as a convenient means for comparison of data. Moreover, E_{inc} is simply related to the Moens–Korteweg–Resal formula (McDonald, 1960) for the calculation of pulse wave velocity (c_o) in a linear isotropic elastic tube

$$c_o = \sqrt{(E_{inc} h / 2R\rho)} \qquad (4.55)$$

where ρ is the density of fluid in the tube (blood); c_o may be used to compare gross elastic properties of intact blood vessels.

The results of various studies in the literature using different techniques for measurement of radius in man and dog are summarized in Table 6. It is not

TABLE 6

Comparison of isotropic incremental elastic moduli (E_{inc}) from various studies

Type of study	Frequency for dynamic experiments (Hz)	p (cm H_2O)	E_{inc} (dynes cm^{-2} × 10^6)			
			AsA	MDTA	AbA	PA
Peterson et al. (1960) Dynamic, In vivo, Dog			7·1 (1)	12·7 (2)		
Bergel (1961a) Static, In vitro, Dog		54 136 218 299	1·2 (6) 4·3 (12) 9·9 (6) 18·1 (5)	1·6 (4) 8·9 (8) 12·4 (4) 18·0 (3)		
Bergel (1961b) Dynamic, In vitro, Dog	2	136	4·7 (10)	10·9 (7)		
Greenfield and Patel† (1962) Dynamic, In vivo, Man	1·6	95	5·6 (10)			
Luchsinger et al. (1962) Dynamic, In vivo, Man		134		9·2 (12)		
Greenfield and Griggs† (1963) Dynamic, In vivo, Man	1·4	20				1·2 (8)
Patel et al. (1963) Dynamic, In vivo, Dog	2 2	134 117		8·7 (6)	14·5 (6)	
Patel et al.† (1964) Dynamic, In vivo, Dog	1.6 1·4	131 25	5·7 (6)			0·8 (12)

TABLE 6—*cont.*

Type of study	Frequency for dynamic experiments (Hz)	p (cm H_2O)	E_{inc} (dynes cm^{-2} × 10^6)			
			AsA	MDTA	AbA	PA
Learoyd and Taylor (1966) Static, *In vitro,* Man		136	7·5 (7)	10·5 (5)		
Gow and Taylor (1968) Dynamic, *In vivo,* Dog	2 2	143 156	3·0 (9)		9·8 (7)	
Attinger *et al.* (1968) Static, *In vitro,* Dog		157	3·5 (4)			
Present study from Section 4B1, Patel *et al.* (1969) Static, *In vivo,* Dog		154	3·6 (14)			

AsA = ascending aorta; MDTA = middle descending thoracic aorta; AbA = abdominal aorta; PA = main pulmonary artery; p = intravascular pressure. The figures in parentheses give the number of specimens studied.

† Since the thickness was not measured in these studies, we used R/h (radius to thickness) ratio from Bergel's study to calculate E_{inc}.

meaningful to comment on small differences in values of E_{inc} in these studies for any comparison would be very crude for the following reasons: (1) Because the initial dimensions were not included in most of these studies the mean intravascular pressure was used to locate the initial state of stress around which the local properties represented by E_{inc} could be compared. Although in general it is true that the larger the pressure, the larger the initial stress in a blood vessel, the actual value of this stress is affected by the geometry of the vessel. Thus, even if two blood vessels of different sizes were made up of exactly the same non-linear elastic material, they will be, for a given intra-vascular pressure, at different states of stress and will, in general, have different values of E_{inc}. (2) In many studies the thickness, h, was not measured and approximate values of h from other studies were used to compute E_{inc}. (3) A wide variety of experimental conditions existed in these studies resulting in variations in local chemical milieu which in turn could affect the value of E_{inc}. (4) Different techniques for measurement of radius would involve different measurement errors.

In spite of these reservations, it is reasonable to conclude from Table 6 that: (1) At a given site in the aorta, E_{inc} increases with pressure (e.g. Bergel, 1961a) indicating non-linear elastic behavior, the vessel becoming stiffer at higher intravascular pressures. (2) The value of E_{inc} increases as one proceeds from the ascending aorta to the abdominal aorta. This trend is consistent with the histological evidence of a decrease in the elastin to collagen ratio in the wall material (which would tend to make the wall stiffer) as one proceeds along the aorta away from the heart (McDonald, 1960). (3) The value of E_{inc} for the pulmonary artery is much lower than that for the aorta; this is, at least in part, due to low intravascular pressure in the pulmonary artery. (4) In general, the static values of E_{inc} are lower than the dynamic values (e.g. see Bergel 1961a,b).

5. NON-LINEAR ELASTIC PROPERTIES

A. THEORETICAL CONSIDERATIONS

(1) *General remarks*

Whereas the incremental response discussed in the preceding section is important in many situations of practical interest, it suffers from the limitation that, for a given arterial segment, the information is useful only around a given state of strain and each state of strain requires a different characterization of the material properties. It is thus important to characterize, if possible, the response of the blood vessel by directly determining its constitutive relation from which the stress or the incremental coefficients at any chosen state of strain can be obtained. Although it would be desirable to obtain the constitutive relation by considering the blood vessel as a curvilinearly orthotropic, non-linearly viscoelastic body, at the present time there is no pertinent theoretical or experimental basis for this. However, we shall present here a theory (see Vaishnav et al., 1972; Young, 1970) which characterizes the aorta as a curvilinearly orthotropic non-linearly elastic body. We shall see that under physiologic loading the non-linearly elastic behavior can be characterized by means of three or seven material parameters depending upon the desired degree of precision.

We shall not give here a full account of the modern theory of non-linear constitutive relations. The general theory is well advanced and reference is made to the authoritative work of Truesdell & Noll (1965) for this.

However, we shall try to give enough details here so that a reader with no special knowledge of the mechanics of material behavior under large deformations can follow the development with reasonable ease.

(2) *Application of theory to a large blood vessel*[†]

Consider a thin-walled blood vessel segment in the form of a circular cylinder as shown in Fig. 1. Under an increasing internal pressure p and uniformly applied longitudinal force F the vessel will gradually change its dimensions. Assuming that the deformed vessel is also a thin-walled circular cylinder, the stretches (extension ratios) λ_θ, λ_z and λ_r will be given by (4.4) to (4.6) as the ratios of the new dimensions to the original dimensions in the undeformed configuration. Because of the curvilinearly orthotropic nature of the aortic segment, an orthogonal grid of coordinate lines corresponding to the polar coordinate system (namely, concentric circles, radial lines and longitudinal generators) embedded in the undeformed body and deforming with the aorta will change dimensions but will remain orthogonal; in other words, no shearing strains will develop in the coordinate surfaces. Thus, under physiologic loading, the deformed configuration can be completely described in terms of the three stretches λ_θ, λ_z and λ_r if the undeformed dimensions are known. Clearly, the value of all three stretches in the undeformed configuration will be unity. As shown in (4.1) to (4.3), the conventional strains γ_θ, γ_z and γ_r will be obtained by subtracting unity from the respective stretches. Thus,

$$\gamma_\theta = \lambda_\theta - 1; \qquad \lambda_\theta = 1 + \gamma_\theta \tag{5.1}$$

$$\gamma_z = \lambda_z - 1; \qquad \lambda_z = 1 + \gamma_z \tag{5.2}$$

$$\gamma_r = \lambda_r - 1; \qquad \lambda_r = 1 + \gamma_r \tag{5.3}$$

Another measure of strain is given by the Green–St. Venant[‡] strains $\bar{\gamma}_\theta$, $\bar{\gamma}_z$ and $\bar{\gamma}_r$ obtained as

$$\bar{\gamma}_\theta = \tfrac{1}{2}(\lambda_\theta^2 - 1); \qquad \lambda_\theta^2 = 1 + 2\bar{\gamma}_\theta \tag{5.4}$$

$$\bar{\gamma}_z = \tfrac{1}{2}(\lambda_z^2 - 1); \qquad \lambda_z^2 = 1 + 2\bar{\gamma}_z \tag{5.5}$$

$$\bar{\gamma}_r = \tfrac{1}{2}(\lambda_r^2 - 1); \qquad \lambda_r^2 = 1 + 2\bar{\gamma}_r \tag{5.6}$$

The Green–St. Venant strains are obtained by taking half the difference between the squared length of an arc element in the deformed and initial configurations, and dividing by the initial squared length; thus, $\bar{\gamma}_\theta = (R^2 - R_o^2)/2R_o^2$ and so on. If the division is carried out using instead the squared deformed length the Almansi–Hamel[‡] strains are obtained. There are many possible measures of strain, too numerous to list here. As do most other

[†] Dr. Vaishnav was responsible for the development of the non-linear theory.
[‡] The terms Lagrangian and Eulerian often used for Green–St. Venant and Almansi–Hamel strains, respectively, are historically incorrect; hence, we prefer the latter terms.

strain measures, those given above vanish when the body is undeformed. Different measures turn out to be useful in different applications and are preferred from different points of view. For a given material a theory may take a simpler form in terms of one type of strain measure than the other. For example, in the theory we present below, the Green–St. Venant strains $\bar{\gamma}_\theta$, $\bar{\gamma}_z$ and $\bar{\gamma}_r$ given by (5.4) to (5.6) will be used, as the resulting theory was found to be more fruitful than the corresponding one based on the more familiar measures γ_θ, γ_z and γ_r given by (5.1) to (5.3). Note that for infinitesimal strains, i.e. when the stretches are approximately equal to unity, the two types of strain are identical.

The problem of defining stresses in a non-linearly elastic material can be approached in two ways. In the first method (Cauchy's method) stresses are expressed directly in terms of strains. In the second method (Green's method) stresses are expressed in terms of the derivatives of a strain energy density function which is a function of strain. As the former method does not depend on the concept of strain energy, it is the more general. On the other hand, if a strain energy density function does exist, the latter method is more economical in the number of constitutive parameters needed. For adiabatic and isothermal deformations at least, it can be proved that a strain energy function does exist. As we have in mind application of the theory to essentially isothermal conditions, we shall follow Green's method of derivation. It should be pointed out here that Patel and Janicki (1970) have demonstrated the existence of a strain energy density function in the middle descending thoracic aorta, the left coronary circumflex artery and the common carotid artery in dogs.

The concept of strain energy may be explained briefly as follows. When the artery is inflated, the external forces responsible for the deformation do work. If the process is adiabatic† or isothermal, and no other energy exchange takes place, then, for a perfectly elastic material (without internal dissipation), the excess of the mechanical work over the increase in kinetic energy is stored in the body as strain energy and is available for doing work when the deformation is allowed to recover. The strain energy is usually expressed in terms of unit mass or unit volume (either in the deformed or the undeformed state) and is then referred to as the strain energy density. The strain energy density for a given elastic body is a function of the state of deformation only.

Let W be the strain energy density (strain energy per unit initial volume) in the aortic segment under physiologic loading. Then W can be expressed as

$$W = W(a, b, c) \tag{5.7}$$

where

$$a = \bar{\gamma}_\theta, \quad b = \bar{\gamma}_z, \quad c = \bar{\gamma}_r \tag{5.8}$$

† i.e. without exchange of heat energy with the surroundings.

are the Green–St. Venant strains given by (5.4) to (5.6). If the shearing strains in the coordinate surfaces were not zero, the list of arguments of W in the parenthesis in (5.7) would have to include these also†. If we assume that W can be approximated by a polynomial in a, b and c, then

$$W = W_o + k_1 a + k_2 b + k_3 c + k_4 a^2 + k_5 b^2 + k_6 c^2 +$$
$$+ k_7 ab + k_8 bc + k_9 ca + k_{10} a^3 + \ldots \quad (5.9)$$

where k_1, k_2, etc. are constants depending upon the elastic properties of the material and W_o is the amount of strain energy density corresponding to the unstrained state and can arbitrarily be set equal to zero. Clearly, the unending polynomial has to be truncated after a finite number of terms. The number of terms that should be retained depends on a variety of considerations. The larger the number of terms retained, the more accurate the representation of material response over a given range of values of a, b and c. Conversely, for a given tolerance in the accuracy of representation, an increase in the number of terms retained would increase the range of applicability. In addition there are practical limits on the number of terms that can be retained, because the larger the number, the larger the minimum experimental effort necessary, and, for a given accuracy of measurement, the more the noise in the values of the material constants. In fact, retaining too many terms would not only be unnecessary, but also misleading.

There has to be some consistent criterion, however, for retaining a certain number of terms. One such criterion would be to retain terms only up to a certain degree in a, b and c. For example, retaining those up to and including those of power two in a, b and c would lead to a theory similar to the classical linear theory of elasticity for a curvilinearly orthotropic body.

As will be shown later, the first order terms in (5.9) can be set equal to zero if it is assumed that the undeformed state is also unstressed. The fourth degree expression for W can then be given as

$$W = k_4 a^2 + k_5 b^2 + k_6 c^2 + k_7 ab + k_8 bc + k_9 ca +$$
$$+ k_{10} a^3 + k_{11} a^2 b + k_{12} a^2 c + k_{13} ab^2 + k_{14} ac^2 +$$
$$+ k_{15} abc + k_{16} b^3 + k_{17} b^2 c + k_{18} bc^2 + k_{19} c^3 +$$
$$+ k_{20} a^4 + k_{21} a^3 b + k_{22} a^3 c + k_{23} a^2 b^2 + k_{24} a^2 bc +$$
$$+ k_{25} a^2 c^2 + k_{26} ab^3 + k_{27} ab^2 c + k_{28} abc^2 + k_{29} ac^3 +$$
$$+ k_{30} b^4 + k_{31} b^3 c + k_{32} b^2 c^2 + k_{33} bc^3 + k_{34} c^4 \quad (5.10)$$

which contains 6 second degree, 10 third degree and 15 fourth degree terms,

† Actually, in that case the Green–St. Venant strains given by (5.4) to (5.6) will not be principal, i.e. they will not be the only non-zero elements of the matrix of the physical components of the Green–St. Venant tensor. For details, see Green and Adkins (1960) and Vaishnav et al. (1972).

a total of 31. Thus, the second-, third- and fourth-order expansions of W would contain 6, 16 and 31 terms, respectively.

The assumption of incompressibility permits further simplification, for it implies that the product of the three principal stretches should equal unity. Using (5.4) to (5.6) and (5.8), the condition of incompressibility may be written as

$$(1+2a)(1+2b)(1+2c) = 1. \tag{5.11}$$

This can be used to determine c when a and b are known. It thus becomes unnecessary to measure c experimentally as it can be computed from the measured values of a and b and the strain energy then computed using (5.10). A better way is to compute the value of c from (5.11) in terms of a and b, substitute in (5.10) and express W solely as a function of a and b. Unfortunately, this does not permit W to retain its simple polynomial character. This can be overcome by solving (5.11) for c, expressing the result in terms of an infinite series in a and b and truncating the result to retain only terms up to order four in a and b. Thus,

$$c \approx -a - b + 2a^2 + 2ab + 2b^2 - 4a^3 - 4a^2b - 4ab^2 - 4b^3 + 8a^4 +$$
$$+ 8a^3b + 8a^2b^2 + 8ab^3 + 8b^4 \tag{5.12}$$

If the approximate expression for c given by (5.12) is used in (5.10) and terms of various degrees in a and b are collected, we get the following expression for W:

$$W = Aa^2 + Bab + Cb^2 + Da^3 + Ea^2b + Fab^2 + Gb^3 + Ha^4 + Ia^3b +$$
$$+ Ja^2b^2 + Kab^3 + Lb^4 \tag{5.13}$$

where $A, B, \ldots, L$ are various combinations of the material constants k_4 through k_{34}; the exact expressions are unimportant. Equation (5.13) could have been written down directly by expressing W as a fourth degree polynomial in a and b, but then the role of the assumption of incompressibility would have been obscured. Moreover, the preceding development derives (5.10); this is the counterpart of (5.13) and can be used as a starting point for a similar investigation of non-linear deformations of compressible orthotropic tissues.

Equation (5.13) involves 12 material constants $A, B, \ldots, L$. By eliminating the fourth degree terms we obtain the expression

$$W = Aa^2 + Bab + Cb^2 + Da^3 + Ea^2b + Fab^2 + Gb^3 \tag{5.14}$$

which contains 7 material constants. Finally, by neglecting the third degree terms also, we obtain

$$W = Aa^2 + Bab + Cb^2 \tag{5.15}$$

which contains only 3 material constants. We shall refer to (5.13), (5.14) and (5.15) as the fourth-order, third-order and second-order expressions for W.

We now derive expressions relating W to the stresses S_θ, S_z and S_r. If a thin-walled arterial segment (see Fig. 1) in equilibrium under an internal pressure p and a longitudinal force F is given a small deformation so that the dimensions R, h and L increase by dR, dh and dL, respectively, then the work done by p as a result of the change in internal radius will be given by the product $2\pi(R-h/2)Lp$, which is the total radial force on the endothelial surface, and $dR-(dh/2)$, which is the increase in the radius of the lumen. Neglecting $h/2R$, small in comparison with unity, and using (2.1) and (2.3), the work done by p during the radial deformation can be shown to be equal to

$$2\pi RLh\left(S_\theta\frac{dR}{R} + S_r\frac{dh}{h}\right).$$

The work done by p and F during the small longitudinal deformation is given by $2\pi RhLS_z(dL/L)$ where S_z is given by (2.2). Assuming no heat exchange, no change in kinetic energy and no internal dissipation during the deformation, the total mechanical work done by p and F can be equated to the increase in strain energy of the arterial segment. Dividing this by the initial volume $(2\pi R_o L_o h_o)$ of the segment and using (4.4) to (4.6), we get

$$dW = \lambda_\theta\lambda_z\lambda_r\left[S_\theta\frac{dR}{R} + S_z\frac{dL}{L} + S_r\frac{dh}{h}\right] \tag{5.16}$$

where dW is the increase in the strain energy per unit initial volume. By making use of (4.16) to (4.18) we can rewrite (5.16) as

$$dW = \lambda_\theta\lambda_z\lambda_r[S_\theta e_\theta + S_z e_z + S_r e_r] \tag{5.17}$$

or

$$dW = \lambda_z\lambda_r S_\theta\,d\lambda_\theta + \lambda_\theta\lambda_r S_z\,d\lambda_z + \lambda_\theta\lambda_z S_r\,d\lambda_r. \tag{5.18}$$

Equation (5.18) can be used to derive the expression for the stresses S_θ, S_z and S_r in terms of W. For a compressible material, W is a function of λ_θ, λ_z, λ_r, since $W = W(a, b, c)$ by (5.7), and a, b and c are functions of λ_θ, λ_z and λ_r through (5.8) and (5.4) to (5.6). Thus,

$$dW = \frac{\partial W}{\partial\lambda_\theta}\,d\lambda_\theta + \frac{\partial W}{\partial\lambda_z}\,d\lambda_z + \frac{\partial W}{\partial\lambda_r}\,d\lambda_r \tag{5.19}$$

which, upon comparison with (5.18), yields

$$S_\theta = \frac{1}{\lambda_r\lambda_z}\frac{\partial W}{\partial\lambda_\theta}$$

$$S_z = \frac{1}{\lambda_\theta\lambda_r}\frac{\partial W}{\partial\lambda_z} \tag{5.20}$$

$$S_r = \frac{1}{\lambda_\theta\lambda_z}\frac{\partial W}{\partial\lambda_r}$$

Equations (5.8) and (5.4) to (5.6) can be used to give the following relations between the partial derivatives of W:

$$\frac{\partial W}{\partial \lambda_\theta} = \lambda_\theta \frac{\partial W}{\partial a}; \quad \frac{\partial W}{\partial \lambda_z} = \lambda_z \frac{\partial W}{\partial b}; \quad \frac{\partial W}{\partial \lambda_r} = \lambda_r \frac{\partial W}{\partial c}. \tag{5.21}$$

The use of (5.21) in (5.20) gives

$$S_\theta = \frac{\lambda_\theta}{\lambda_z \lambda_r} \frac{\partial W}{\partial a}$$

$$S_z = \frac{\lambda_z}{\lambda_\theta \lambda_r} \frac{\partial W}{\partial b} \tag{5.22}$$

$$S_r = \frac{\lambda_r}{\lambda_\theta \lambda_z} \frac{\partial W}{\partial c}$$

These expressions are valid for any form of W if the material is compressible. In particular, one may use (5.10) for W. However, we are concerned here with an incompressible material for which W is a function only of λ_θ and λ_z or equivalently, of a and b. To account for this we use the incremental condition of incompressibility given by (4.19). Accordingly,

$$d\lambda_r = -\lambda_r \left(\frac{d\lambda_\theta}{\lambda_\theta} + \frac{d\lambda_z}{\lambda_z} \right). \tag{5.23}$$

Upon using (5.23) in (5.18) we get

$$dW = \lambda_z \lambda_r (S_\theta - S_r) \, d\lambda_\theta + \lambda_\theta \lambda_r (S_z - S_r) \, d\lambda_z. \tag{5.24}$$

As W is now a function of λ_θ and λ_z only,

$$dW = \frac{\partial W}{\partial \lambda_\theta} \, d\lambda_\theta + \frac{\partial W}{\partial \lambda_z} \, d\lambda_z \tag{5.25}$$

which, upon comparison with (5.24) yields

$$S_\theta - S_r = \frac{1}{\lambda_z \lambda_r} \frac{\partial W}{\partial \lambda_\theta} = \lambda_\theta \frac{\partial W}{\partial \lambda_\theta} \tag{5.26}$$

$$S_z - S_r = \frac{1}{\lambda_\theta \lambda_r} \frac{\partial W}{\partial \lambda_z} = \lambda_z \frac{\partial W}{\partial \lambda_z} \tag{5.27}$$

The rightmost sides of (5.26) and (5.27) arise from the fact that for incompressible materials $\lambda_\theta \lambda_z \lambda_r = 1$. Use of (5.21) in (5.26) and (5.27) gives

$$S_\theta - S_r = \lambda_\theta^2 \frac{\partial W}{\partial a} = (1 + 2a) \frac{\partial W}{\partial a} \tag{5.28}$$

$$S_z - S_r = \lambda_z^2 \frac{\partial W}{\partial b} = (1 + 2b) \frac{\partial W}{\partial b} \tag{5.29}$$

which are the stress-strain relations for large deformations of an incompressible material. We compare (5.28) and (5.29) with (5.22) and note that, whereas for a compressible material all three stresses are determined completely from the knowledge of W as a function of the strains, only the stress differences are determined completely from the knowledge of W as a function of strains in the case of an incompressible material. By rewriting (2.7) as $S_h = S_r + \frac{1}{3}(S_\theta - S_r) + \frac{1}{3}(S_z - S_r)$, we see that knowledge only of the stress differences $S_\theta - S_r$ and $S_z - S_r$, leaves a part of the hydrostatic stress undetermined. This is not surprising, for hydrostatic stress causes no strain in an incompressible material and cannot change the strain energy and hence it cannot be determined from the energy either. In practice, the indeterminacy can be removed by knowing some stress boundary condition.

Specifically, we may use (5.13), (5.14) or (5.15) in (5.28) and (5.29). From (5.13) we have

$$
\begin{aligned}
S_\theta - S_r = {} & 2Aa + Bb + (4A + 3D)a^2 + (2B + 2E)ab + Fb^2 + \\
& + (6D + 4H)a^3 + (4E + 3I)a^2 b + (2F + 2J)ab^2 + \\
& + Kb^3 + 8Ha^4 + 6Ia^3 b + 4Ja^2 b^2 + 2Kab^3
\end{aligned}
\tag{5.30}
$$

$$
\begin{aligned}
S_z - S_r = {} & Ba + 2Cb + Ea^2 + (2B + 2F)ab + (4C + 3G)b^2 + \\
& + Ia^3 + (2E + 2J)a^2 b + (4F + 3K)ab^2 + \\
& + (6G + 4L)b^3 + 2Ia^3 b + 4Ja^2 b^2 + 6Kab^3 + 8Lb^4
\end{aligned}
\tag{5.31}
$$

Equations (5.30) and (5.31) are the desired stress-strain relations based on the fourth-order strain energy density function. Those for the third- and second-order expressions, (5.14) and (5.15), respectively, can be obtained by setting appropriate constants in (5.30) and (5.31) equal to zero. It should be pointed out that the stress differences $S_\theta - S_r$ and $S_z - S_r$ in (5.30) and (5.31) are polynomial functions in a and b, and that all the coefficients are based on the 12 coefficients describing W in (5.13). Had the existence of a strain energy density function not been assumed, it would have been necessary to express both $S_\theta - S_r$ and $S_z - S_r$ as polynomials of an appropriate degree in a and b. For a representation equivalent to that in (5.30) and (5.31), a total of 26 independent material constants would have been required. In the present formulation the terms in b^4 and a^4 are missing from (5.30) and (5.31), respectively. A consistent direct fourth-degree expansion of $S_\theta - S_r$ and $S_z - S_r$ in powers of a and b would require inclusion of all the fourth-degree terms in the expressions for the stress differences. This would require a total of 28 material constants against 12 in the present theory using W.

If the material constants are known, the form of stress-strain relations given by (5.30) and (5.31) is preferable. On the other hand, the terms may with advantage be rearranged as given below if the material constants are to be evaluated:

$$S_\theta - S_r = A(2a + 4a^2) + B(b + 2ab) + D(3a^2 + 6a^3) + E(2ab + 4a^2b) +$$
$$+ F(b^2 + 2ab^2) + H(4a^3 + 8a^4) + I(3a^2b + 6a^3b) +$$
$$+ J(2ab^2 + 4a^2b^2) + K(b^3 + 2ab^3) \tag{5.32}$$

$$S_z - S_r = B(a + 2ab) + C(2b + 4b^2) + E(a^2 + 2a^2b) + F(2ab + 4ab^2) +$$
$$+ G(3b^2 + 6b^3) + I(a^3 + 2a^3b) + J(2a^2b + 4a^2b^2) +$$
$$+ K(3ab^2 + 6ab^3) + L(4b^3 + 8b^4) \tag{5.33}$$

By setting the constants H, I, J, K and L equal to zero in (5.32) and (5.33) the stress-strain relations for the third-degree expression in W follow. Upon further setting D, E, F and G equal to zero, those for the second-degree expression in W follow.

(3) *Relation with the incremental elastic theory*

It is easy to compute the incremental response of a material whose stress-strain response under large deformations is described by (5.32) and (5.33). As mentioned before, the incremental stresses P_θ, P_z and P_r are differentials of S_θ, S_z and S_r, respectively. Thus,

$$P_\theta - P_r = \frac{\partial(S_\theta - S_r)}{\partial a} da + \frac{\partial(S_\theta - S_r)}{\partial b} db \tag{5.34}$$

$$P_z - P_r = \frac{\partial(S_z - S_r)}{\partial a} da + \frac{\partial(S_z - S_r)}{\partial b} db \tag{5.35}$$

Now, from (4.16) to (4.18), (5.4), (5.5) and (5.8) it can be seen that

$$da = (1 + 2a)e_\theta; \quad db = (1 + 2b)e_z. \tag{5.36}$$

Thus, from (5.32) to (5.35) we have the incremental relations

$$P_\theta - P_r = \beta_{\theta\theta}e_\theta + \beta_{\theta z}e_z \tag{5.37}$$
$$P_z - P_r = \beta_{z\theta}e_\theta + \beta_{zz}e_z \tag{5.38}$$

where

$$\beta_{\theta\theta} = (1 + 2a)[A(2 + 8a) + 2Bb + D(6a + 18a^2) + E(2b + 8ab) +$$
$$+ 2Fb^2 + H(12a^2 + 32a^3) + I(6ab + 18a^2b) +$$
$$+ J(2b^2 + 8ab^2) + 2Kb^3] \tag{5.39}$$

$$\beta_{\theta z} = \beta_{z\theta} = (1 + 2a)(1 + 2b)(B + 2Ea + 2Fb + 3Ia^2 + 4Jab + 3Kb^2) \tag{5.40}$$

$$\beta_{zz} = (1 + 2b)[2Ba + C(2 + 8b) + 2Ea^2 + F(2a + 8ab) +$$
$$+ G(6b + 18b^2) + 2Ia^3 + J(2a^2 + 8a^2b) +$$
$$+ K(6ab + 18ab^2) + L(12b^2 + 32b^3)]. \tag{5.41}$$

The equality $\beta_{\theta z} = \beta_{z\theta}$ (obtained here for an incompressible material) does not in general hold for the incremental relations of compressible materials.

Equations (5.37) and (5.38) can be inverted to express the incremental strains in terms of the incremental stresses. Thus,

$$e_\theta = (\beta_{zz}/\beta)(P_\theta - P_r) - (\beta_{\theta z}/\beta)(P_z - P_r) \tag{5.42}$$

$$e_z = (-\beta_{\theta z}/\beta)(P_\theta - P_r) + (\beta_{\theta\theta}/\beta)(P_z - P_r) \tag{5.43}$$

where

$$\beta = \beta_{\theta\theta}\beta_{zz} - \beta_{\theta z}^2. \tag{5.44}$$

We may collect the terms in P_θ, P_z and P_r in (5.42) and (5.43) and compare them with (4.28) to (4.30) where the coefficients C_{ij} are now real. We then have

$$
\begin{aligned}
C_{rr} &= (\beta_{zz} + \beta_{\theta\theta} - 2\beta_{\theta z})/\beta \\
C_{\theta\theta} &= \beta_{zz}/\beta \\
C_{zz} &= \beta_{\theta\theta}/\beta \\
C_{r\theta} &= C_{\theta r} = (\beta_{\theta z} - \beta_{zz})/\beta \\
C_{zr} &= C_{rz} = (\beta_{\theta z} - \beta_{\theta\theta})/\beta \\
C_{\theta z} &= C_{z\theta} = -\beta_{\theta z}/\beta.
\end{aligned}
\tag{5.45}
$$

As β_{ij} are known in terms of $A, \ldots, L$, through (5.39) to (5.41), C_{ij} can be obtained in terms of $A, \ldots, L$ through (5.45). Similarly, using (4.47) and (4.50) after omitting primes and setting double-primed quantities equal to zero, we can obtain E_r, E_θ, E_z, $\sigma_{\theta z}, \ldots, \sigma_{r\theta}$, in terms of C_{ij}, and through (5.45) in terms of β_{ij}. Thus,

$$E_\theta = \beta/\beta_{zz}; \quad E_z = \beta/\beta_{\theta\theta}; \quad E_r = \beta/(\beta_{\theta\theta} - \beta_{zz} - 2\beta_{\theta z})$$

$$\sigma_{r\theta} = (\beta_{zz} - \beta_{\theta z})/\beta_{zz}$$

$$\sigma_{\theta r} = (\beta_{zz} - \beta_{\theta z})/(\beta_{\theta\theta} + \beta_{zz} - 2\beta_{\theta z})$$

$$\sigma_{\theta z} = \beta_{\theta z}/\beta_{\theta\theta}; \quad \sigma_{z\theta} = \beta_{\theta z}/\beta_{zz} \tag{5.46}$$

$$\sigma_{zr} = (\beta_{\theta\theta} - \beta_{\theta z})/(\beta_{\theta\theta} + \beta_{zz} - 2\beta_{\theta z})$$

$$\sigma_{rz} = (\beta_{\theta\theta} - \beta_{\theta z})/\beta_{\theta\theta}.$$

Again, using (5.39) to (5.41) in (5.46), $E_\theta, \ldots, \sigma_{rz}$, can be obtained in terms of $A, \ldots, L$. In (5.46) we have the interesting relations

$$\sigma_{r\theta} + \sigma_{z\theta} = \sigma_{rz} + \sigma_{\theta z} = \sigma_{\theta r} + \sigma_{zr} = 1. \tag{5.47}$$

These relations are borne out in the numerical results given in Table 4.

Finally, we write down the equations expressing β_{ij} in terms of C_{ij} and also of $E_\theta, \ldots, \sigma_{rz}$:

$$\beta_{\theta\theta} = C_{zz}/\Delta = 1/E_z\Delta$$

$$\beta_{\theta z} = -C_{\theta z}/\Delta = -\sigma_{\theta z}/E_z\Delta = -\sigma_{z\theta}/E_\theta\Delta \tag{5.48}$$

$$\beta_{zz} = C_{\theta\theta}/\Delta = 1/E_\theta\Delta$$

where

$$\Delta = C_{\theta\theta}C_{zz} - C_{z\theta}^2 = (1/E_\theta E_z)(1 - \sigma_{z\theta}\sigma_{\theta z}) = 1/\beta. \tag{5.49}$$

4*

Equations (5.39) to (5.41) and (5.48) with (5.49) can be used to obtain the constitutive constants $A, \ldots, L$ from the incremental moduli at sufficient numbers of states of strain.

(4) *Further discussion of certain aspects of the constitutive relations*

(a) In deriving (5.13) it was stated that the terms of degree one in a and b can be set equal to zero if it is assumed that the undeformed configuration is stress-free. This can now be proved by retaining such terms in W, computing the stress differences $S_\theta - S_r$ and $S_z - S_r$ from (5.28) and (5.29) and setting $S_\theta = S_z = S_r = a = b = 0$. Specifically, for the second-order expression we would have

$$W = A_o a + B_o b + A a^2 + B a b + C b^2 \tag{5.50}$$

$$S_\theta - S_r = A_o + 2A_o a + 2Aa + Bb + 4Aa^2 + 2Bab \tag{5.51}$$

$$S_z - S_r = B_o + 2B_o b + 2Cb + Ba + 4Cb^2 + 2Bab \tag{5.52}$$

For $a = b = 0$, $S_\theta - S_r = A_o$ and $S_z - S_r = B_o$, and if $S_\theta = S_z = S_r = 0$, $A_o = B_o = 0$. The same is true for the higher order expressions.

(b) If the material were transversely isotropic in the θz surface, i.e. its properties were identical in all directions in the θz surface, then the following equalities among the constants in (5.13) would obtain

$$A = C, E = F, D = G, H = L, I = K. \tag{5.53}$$

Thus the second-order theory would need only two constants, the third-order theory four constants and the fourth-order theory seven constants. If the material were completely isotropic, no further simplification beyond that given by (5.53) would result within the framework of the present formulation, and it would be preferable to use (5.10) as the starting point for reduction. Finally, if the material were transversely isotropic in the $r\theta$ plane, (5.13) would not indicate this. For this a formulation similar to (5.13) should be obtained from (5.10) in terms of the Green–St. Venant strains a and c by eliminating b, and then imposing equalities among the constants as in (5.33).

(c) In cardiovascular mechanics, it is important to know the distribution of S_r through the wall thickness. It is also important for the analysis of the failure of a blood vessel under stress, to know the distribution of W, S_θ, S_z and S_r through the thickness. As a first approximation, we may use the material constants obtained with the thin-wall assumption and compute the distribution of S_r by using the following formula (Green and Adkins, 1960):

$$S_r = r_o \int^r (S_\theta - S_r) \frac{dr}{r} \tag{5.54}$$

where r_o is the outside radius of the blood vessel in the deformed state and $S_\theta - S_r$ is computed from (5.30) where a and b are now the local values of the

Green–St. Venant strains in the θ and z directions. Assuming that λ_z is constant through the thickness, $b = \frac{1}{2}(\lambda_z^2 - 1)$ is also constant. From the requirement of preservation of tissue volume, the local value of a at a particle with radial coordinate r in the deformed configuration can be obtained by

$$a = \frac{1}{2}\left[\frac{r^2}{\{R^2/(1+2a_m)\}+(1+2b)^{\frac{1}{2}}(r^2-R^2)} - 1\right] \qquad (5.55)$$

where a_m is the value of a at $r = R$. If a is known as a function of r, (5.54) gives the distribution of S_r through the thickness, and consequently, (5.30), (5.31) and (5.13) will yield the distributions of W, S_θ and S_z. Simon et al. (1970) obtained a distribution of S_r and S_θ through the thickness, based on a constitutive relation described below. Unfortunately, as their theory did not include stresses in the longitudinal direction, no analysis of the distribution of S_z or W through the thickness was possible.

(5) *Relation of the proposed constitutive relations to some other constitutive relations*

A direct comparison of various non-linear constitutive relations is, in general, difficult because of the possible variety of formulation. We shall however comment below on a few typical relations proposed for arterial tissue.

(a) *Mooney and Neo-Hookean materials.* One of the most celebrated constitutive equations applied to large elastic deformations of isotropic incompressible rubber-like materials is due to Mooney (1940) and has been used by Ling (1970) to describe the lower part of the pressure-radius curve of a canine thoracic aorta. The strain energy density function of a Mooney material is given by

$$W = \alpha_1(I_1 - 3) + \alpha_2(I_2 - 3) \qquad (5.56)$$

where α_1 and α_2 are material constants of I_1 and I_2 are strain invariants given by

$$I_1 = \lambda_\theta^2 + \lambda_z^2 + \lambda_r^2 = (1+2a)+(1+2b)+(1+2a)^{-1}(1+2b)^{-1} \qquad (5.57)$$

$$I_2 = \lambda_\theta^2\lambda_z^2 + \lambda_z^2\lambda_r^2 + \lambda_r^2\lambda_\theta^2 = (1+2a)(1+2b)+(1+2a)^{-1}+(1+2b)^{-1} \qquad (5.58)$$

where in (5.57) and (5.58) the incompressibility condition $\lambda_\theta^2\lambda_z^2\lambda_r^2 = 1$ has been used. On expanding the expressions $(1+2a)^{-1}$ and $(1+2b)^{-1}$ in terms of powers of a and b and retaining only those of order two in a and b, we get

$$I_1 = I_2 = 3 + 4(a^2 + ab + b^2). \qquad (5.59)$$

Substituting (5.59) in (5.56) we get

$$W = 4(\alpha_1 + \alpha_2)(a^2 + ab + b^2). \qquad (5.60)$$

Comparison of (5.15) with (5.60) shows that the former would yield the latter if

$$A = B = C = 4(\alpha_1 + \alpha_2). \qquad (5.61)$$

We note that if we use as the starting point the strain energy density function of the so-called Neo-Hookean material (Treloar, 1958), namely,

$$W = (\alpha_1 + \alpha_2)(I_1 - 3) \qquad (5.62)$$

we again obtain (5.60). Thus in terms up to order two in a and b, the Mooney material, the Neo-Hookean material and the isotropic special case of the second degree expression† for W given here, viz. (5.15), are all equivalent.

(b) *Isotropic compressible theory of Tickner and Sacks.* Tickner and Sacks (1967) suggested the following expression for the strain energy density of a blood vessel:

$$W = \alpha_1(I_1 - 3) + \alpha_2(I_2 - 3) + \alpha_3(I_3 - 1) + \alpha_4(I_1 - 3)^2 + \alpha_5(I_2 - 3)^2 +$$
$$+ \alpha_6(I_3 - 1)^2 + \alpha_7(I_1 - 3)^3 + \alpha_8(I_2 - 3)^3 + \alpha_9(I_3 - 1)^3 \qquad (5.63)$$

where $\alpha_1, \ldots, \alpha_9$ are material constants, I_1 and I_2 are given by (5.57) and (5.58) and I_3 is the third strain invariant given by

$$I_3 = \lambda_\theta^2 \lambda_z^2 \lambda_r^2 \qquad (5.64)$$

which equals unity for incompressible materials. As I_1, I_2 and I_3 are symmetric functions of λ_θ, λ_z and λ_r, it is clear that (5.63) represents an isotropic material. Also, as $I_3 - 1$ appears explicitly in (5.63), it represents a compressible material. As an artery is an incompressible orthotropic body (5.63) is not truly applicable. It may be mentioned, however, that Tickner and Sacks' work was the first occasion on which the modern theory of non-linear elasticity was used to develop a fully three-dimensional theory of arterial elasticity.

(c) *Work of Simon* et al. Simon *et al.* (1970) properly considered the aorta as an incompressible orthotropic material and used as their starting point the following expression for the strain energy density function:

$$W = W(I_1, b) \qquad (5.65)$$

where I_1 is given by (5.57) and b by (5.8) and (5.5). Since, for an incompressible material, I_1 is a function of λ_θ and λ_z only, and b is a function of λ_z only, (5.65) effectively expresses W as a function of λ_θ and λ_z, and is, thus, a correct starting point. However, they only carried out experiments for a fixed value of b, which, can of course, yield only partial information on the non-linear elastic properties of the aorta. They found that the exponential form for $\partial W/\partial I_1$ proposed by Fung (1967) from uniaxial tensile test data

† Although not shown here, it can be proved that $A = B = C$ for the isotropic case.

on the mesentery was applicable to their data for constant length inflation experiments. They evaluated the constants $\bar{A}$ and k in the expression

$$\frac{\partial W}{\partial I_1} = \bar{A} \exp(kI_1) \tag{5.66}$$

for a constant λ_z. Unfortunately, we have found no convenient way of correlating their expression with ours.

B. EXPERIMENTAL VERIFICATION

(1) *Methods*

Experiments were conducted *in vitro* on specimens from four dogs (average weight 28 kg) to test the applicability of the non-linear theory to a canine aorta (for details, see Vaishnav et al., 1972). The experiments involved measuring the dimensions of an aortic segment in the unstressed state and in 27 other states corresponding to various degrees of circumferential and longitudinal stretches within physiologic limits. From the knowledge of the circumferential, longitudinal and radial stresses in the stressed states it was possible to compute the values of the constitutive parameters for the second-degree (3-constant), third-degree (7-constant) and the fourth-degree (12-constant) expressions in W.

The instruments and the experimental arrangement in these experiments were essentially the same as those described in Section 4 for the measurement of static elastic incremental constants, except that in the present case the experiments were performed *in vitro*. The segment was approximately 8 cm long at a pressure of 150 cm H_2O. As before, to remove the effects of hysteresis, the segment was subjected to two cycles of loading and unloading prior to the start of the actual experiment. The main experiment consisted of measuring p, R, F, L relationships as the segment was inflated from 30 cm H_2O to 180 cm H_2O at average constant lengths of 7·88, 8·03 and 8·18 cm. At the end the unstressed dimensions and the volume of the segment were determined.

From these data stresses S_θ, S_z and S_r were calculated using equations (2.1) to (2.3); λ_θ and λ_z using (4.4) and (4.5); and a and b using (5.4), (5.5) and (5.8). The experiments covered an average range of λ_θ from 1·10 to 1·65, and of λ_z from 1·47 to 1·53. The average maximum values of $S_\theta - S_r$ and $S_z - S_r$ were $2·13 \times 10^6$ dynes cm^{-2} and $1·47 \times 10^6$ dynes cm^{-2}, respectively.

Using (5.32) and (5.33) for each set of known values of a, b, $S_\theta - S_r$ and $S_z - S_r$ two equations were obtained in the 3, 7 or 12 material parameters depending upon the theory used. As more equations were available than the number of constants to be evaluated in each case, they were solved by the method of least squares.

(2) Results and discussion

For the 3-constant theory based on (5.15) the following average values ($\pm$ SEM) were obtained for the material constants:

$$A = 0.372\,(\pm 0.030); \quad B = 0.219\,(\pm 0.019); \quad C = 0.288\,(\pm 0.038)$$

where the units are (dynes cm$^{-2} \times 10^6$). In spite of the fact that the values are averaged over four dogs the constants show a rather narrow spread. The parameter A is the coefficient of a^2 in (5.15) and thus dominates the elastic properties in the θ direction. Similarly, the parameter C dominates the elastic properties in the z direction. The parameter B controls the interaction of the responses in the θ and z directions. By an analysis of (5.46) using (5.39) to (5.41) and (5.44) it can be shown that the initial elastic moduli for a material governed by (5.15) are: $E_\theta = (4AC - B^2)/2C$, $E_z = (4AC - B^2)/2A$, $E_r = (4AC - B^2)/2(A - B + C)$. Using the above values of A, B and C we can obtain the initial values of the moduli E_θ, E_z and E_r as 0.663, 0.512 and 0.433 (dynes cm$^{-2} \times 10^6$), respectively, thus indicating that the vessel is initially anisotropic and is approximately 30 per cent and 53 per cent stiffer in the θ direction than in the z and r directions, respectively. Relative stiffnesses at any other state of strain will, of course, depend on the values of a and b in that state. In a similar manner, initial values of the Poisson's ratios were computed and found to be 0.29, 0.38, 0.62. 0.40, 0.60 and 0.71 for $\sigma_{\theta z}$, $\sigma_{z\theta}$, $\sigma_{r\theta}$, $\sigma_{\theta r}$, σ_{zr} and σ_{rz}, respectively. The numerical values for the elastic moduli and the Poisson's ratios are computed here only to give a feeling for the role of A, B and C.

To obtain an estimate of the goodness of fit of the 3-constant theory, the stress differences $S_\theta - S_r$ and $S_z - S_r$ were computed for each dog at each state of strain using (5.32) and (5.33), and compared with their measured values. When plotted against each other, with the computed stress differences on the ordinate and the measured differences on the abscissa the ideal result would be a straight line with unit slope, zero intercept on the ordinate and unit correlation coefficient. The average values obtained were:

$$S_\theta - S_r: \; c.c. = 0.997, \; m = 0.930, \; C = 0.095 \; (\text{dynes cm}^{-2} \times 10^6)$$
$$S_z - S_r: \; c.c. = 0.987, \; m = 0.730, \; C = 0.276 \; (\text{dynes cm}^{-2} \times 10^6)$$

where m is the slope, C is the intercept and $c.c.$ is the correlation coefficient. We observe that the correlation coefficients are very good in both cases. The values of m and C for $S_z - S_r$ are not good; this is probably attributable to the rather narrow range of λ_z values used in the experiments. It is thus seen that the 3-constant theory gives a good fit in the θ direction but not in the z direction.

For the 7-constant theory based on (5.14), the following average values ($\pm$ SEM) were obtained for the material parameters:

$$A = 0\cdot412\ (\pm0\cdot066); \quad B = -0\cdot067\ (\pm0\cdot131); \quad C = 0\cdot191\ (\pm0\cdot059);$$
$$D = -0\cdot055\ (\pm0\cdot036); \quad E = 0\cdot162\ (\pm0\cdot051); \quad F = 0\cdot179\ (\pm0\cdot103);$$
$$G = 0\cdot099\ (\pm0\cdot087)$$

where the units are (dynes $cm^{-2} \times 10^6$). Although the constants do not show the narrow spread characteristic of the 3-constant theory, the 7-constant theory fits the experimental data much better as can be seen by the average values given below for the correlation coefficient, c.c., slope, m, and intercept, C, on the ordinate axis for graphs with the computed stress differences as the ordinate and the experimental values as the abscissa:

$$S_\theta - S_r: \ c.c. = 0\cdot998,\ m = 0\cdot997,\ C = 0\cdot0027\ (\text{dynes cm}^{-2} \times 10^6)$$
$$S_z - S_r: \ c.c. = 0\cdot993,\ m = 0\cdot991,\ C = 0\cdot0082\ (\text{dynes cm}^{-2} \times 10^6)$$

The results show that the 7-constant theory fits the experimental results very well. The 12-constant theory was also tried and found to fit the data still better, but the marginal improvement in the quality of fit was not judged to be of sufficient importance to recommend the use of the 12-constant theory; consequently, we shall not discuss it further.

Finally, the values of the incremental moduli, E_θ, E_z and E_r were computed using the 3-constant and the 7-constant theories and equations (5.46), (5.39) to (5.41) and (5.44). The values were compared with those obtained directly using the method outlined in Section 4. A comparison of the moduli from four dogs showed that on the average the 3- and 7- constant theories agreed with direct measurements to within the percentages listed below:

	E_θ	E_z	E_r
3-constant theory	8	22	20
7-constant theory	1	2	1

As can be seen, agreement with the 7-constant theory is good.

The values of strain energy density (SED) were computed using the average values of the non-linear constitutive coefficients from the 3- and 7-constant theories in (5.15) and (5.14), respectively. For a state of strain corresponding to stretches of $\lambda_\theta = 1\cdot62$ and $\lambda_z = 1\cdot41$, the values of SED were found to be 403×10^3 and 362×10^3 dynes cm^{-2} for the 3- and 7-constant theories, respectively. They compare favorably with the average value $352(\pm 26\ \text{SEM}) \times 10^3$ dynes cm^{-2} of SED obtained by Patel and Janicki (1970), for the same state of strain, using direct integration of external work done on eight segments of the middle descending thoracic aorta of dogs.

In conclusion, we have experimentally tested the 3-, 7- and 12-constant non-linearly elastic theories. The 7-constant theory appears to be satisfactory for most practical purposes.

6. Summary and Future Research

In this chapter we have reviewed various techniques used in the last decade to characterize the mechanical properties of a large blood vessel such as the aorta. The studies mainly fall into four categories: (1) Study of general material properties, e.g. incompressibility and the elastic symmetry of the arterial wall; (2) The role of vascular tethering; (3) Determination of incremental viscoelastic coefficients; (4) Development of non-linear elastic theory. The theoretical material is, wherever possible, supported by experimental data from our laboratory. Pertinent data from the literature are also discussed, with comparisons among various studies when appropriate. This should provide a rational basis for the characterization of the mechanical properties of the circulatory system in health and disease.

In addition to the systematic exposition of the various approaches to the study of blood vessels, we wish also to suggest areas for future research. Again restricting ourselves to large blood vessels, these are summarized below: (1) A non-linear viscoelastic theory should be developed to characterize the wall material. The incremental viscoelastic constants can then be obtained from this theory as needed. One could also study the effect of disease and various pharmacological agents on these constants. (2) Since the ultimate goal of this research is application to man, one will need to develop methods to use these concepts in intact man. (3) As mentioned before, the blood vessel wall is non-homogeneous and consists of collagen, smooth muscle and elastic fibers embedded in a gelatinous matrix. It will be important to incorporate this feature in future considerations to permit characterization of local material properties through the wall as well as calculation of stress distributions through the wall. The knowledge of wall stresses is important since they control the nutrition of the vessel wall (through the regulation of blood flow in the *vasa-vasorum*) as well as the passage of various materials from the blood stream into the vessel wall.

Acknowledgement

We are grateful to Dr. D. L. Fry for his help and criticisms throughout this research. We thank Messrs. J. S. Janicki, J. T. Young and T. E. Carew for collaboration in various aspects of the research; Professor H. B. Atabek and Dr. J. T. Flaherty for a critical review of the manuscript; Mrs. V. M. Fry for technical illustrations; Mrs. C. Floyd for editing and typing the manuscript and Messrs. J. M. Pearce, F. Plowman, L. Brown and G. Johnson for technical assistance. We also thank the American Heart Association Inc. for permission to reproduce illustrations and tables from previous publications. The development of the non-linear theory was based on work performed under NSF Grants No. GK–782, GK–2802 and GK–23747 for which thanks are acknowledged to the National Science Foundation.

SYMBOLS USED IN THE TEXT

$A, \ldots, L$	Constitutive parameters in the non-linear theory. See (5.13).
A_{ij}, B_{ij}	Elastic coefficients relating strains $\gamma_r, \ldots, \gamma_{z\theta}$ and stresses $S_r, \ldots, S_{z\theta}$. See (2.9) and (2.10).
a, b, c	Same as $\bar{\gamma}_\theta$, $\bar{\gamma}_z$ and $\bar{\gamma}_r$, respectively.
C_{ij}	Complex incremental constitutive coefficients. See (4.28) to (4.30).
$C'_{\theta\theta}, C''_{\theta\theta}$	The real part and the negative of the imaginary part of $C_{\theta\theta}$. Similarly, for C_{zz} and C_{rr}.
E_θ, E_z, E_r	Complex circumferential, longitudinal and radial incremental moduli.
E'_θ, E''_θ	Real and imaginary parts of E_θ. Similarly for E_z and E_r.
e_θ, e_z, e_r	Incremental strains in the θ, z and r directions, respectively.
F	Longitudinal force on the vessel segment in addition to that due to p.
$\bar{F}, X$	Force per unit endothelial area and the corresponding displacement in the longitudinal tethering experiment.
G	Shear modulus of elasticity.
h	Thickness of the arterial wall.
h_o	Thickness of the arterial wall in the unstressed state.
j	Square root of -1.
K_R, η_R	Elastic and viscous coefficients of the model representing the plug-instrument assembly in the longitudinal tethering experiments.
k	Bulk modulus of elasticity.
L	Length of the arterial segment.
L_o	Length of the arterial segment in the unstressed state.
$M_V, M_A, K_1, K_2, \\ \eta_1, \eta_2$	Parameters of the Patel–Fry model for longitudinal tethering. See Fig. 5.
P_θ, P_z, P_r	Incremental stresses in the θ, z and r directions, respectively.
$P_{\theta\theta}$, etc.	Various combinations of P_θ, P_z and P_r. See (4.42).
p	Intravascular pressure.
R	Midwall radius of the arterial segment.
R_o	Midwall radius of the segment in the unstressed state.

r, θ, z	Polar cylindrical coordinates of any point in the vessel wall.
S_d	Deviatoric stress.
S_h	Hydrostatic stress.
S_θ, S_z, S_r	Normal stresses in the circumferential, longitudinal and radial directions, respectively.
$S_{\theta z}, S_{r\theta}, S_{rz}$, etc.	Shear stresses on various faces of an element of aortic wall. $S_{\theta z}$ indicates that the shear stress is acting in z direction on a plane perpendicular to θ axis, similarly for $S_{r\theta}$ and S_{rz}.
V	Volume of the arterial wall (tissue volume).
V_o	Volume of the arterial wall in the unstressed state (tissue volume).
W	Strain energy density function (per unit volume in the undeformed configuration).
β_{ij}	Incremental constitutive coefficients. See (5.37) and (5.38).
$\gamma_r, \gamma_\theta, \gamma_z$	Elongating strains in the r, θ and z directions, respectively.
$\gamma_{\theta z}, \gamma_{r\theta}, \gamma_{rz}$	Shear strains. See Fig. 2.
$\bar{\gamma}_\theta, \bar{\gamma}_z, \bar{\gamma}_r$	Green–St. Venant strains in the θ, z and r directions, respectively. See (5.4) to (5.6).
$\Delta R, \Delta p, \Delta L, \Delta F$	Complex incremental changes in R, p, L and F respectively.
$\Delta p', \Delta F', \Delta L'$	Real parts of Δp, ΔF and ΔL.
$\Delta p'', \Delta F'', \Delta L''$	Imaginary parts of Δp, ΔF and ΔL.
ΔV	Change in wall volume of the arterial segment.
η_θ	Viscous coefficient of the model of Fig. 10.
$\lambda_\theta, \lambda_z, \lambda_r$	Stretches or extension ratios in the θ, z and r directions, respectively.
ϕ, α, ψ	Angles by which Δp, ΔF and ΔL lead ΔR.
$\sigma_{\theta z}$, etc.	Complex Poisson's ratios for an orthotropic material. See (4.48).
$\sigma'_{\theta z}, \sigma''_{\theta z}$, etc.	Real and imaginary parts of $\sigma_{\theta z}$, etc.
Ω	Relative angular rotation between the ends of the vessel segment under inflation.
ω	Circular frequency in radians s^{-1}.

REFERENCES

Anliker, M., Moritz, W. E. and Ogden, E. (1968). Transmission characteristics of axial waves in blood vessels. *J. Biomech.* **1**, 235–246.

Apter, J. T. (1967). Correlation of visco-elastic properties with microscopic structure of large arteries: IV. Thermal responses of collagen, elastin, smooth muscle, and intact arteries. *Circulation Res.* **21**, 901–918.

Apter, J. T. and Marquez, E. (1968). A relation between hysteresis and other visco-elastic properties of some biomaterials. *Biorheology* 5, 285–301.

Apter, J. T., Marquez, E. and Janas, M. (1970). Dynamic viscoelastic anisotropy of canine aorta correlated with aortic wall composition. *J. Assoc. Advan. of Med. Instrum.* 4, 15–21.

Atabek, H. B. (1968). Wave propagation through a viscous fluid contained in a tethered, initially stressed, orthotropic elastic tube. *Biophys. J.* 8, 626–649.

Attinger, F. M. L. (1968). Two-dimensional *in-vitro* studies of femoral arterial walls of the dog. *Circulation Res.* 22, 829–840.

Attinger, E., Anne, A., Mikami, T. and Sugawara, H. (1968). Modeling of pressure-flow relations in arteries and veins. *In* "Hemorrheology" (A. L. Copley, ed.), p. 255, Pergamon Press, New York.

Attinger, E. O. (1964). "Pulsatile Blood Flow" p. 15, McGraw-Hill, New York.

Azuma, T., Hasegawa, M. and Matsuda, T. (1970). Rheological properties of large arteries. *In* "Proceedings of the Fifth International Congress on Rheology" (S. Onogi, ed.), pp. 129–141, University of Tokyo Press, Tokyo and University Park Press, Baltimore.

Bergel, D. H. (1960). The visco-elastic properties of the arterial wall. Ph.D. Thesis, University of London.

Bergel, D. H. (1961a). The dynamic elastic properties of the arterial wall. *J. Physiol.* 156, 458–469.

Bergel, D. H. (1961b). The static elastic properties of the arterial wall. *J. Physiol.* 156, 445–457.

Biot, M. A. (1965). "Mechanics of Incremental Deformations", pp. 67, 89, 337, John Wiley and Sons, New York.

Blatz, P. J., Chu, B. M. and Wayland, H. (1969). On the mechanical behavior of elastic animal tissue. *Trans. Soc. Rheol.* 13, 83–102.

Burton, A. C. (1962). Physical principles of circulatory phenomena: the physical equilibria of the heart and blood vessels. *In* "Handbook of Physiology, Section 2, Circulation" (W. F. Hamilton and P. Dow, eds.), Vol. I, pp. 85–106, American Physiological Society, Washington, D. C.

Carew, T. E., Vaishnav, R. N. and Patel, D. J. (1968). Compressibility of the arterial wall. *Circulation Res.* 23, 61–68.

Cox, R. H. (1968). Wave propagation through a Newtonian fluid contained within a thick-walled, viscoelastic tube. *Biophys. J.* 8, 691–709

Dobrin, P. B. and Doyle, J. M. (1970). Vascular smooth muscle and the anisotropy of dog carotid artery. *Circulation Res.* 27, 105–119.

Dobrin, P. B. and Rovick, A. A. (1969). Influence of vascular smooth muscle on contractile mechanics and elasticity of arteries. *Am. J. Physiol.* 217, 1644–1651.

Fry, D. L. (1969). Certain chemorheologic considerations regarding the blood vascular interface with particular reference to coronary artery disease. *In* "Research on Acute Myocardial Infarction" (S. Bondurant, ed.), pp. IV-38–IV-59, American Heart Association, New York.

Fry, D. L., Patel, D. J. and de Freitas, F. M. (1962). Relation of geometry to certain aspects of hydrodynamics in larger pulmonary arteries. *J. Appl. Physiol.* 17, 492–496.

Fung, Y. C. B. (1967). Elasticity of soft tissues in simple elongation. *Am. J. Physiol.* 213, 1532–1544.

Fung, Y. C. B. (1968). Biomechanics. Its scope, history, and some problems of continuum mechanics in physiology. *Appl. Mech. Rev.* 21, 1–20.

Gow, B. S. and Taylor. M. G. (1968). Measurement of viscoelastic properties of arteries in the living dog. *Circulation Res.* **23**, 111–122.

Green, A. E. and Zerna, W. (1968). "Theoretical Elasticity", 2nd Ed., p. 155, University Press, Oxford.

Green, A. E. and Adkins, J. E. (1960). "Large Elastic Deformations and Nonlinear Continuum Mechanics", p. 29. University Press, Oxford.

Greenfield, J. C., Jr. and Griggs, D. M. Jr., (1963). Relation between pressure and diameter in main pulmonary artery of man. *J. Appl. Physiol.* **18**, 557–559.

Greenfield, J. C., Jr. and Patel, D. J. (1962). Relation between pressure and diameter in the ascending aorta of man. *Circulation Res.* **10**, 778–781.

Hardung, V. (1962). Propagation of pulse waves in visco-elastic tubings. *In* "Handbook of Physiology, Section 2, Circulation", (W. F. Hamilton and P. Dow, eds.), Vol. 1, pp. 107–135, American Physiological Society, Washington, D.C.

Hardung, V. (1964). Significance of anisotropy and inhomogeneity in the determination of the elasticity of blood vessels. *Angiologica* **1**, 185–196.

Iberall, A. S. (1967). Anatomy and steady flow characteristics of the arterial system with an introduction to its pulsatile characteristics. *Math. Biosci.* **1**, 375–395.

Janicki, J. S. and Patel, D. J. (1968). A force gauge for measurement of longitudinal stresses in a blood vessel *in situ*. *J. Biomech.* **1**, 19–21.

Jeffreys, H. and Jeffreys, B. S. (1962). "Methods of Mathematical Physics", 3rd Ed., p. 114, University Press, Cambridge.

Lawton, R. W. (1954). The thermoelastic behavior of isolated aortic strips of the dog. *Circulation Res.* **2**, 344–353.

Learoyd, B. M. and Taylor, M. G. (1966). Alterations with age in the viscoelastic properties of human arterial walls. *Circulation Res.* **18**, 278–291.

Lee, J. S., Frasher, W. G., Jr., and Fung, Y. C. B. (1967). Two-dimensional finite-deformation experiments on dogs' arteries and veins. Rep. No. AFOSR 67-1980, Bioengineering. University of California, San Diego.

Ling, S. C. (1970). Modeling the non-linear behavior of arteries. American Institute of Aeronautics and Astronautics (AIAA), Third Fluid and Plasma Dynamics Conference.

Love, A. E. H. (1927). "A Treatise on the Mathematical Theory of Elasticity", 4th Ed., p. 161, Dover Publications, New York.

Luchsinger, P. C., Sachs, M. and Patel, D. J. (1962). Pressure-radius relationship in large blood vessels of man. *Circulation Res.* **11**, 885–888.

Mallos, A. J. (1962). An electrical caliper for continuous measurement of relative displacement. *J. Appl. Physiol.* **17**, 131–134.

McDonald, D. A. (1960). "Blood Flow in Arteries", pp. 4, 146, 155, 162, Williams and Wilkins, Baltimore.

Mooney, M. (1940). A theory of large elastic deformation. *J. Appl. Physics* **11**, 582–592.

Nash, W. A. (1957). "Theory and Problems of Strength of Materials", p. 54, Schaum Publishing Co., New York.

Patel, D. J. (1969). Mechanical properties of large blood vessels. *In* "The Pulmonary Circulation and Interstitial Space", (A. P. Fishman and H. H. Hecht, eds.), pp. 355–360, The University of Chicago Press, Chicago.

Patel, D. J., Austen, W. G., Greenfield, J. C., Jr., and Tindall, G. T. (1964a). Impedance of certain large blood vessels in man. *Ann. N.Y. Acad. Sci.* **115**, 1129–1139.

Patel, D. J., de Freitas, F. M., Greenfield, J. C., Jr., and Fry, D. L. (1963). Relationship of radius to pressure along the aorta in living dogs. *J. Appl. Physiol.* **18,** 1111–1117.

Patel, D. J., de Freitas, F. M. and Mallos, A. J. (1962). Mechanical function of the main pulmonary artery. *J. Appl. Physiol.* **17,** 205–208.

Patel, D. J. and Fry, D. L. (1964). *In situ* pressure-radius-length measurements in ascending aorta in anesthetized dogs. *J. Appl. Physiol.* **19,** 413–416.

Patel, D. J. and Fry, D. L. (1966). Longitudinal tethering of arteries in dogs. *Circulation Res.* **19,** 1011–1021.

Patel, D. J. and Fry, D. L. (1969). The elastic symmetry of arterial segments in dogs. *Circulation Res.* **24,** 1–8.

Patel, D. J., Greenfield, J. C., Jr. and Fry, D. L. (1964b). *In vivo* pressure-length-radius relationship of certain blood vessels in man and dog. *In* "Pulsatile Blood Flow", (E. O. Attinger, ed.), pp. 293–305, McGraw-Hill, New York.

Patel, D. J. and Janicki, J. S. (1966). Catalogue of some dynamic analogies used in pulmonary and vascular mechanics. *Med. Res. Engr.* **5,** 30–33.

Patel, D. J. and Janicki, J. S. (1970). Static elastic properties of the left coronary circumflex artery and the common carotid artery in dogs. *Circulation Res.* **27,** 149–158.

Patel, D. J., Janicki, J. S. and Carew, T. E. (1969). Static anisotropic elastic properties of the aorta in living dogs. *Circulation Res.* **25,** 765–779.

Patel, D. J., Mallos, A. J. and Fry, D. L. (1961). Aortic mechanics in the living dog. *J. Appl. Physiol.* **16,** 293–299.

Patel, D. J., Schilder, D. P. and Mallos, A. J. (1960). Mechanical properties and dimensions of the major pulmonary arteries. *J. Appl. Physiol.* **15,** 92–96.

Patel, D. J., Tucker, W. K. and Janicki, J. S. (1970). Dynamic elastic properties of the aorta in radial direction. *J. Appl. Physiol.* **28,** 578–582.

Peterson, L. H., Jensen, R. E. and Parnell, J. (1960). Mechanical properties of arteries *in vivo*. *Circulation Res.* **8,** 622–639.

Remington, J. W. (1963). The physiology of the aorta and major arteries. *In* "Handbook of Physiology, Section 2, Circulation", (W. F. Hamilton and P. Dow, eds.), Vol. II, pp. 799–838, American Physiological Society, Washington, D.C.

Roach, M. R. and Burton, A. C. (1957). The reason for the shape of the distensibility curves of arteries. *Can. J. Biochem. Physiol.* **35,** 681–690.

Simon, B. R., Kobayashi, A. S., Strandness, D. E. and Wiederhielm, C. A. (1970). Large deformation analysis of the arterial cross section. *In* "Proceedings of the 23rd Annual Conference on Engineering in Medicine and Biology", Vol. 12, p. 10, The Alliance for Engineering in Medicine and Biology, Washington, D.C.

Sokolnikoff, I. S. (1956). "Mathematical Theory of Elasticity", 2nd Ed., p. 58, McGraw-Hill, New York.

Tickner, E. G. and Sacks, A. H. (1967). A theory for the static elastic behavior of blood vessels. *Biorheology* **4,** 151–168.

Timoshenko, S. and Goodier, J. N. (1970). "Theory of Elasticity", 3rd Ed., p. 71, McGraw-Hill, New York.

Treloar, L. R. G. (1958). "The Physics of Rubber Elasticity", 2nd Ed., p. 66, University Press, Oxford.

Truesdell, C. and Noll, W. (1965). The non-linear field theories of mechanics. *In* "Encyclopedia of Physics", (S. Flugge, ed.), Vol. III, Springer-Verlag, Berlin.

Vaishnav, R. N., Young, J. T., Janicki, J. S. and Patel, D. J. (1972). Non-linear anistropic elastic properties of the canine aorta. *Biophys. J.* (in press).

Weiner, F., Morkin, E., Skalak, R. and Fishman, A. P. (1966). Wave propagation in the pulmonary circulation. *Circulation Res.* **19**, 834–850.

Wolinsky, H. and Glagov, S. (1964). Structural basis for the static mechanical properties of the aortic media. *Circulation Res.* **14**, 400–413.

Wolinsky, H. and Glagov, S. (1967). A lamellar unit of aortic medial structure and function in mammals. *Circulation Res.* **20**, 99–111.

Womersley, J. R. (1957a). An elastic tube theory of pulse transmission and oscillatory flow in mammalian arteries. WADC Tech. Rept. TR. 56–614.

Womersley, J. R. (1957b). Oscillatory flow in arteries: the constrained elastic tube as a model of arterial flow and pulse transmission. *Phys. Med. Biol.* **2**, 177–187.

Young, J. T. (1970). Determination of constitutive constants of canine aorta under large deformations. M. S. Thesis. Catholic University of America, Washington, D.C.

Young, T. (1808). The Croonian Lecture. On the functions of the heart and arteries. *Phil. Trans.* **99**, 1–31.

Chapter 12

The Influence of Vascular Smooth Muscle on the Viscoelastic Properties of Blood Vessels

B. S. GOW

Department of Physiology, University of Sydney,
Sydney, Australia

1. INTRODUCTION

A. GENERAL PROPERTIES OF BLOOD VESSELS

Apart from the reservoir function of the large arteries and veins, blood vessels are primarily conduits for transporting blood. Their endothelial lining forms a compatible interface separating the blood from the mass of elastic and collagen fibres, smooth muscle cells and ground substance which constitute the vessel walls. Pease and Paule (1960) have shown the smooth muscle cell to be the only cell type in the aortic media and concluded that it must be responsible for laying down the other structures; these structures have passive viscoelastic properties. The presence of contractile components introduces complexity into an otherwise simple relationship between pressure and vessel diameter. Not only does vascular smooth muscle vary the calibre, wall thickness and the distensible properties of blood vessels but it is primarily responsible for much of their complicated, time-dependent, mechanical behaviour.

A comprehensive treatment of the elastic properties of blood vessels has not been intended except where the elastic properties are related to vasomotor changes. There are a number of reviews available which deal with both elastic and time-dependent behaviour of blood vessels, (Reuterwall, 1921; Wezler and Sinn, 1953; Burton, 1954; Kapal, 1954; Sinn, 1956; Meyer, 1958; Bergel, 1960). Alexander (1963), Bader (1963) and Remington (1963) have reviewed many of the mechanical properties of veins and arteries in their respective chapters in the "Handbook of Physiology". More recently Bergel (1966) discussed stress-strain properties of blood vessels. McDonald (1968) covered the subject of arterial elasticity in his review on haemodynamics as did Johnson (1969) the following year. Recent reviews on the mechanical properties of veins are those of Thron (1967) and Attinger (1969).

Studies of the mechanical properties of blood vessels can be divided into those done *in vitro* and those done *in vivo*. By far the majority of experiments have been done *in vitro* and, while having the advantage of ease of controlling the variables, have the disadvantages common to all experiments done *in vitro*, that of difficulty in extrapolating the results to the living animal. This difficulty is increased by the fact that many workers have used strips and rings of arterial or venous wall rather than intact vessels. Some workers, who have used excised arteries obtained sigmoid pressure-volume relationships because they allowed isolated segments to lengthen on inflation. This sigmoidal relationship was subsequently shown to be an artifact (Bergel, 1961a) for arteries are tethered longitudinally *in vivo*. Of those experiments done *in vivo* insufficient data was often recorded; for example, measurement of arterial elasticity requires corresponding measurements of stress and strain, not simply pressure and volume (or radius) changes, nor simply changes in force and length.

In recent years the introduction of improved techniques for the measurement of arterial diameter (Peterson *et al.*, 1960; Mallos, 1962; Gow, 1966; Pieper and Paul, 1968) has permitted studies of arterial viscoelastic properties within the living animal. These conditions demand a device with a high frequency response and a low mechanical impedance. Such criteria are not met in some of the existing instruments, while in others inadequate procedures were used to test their dynamic accuracy.

The work of Patel and his collaborators has provided valuable information regarding the geometry and elastic properties of the major pulmonary artery (Patel *et al.*, 1960) and systemic arteries (Patel *et al.*, 1963). Recent measurements of veins and venous reservoirs made with a number of devices described by Guntheroth (1969) have provided new and useful information. On the micro scale, one is impressed with the ingenious flying spot technique of Johnson and Greatbatch (1966) and the closed-circuit TV system of Wiederhielm (1965a).

Since most studies of arterial elasticity have been made on excised vessels it cannot be assumed that the state of contraction of smooth muscle in the wall is the same as it was in the living animal. Comparison of results of Patel *et al.* (1963) from arteries in living dogs with those from excised vessels (Bergel, 1961b) suggested that living arteries had a higher elastic modulus than excised ones. Although Lee *et al.* (1968) concluded that the longitudinal elastic properties of the carotid artery were little affected by its excision, this conclusion does not necessarily apply to circumferential elasticity. In the same year Gow and Taylor (1968) obtained results from living dogs which, for the aorta, agreed well with those of Bergel. Resolution of this disagreement between Patel's results and those of Bergel, and Gow and Taylor was achieved following a recent investigation of Patel *et al.* (1969) in which new data gave excellent agreement with those of other workers. The reason for the former disparity in the respective findings was related among other things, to problems associated with diameter measurement and is discussed fully by Patel *et al.* (1969). Hence for the aorta at least, it would appear, as Bergel suggested, that the elastic properties are little affected by loss of vascular tone. Whether this is true for muscular arteries and other blood vessels remains to be demonstrated.

In most investigations of pressure–volume or pressure–radius relationships there is some manipulation of the vessel and disturbance of its environment. What effect this has on the intrinsic level of vasomotor tone in the vessel awaits studies using sophisticated techniques. Such a technique for measuring aortic diameter is one using the diameter gauge of Pieper and Paul (1969) which allows pressure and diameter measurement without exposure of the exterior of the vessel; although it should be noted that, with this particular device, it is not clear what the effects of mechanical stimulation of the endothelium would be. Finally, it has been assumed that blood vessels are tubes whose distensible properties are determined by the structures lying between the adventitia and the lumen. This is a reasonable concept when applied to the aorta and its major branches. However, as far as arterioles are concerned, Fung (1966) has suggested that a more appropriate model might be a system of branching tunnels within a gel. The contribution of perivascular tissue to the distensible properties of small blood vessels is poorly understood and deserves attention in future.

Before considering the effects of alterations in vasomotor tone on the mechanical properties of arteries and veins it is relevant to discuss a few points regarding their structure and mechanical behaviour.

B. MECHANICAL STRUCTURE AND ELASTIC PROPERTIES OF ARTERIES AND VEINS

(1) Systemic arteries

The histological structure of blood vessels is covered in standard text-books and also in books dealing predominantly with blood vessels (Luisada, 1961; Abrahamson, 1962). The walls of arteries and veins are classically described in terms of concentric zones: intima, internal elastic lamina, media, external elastic lamina and adventitia. From the point of view of stress-bearing, the media and perhaps the adventitia are the most important. The media is of special interest here since it contains the vascular smooth muscle. The media of an elastic artery is composed of a series of concentric elastic lamellae connected by obliquely orientated smooth muscle fibres. In adjacent interlamellar spaces the muscle fibres often run in reverse direction giving the wall a herringbone appearance (Benninghoff, 1927, 1930). Wolinsky and Glagov (1967) found that over a wide range of species and body weight the number of lamellae in the aortic media was roughly proportional to the diameter of the aorta. On the basis of their data and the Frank equation (stress $= pr_i/h$, where p is pressure, r_i inner radius and h wall thickness) it can be shown that, at a given pressure, stress will be roughly the same in the aortae of all species.

The stress-strain properties of aortic tissue are rubber-like, (Lawton, 1954;

King, 1957) time-dependent and non-linear (Roy, 1880). As the mean distending pressure increases the wall strain increases, the distensibility ($\Delta V/\Delta p$) falls and the elastic modulus of the wall increases (Bergel, 1961a). The non-linear relationship of pressure to diameter (or volume) and strain-dependency of the elastic modulus follows as the consequence of having both extensible (elastin) and relatively inextensible (collagen) components in the wall (Roach and Burton, 1957). The popular analogy of the rubber balloon in the string-bag to explain the change in slope of the pressure-radius relationship is probably not a good one, if taken literally, for it suggests that the stress is borne solely by adventitial collagen fibres at physiological pressures. The histologic evidence obtained by Wolinsky and Glagov (1964) from sections of arteries fixed at various distending pressures suggests that the interlamellar collagen is important in stress-bearing at higher pressures. These workers did not consider the contribution of smooth muscle to this "two phase" system, yet it seems likely from other evidence (Goto and

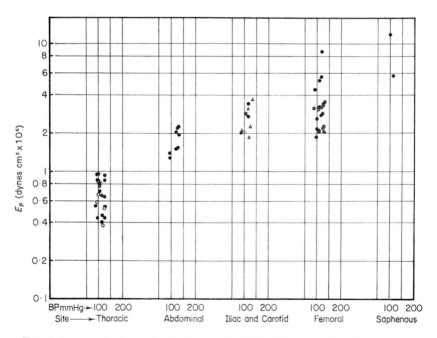

FIG. 1. Increase in dynamic elastic modulus (E_p) of the arterial wall as one moves peripherally. ($E_p = \bar{D}_o |p|/|D_o|$) where $\bar{D}_o$ is the mean diameter at a given pressure, $|p|/|D_o|$ is the ratio of the first harmonic of pressure to that of diameter obtained from Fourier analyses of pressure and corresponding diameter pulse waves from all sites except the carotid arteries, in which case $|p|/|D_o|$ was obtained from power spectrum analysis of randomly varying pressure and diameter waves.

Kimoto, 1966; Laszt, 1968; Dobrin and Rovick, 1969) that in contracting, the muscle transfers the circumferential tension from the collagen to itself and elastin (into which it inserts) thus increasing the extensibility of the wall.

The wall material shows different moduli of elasticity (orthogonal aniso-tropy) depending on whether the strain is circumferential, longitudinal or radial (Lambossy and Müller, 1954; Tickner and Sacks, 1964; Hardung, 1964; Patel and Fry, 1969; Patel et al., 1969; see also Patel and Vaishnav, Chapter 11 in this volume). As one moves peripherally along the aorta its distensibility falls and the circumferential elastic modulus of the wall increases (Bergel, 1961a; Remington, 1963; Patel et al., 1963; Learoyd and Taylor, 1966; Gow and Taylor, 1968). The non-uniform elasticity of the aorta and major branches measured in living dogs is demonstrated in Fig. 1 using values of E_p; see equation (1.3). The haemodynamic consequences of this non-uniformity have been discussed in detail by Taylor (1964, 1967). The increasing stiffness along the length of the aorta and its branches is well correlated with the rise in the relative collagen content and fall in relative elastin content (Harkness et al., 1957; Cleary, 1963), the former protein having a Young's modulus approximately one thousand times greater than the latter. Not only does the content of collagen exceed elastin in the smaller arteries but the relative quantity of smooth muscle increases as well. The elastin lamellae disappear and the smooth muscle cells form a flat helix ("Ringmuskeln", Benninghoff, 1930) which gives the appearance of a circumferential orientation.

(2) *Pulmonary arteries*

The main pulmonary artery and its major branches, in contrast to the aorta, have no elastic lamellae, the elastin fibres having a sparse distribution. The fibres are short and separated by other slender elastin fibres which terminate in club-like expansions (Harris and Heath, 1962). The major pulmonary artery has a relatively thin wall, its medial thickness being 40–70 per cent of that of the aorta. A single record (Patel et al., 1960) shows this vessel to have a slightly non-linear pressure diameter relationship convex to the diameter axis over the dynamic range of approximately 10–40 mmHg. At a mean pressure of 18·5 mmHg the outside diametrical variation was ± 8 per cent about the mean diameter with each cardiac cycle. This constitutes a 50 per cent variation (relative to diastolic dimensions) in lumenal cross-sectional area assuming isovolumetric wall strain and a ratio of wall thickness to vessel outer radius (γ) equal to 0·1. The elastic modulus E_p, calculated from data of Patel et al. (1960) was $0·103 \times 10^6$ dynes cm^{-2} which is roughly one-sixth of that of the descending aorta. Using equation (1.3) in Section C and assuming $\gamma = 0·1$, one obtains a velocity of 207 cm s^{-1} at a mean pressure of 18·5 mmHg which agrees well with the measured value of 230 cm s^{-1} obtained by Attinger (1963). Whether the pulmonary tree has non-uniform elastic properties like those of the systemic tree has not been substantiated although preliminary results by Morris (1965) suggest little change in the elastic composition between the major pulmonary artery and the lower lobe branch. In smaller arteries of about 5 mm in diameter, 16–20 concentric elastic lamellae are seen (Brenner, 1935). Transition from elastic to muscular vessels occurs in small arteries (100–1000 μm diameter) compared to the systemic system where the transition occurs at the third order of branching, namely the aorta (elastic)-iliac (intermediate)-femoral (muscular).

(3) *Veins*

Unlike arteries, veins have valves, thinner walls, lower distending pressures, and are often in a collapsed state. Their media consists essentially of spirally arranged smooth muscle with few elastin fibres. It is this relative lack of elastin fibres which constitutes the major structural difference between arteries and veins. In some medium-sized veins the innermost muscle fibres in the media are oriented longitudinally (Ham and Leeson, 1961). Veins in the limbs have a thicker media than elsewhere which is consistent with the higher hydrostatic pressures developed in this part of the venous system. In large veins there is little smooth muscle in the media. The adventitia is thicker than the media and contains both collagen and elastin fibres. Like the smaller veins the inner layer of muscle is longitudinally disposed.

Veins, like arteries, have a typical non-linear force–length, pressure–volume, or pressure–diameter relationship (Alexander, 1963) convex to the length, volume or diameter axis, respectively. At low pressures the veins are very distensible (being collapsed) with large volume changes resulting from very small pressure changes. Once the vein becomes circular in cross-section the distensibility drops markedly, small changes in volume then resulting from relatively large changes in pressure. Veins differ from thin, latex rubber tubes (which might be thought to provide analogous mechanical behaviour at low pressures) in that the transition from an oval to circular cross-section occurs without change in the perimeter of the rubber tube whereas in veins there is bending, circumferential stretching and increases in perimeter (Moreno *et al.*, 1970). Like arteries the elastic modulus of veins is strain-dependent and hence pressure-dependent. This was well demonstrated by Attinger (1969) who compared the elasticity of the combined superior and inferior vena cava with that of the pulmonary artery and aorta. Above 7 mmHg the large veins have a higher elastic modulus than either systemic or pulmonary arteries at their normal distending pressures. This is probably not of great physiological importance since the distending pressures in these particular veins are normally close to zero. The comparison shows convincingly that a vessel of low elastin content has a low distensibility. Because of this difference in collagen and elastin content it is conceivable that the effects of smooth muscle contraction on the elasticity of veins might well be different to those in arteries. However, a qualitative difference in the static elastic behaviour of veins and arteries was not so apparent when transverse strips of rabbit vena cava and aorta were studied following relaxation with papaverine (Pürschel *et al.*, 1969). The difference was mainly one in slope of the tension–length curves, since, when suitably scaled, a linear relationship between wall stress in the vena cava and wall stress in the aorta was obtained at equivalent strains.

C. THE RELATIONSHIP OF THE MECHANICAL PROPERTIES OF ARTERIES TO CIRCULATORY DYNAMICS

Pulsatile pressure and flow in the arterial system are conveniently related in the frequency domain by the quantity vascular impedance. This complex mathematical quantity determines the pulsatile cardiac work (Taylor, 1967; O'Rourke, 1967). At all but the lowest frequencies the circulation presents a low impedance to ventricular outflow, such a situation resulting from wave reflection, a low elastic modulus of the most proximal portions of the systemic and pulmonary trees, and the existence of branched terminations (Taylor, 1966a). At frequencies above about twice the resting heart rate the impedance modulus approximates that predicted by the wave velocity (McDonald, 1960; Bergel and Milnor, 1965).

In the absence of reflections, the wave velocity is classically related to the elastic modulus of the tube by the Moens–Korteweg equation. Bergel (1961a) modified this equation to take account of the finite wall thickness of arteries and a Poisson's ratio of 0·5, and also used a circumferential incremental elastic modulus defined as follows:

$$E_{inc} = (\Delta p \bar{r}_o / \Delta r_o)\{1\cdot5 r_i^2 / [r_o^2 - r_i^2]\} \tag{1.1}$$

where Δp and Δr_o are the corresponding changes in pressure and outer radius at a mean outer radius, $\bar{r}_o$; r_i is the inside radius. The wave velocity (c) can be computed from:

$$c = \{\Delta p \bar{r}_o / \Delta r_o [1\cdot5(1-\gamma)^2 / 1 - (1-\gamma)^2 \rho][2(2-\gamma)/3]\}^{\frac{1}{2}} \tag{1.2}$$

where γ is the ratio of wall thickness, h, to outer radius, r_o, and ρ is the density of the fluid (blood).

The above equation reduces to

$$c = (1-\gamma)(E_p/2\rho)^{\frac{1}{2}} \tag{1.3}$$

where E_p $(= \Delta p \bar{r}_o / \Delta r_o)$ is the convenient pressure–strain elastic modulus of Peterson *et al.* (1960). For smaller isovolumetric wall strains it can be shown that

$$\Delta r_o r_o = \Delta r_i r_i \quad \text{and} \quad \Delta V/V = 2\Delta r_i/r_i$$

where V is volume of a segment and r_i the inside radius; substitution into (1.3) gives

$$c = [V\Delta p/\rho\Delta V]^{\frac{1}{2}} \tag{1.4}$$

which is the well-known volume elasticity equation used by Bramwell and Hill (1922) and as such is a useful measure of the distensible properties of a blood vessel.

D. THE POSSIBLE EFFECTS OF CHANGE IN SMOOTH MUSCLE TONE ON VESSEL ELASTICITY

The extent to which blood vessel elasticity is influenced by smooth muscle contraction will first depend on what parameter of elasticity we choose to observe and second, on whether the elasticity of the constricted and relaxed vessels is compared at equivalent strains or at equivalent mean distending pressures. With regard to elastic parameters the simplest one is the extensibility index $\Delta l/\Delta F$, where l and F are length and force respectively; this, while being readily obtainable from a strip of tissue, is difficult to relate to the elastic behaviour of an intact and tethered blood vessel. The similar indices $\Delta r/\Delta p$ and $\Delta V/\Delta p$ are useful in the venous circulation since here it is important to know the volume change resulting from a given pressure change. However, these indices are markedly strain dependent and of limited value unless the mean pressure and absolute volume are also known.

(1) *The use of an elastic modulus*

The above indices are by themselves inadequate to quantitate arterial elasticity completely, for in order to relate the mechanical properties of arteries to pulsatile phenomena we require an elastic modulus and measurements of relative wall thickness (γ). However, an elastic modulus in its strict definition relates stress to strain in a homogeneous and isotropic substance. A histological examination of arterial tissue shows it to be made up of different structures each with its own orientation and extensibility, and hence the wall can be expected to be anisotropic. However, the anisotropy is limited to three orthogonal planes (orthotropicity, Patel and Fry, 1969) and is discussed in detail by Patel and Vaishnav in Chapter 11 of this volume. Despite the orthotropicity many workers have used a circumferential incremental elastic modulus (see (1.1)) to quantitate the elastic behaviour of arteries (Krafka, 1939, 1940; Bergel, 1961a, b; Horeman and Noordergraaf, 1958; Attinger *et al.*, 1966; Hinke, 1965; Jaeger, 1966; Gow and Taylor, 1968; Dobrin and Rovick, 1969). This modulus is based on an incompressible wall, a Poisson's ratio of 0·5, isotropic properties and no change in length of the segment. Not all of these assumptions are valid. The wall is incompressible however, and the mean Poisson's ratio is 0·5 (Carew et al., 1968). However, the Poisson's ratios in the three orthogonal directions are different; for instance, that relating circumferential to longitudinal strain is about 0·3 (Dobrin and Doyle, 1970). Changes in length of the aorta may occur with each pulse or with pulmonary inflation (Patel et al., 1961) or in the peripheral vessels, with movement of the head and limbs relative to the trunk. However, in defence of this modulus for the subject of this chapter, I noted that Attinger (1968) and Dobrin and Doyle (1970) found that circumferential elasticity was not markedly affected by the small longitudinal changes occurring as the result of vasoconstriction, provided that strain was small; this is true of most pulsatile strains. Secondly, Patel et al. (1969) consider it a useful quantity to compare the results of different investigators, and of greater importance, the modulus was found by them to predict accurately pulse wave (foot-to-foot) velocity in the mid-descending aorta. Moreover, Bergel (1961b) had previously shown that the wave velocity calculated from (1.2) agreed with measured values in the aorta, femoral and carotid arteries. It should be emphasized that the dynamic incremental elastic modulus is a function of mean pressure, frequency of the applied stress (Hardung, 1953; Bergel, 1961b; Gow, 1969, 1970) as well as depending on the site in the vascular tree and the animal species. Clearly these variables must be listed when reporting the modulus.

Recently, Dobrin and Rovick (1969) showed that if the elastic modulus was plotted as a function of strain then constricted vessels were stiffer than relaxed ones but when plotted as a function of transmural pressure, the converse was true. As far as the conduit arteries are concerned the prime determinant of calibre, hence strain, is the mean distending pressure and, from a haemodynamic point of view, it is important to know the effects of smooth muscle contraction on the elastic modulus as a function of pressure. Hence in Section 3 the question whether vasoconstriction increases or decreases the elastic modulus of vessel has been answered on the basis of the same mean transmural pressure before and after changes in vasomotor tone. Following vasoconstriction the vessel has a thicker wall. If a relaxed and a constricted vessel expand equally when subjected to the same pressure change than one concludes that the thicker walled vessel has the lower elastic modulus. This conclusion also follows from an examination of (1.1) where it can be seen that E_{inc} is a function of the product $r_o r_i^2$. Since for isovolumetric strain $r_o^2 - r_i^2$ remains constant it follows that unless large changes occur in $\Delta p/\Delta r_o$ in the opposite sense to the mean diameter change, the elastic modulus decreases during vasoconstriction and increases during vasodilatation.

Although E_{inc} is a popular haemodynamic parameter it should be realized that in vascular tissue where stress and strain are non-linearly related an incremental modulus calculated at some given pressure is not comparable to that calculated in another animal with the same mean blood pressure unless γ is the same. One readily reaches this conclusion on realizing that two vessels made of the same material but of different radii have different wall stresses ($S = pr_i/h$, Lamé approximation). The wall stress will be higher in the larger diameter vessel but because of the non-linearity, the strain will be disproportionately less and hence a higher elastic modulus will be calculated. However γ is relatively constant for the aorta at 100 mmHg in a number of animal species (Wolinsky and Glagov, 1967) and hence the errors in E_{inc} may not be as large as might have been anticipated. Notwithstanding its probable limitations as an elastic modulus representing a given vascular tissue it can be used to evaluate whether the vessel wall increases in stiffness during a vasomotor change. The extent to which it quantitates the alteration in stiffness following a vasomotor change should be tested by observing whether it predicts wave velocity following vasodilatation and constriction. Since errors in the foot-to-foot or phase velocity measured over short distances are unavoidable, some difficulty might be experienced in arriving at a firm conclusion either way, especially if the changes in elasticity were small. Because wave velocity is also a function of α†, the testing of this modulus would be made easier if measurements of elasticity, constrictor tone and phase velocity were confined to the largest arteries. Unfortunately, the effects of smooth muscle are minimal in the largest vessels.

(2) *The effects of smooth muscle contraction on elasticity as a function of strain*

While the main interest in this chapter has been elasticity changes in vessels held at constant mean transmural pressure, one should consider, if only briefly, the possible effects of alterations in vasomoter tone on the elasticity of vessels as a function of strain as done by some workers. When a vessel constricts at a constant transmural pressure the wall stress diminishes; first, because the wall thickness increases, second, because of the reduction in radius and the consequences predicted by the Lamé approximation ($S = pr_i/h$). This change in vessel geometry complicates the situation since, if one accepts the possibility of a contribution of myogenic tone to the total contraction (Bayliss, 1902; Folkow, 1964), a reduction in wall stress can be presumed to allow the smooth muscle to relax partially. Hence the degree of contraction of the muscle in this situation for a given stimulus will

† α (Womersley, 1955) $= r_i (2\pi f/v)^{\frac{1}{2}}$ where r_i, f and v are inner radius, frequency and kinematic viscosity respectively.

presumably be different from that where a vessel segment is allowed to contract against a constant load.

When considering the elasticity changes accompanying alterations in vasomotor tone as a function of strain, it is of paramount importance to realize that in contracting and changing the orientation of structural elements and the external dimensions of a vessel, the muscle has, from the physical standpoint, transformed the wall material into a different substance. Hence the unstressed dimensions of a constricted vessel segment are irrelevant when calculating strains for the same segment following muscle relaxation and, should it be desired to calculate a Young's modulus for the material in some given state, one must use the individual unstressed dimensions for the control and constricted or relaxed segments. In this regard, Attinger (1968) showed that constricted dog carotid artery rings had a higher modulus than in the control state when the dimensions of the control segment were used to calculate strains in both situations. However, when the strain values for the constricted state were calculated from the unstressed length of the constricted specimen the opposite conclusion, and I believe the correct one, was obtained, i.e. the constricted artery has a lower modulus of elasticity.

E. CONCLUSION

The effects of smooth muscle on the mechanical properties of blood vessels can be expected to be different in arteries, veins and arterioles where the relative composition and orientation of other passive elements differ. Changes in viscoelastic properties of contracting vascular smooth muscle itself are probably best studied in arterioles where this tissue predominates. In larger vessels, especially conduit arteries, the relative contribution to the total mass of tissue in the wall is much less and hence it has been postulated that the muscle modifies the passive elastic behaviour of the elastin and collagen fibres. Unfortunately the way in which the muscle interacts with these passive elements is poorly understood.

It is evident that there are severe limitations to the concept of an elastic modulus applied to a substance such as a blood vessel which contains an element capable of actively altering its dimensions and the internal orientation of its structural components. The only hope of supplying the theoretician with useful elastic constants probably relies on there being only small changes in vasomotor tone in the conduit arteries and insignificant consequent effects on viscoelastic properties; that this is probably so for the aorta can be seen from the agreement of *in vivo* measurements made by Patel *et al.* (1969) and Gow and Taylor (1968) with those of excised vessels (Bergel, 1961b) where presumably the smooth muscle tone in the excised vessels had been lost. These changes and those in smaller conduit vessels are discussed in detail in Sections 3 and 4.

2. TIME- AND FREQUENCY-DEPENDENT BEHAVIOUR OF VASCULAR TISSUES

A. INTRODUCTION

In view of the heterogeneous collection of cellular and fibrous elements and mucopolysaccharide making up the vascular wall it is not surprising that the strain behaviour of these tissues depends on the time course and history of stress application. It would also not be surprising if this behaviour was modified in some way by the contraction or relaxation of the smooth muscle cells. Biological substances in general display time-dependent behaviour (Stacy et al., 1955). This is well demonstrated in a number of papers on tissue elasticity edited by Remington (1957). (This book contains a useful glossary of rheological terms prepared by Randall and Stacy.) Time- and frequency-dependency are characteristics of substances possessing elasticity and viscosity and perhaps plasticity, although the latter term implies a finite yield stress, above which the material flows. In this discussion the fluid-like properties of vascular wall are described solely in terms of the viscous behaviour and the term plasticity is not used.

Viscoelastic materials are characterized by stress relaxation, creep and hysteresis. These properties are demonstrated in the simplest viscoelastic models comprising a single spring (pure elastic behaviour) and a dashpot (pure viscous behaviour) in parallel configuration (Kelvin–Voigt element) and in series (the Maxwell element). When a force is applied to the Kelvin–Voigt element the spring is prevented from extending instantaneously to its appropriate length because of the viscous drag of the dashpot. Instead, the length of the combination "creeps" exponentially until the spring has extended sufficiently to oppose the force. On the other hand, if the Maxwell element is extended to some given length, a force will instantly appear across the spring; the dashpot will then extend exponentially and the force will decay. This is the nature of stress relaxation. An exponential decay of stress in a viscoelastic substance may be quantified in terms of a "time constant". An analogous quantity is commonly used in electrical engineering and gives the time course of voltage decay on a capacitance (C) in parallel with a resistance (R); it is defined in the following expression

$$E = E_o \exp\left(-t/RC\right) \tag{2.1}$$

as $1/RC$ where E and E_o are the instantaneous and initial voltages respectively. In terms of the above elements $1/C$ and R are analogous to elasticity and viscosity. When force is plotted against extension for the Kelvin–Voigt element during cyclic stretch and release, the tension–length relationship traced out during extension does not coincide with that of retraction and a loop is traced out (Fig. 2). If the substance has Newtonian viscous properties and the stretch is sinusoidally applied, the loop will be elliptical, with its long axis coincident with the stress–strain relationship for the elastic component. The wider the ellipse the higher is the viscous contribution to the overall properties. The relationship between force (F) and extension (x) can be represented by a first-order differential equation:

$$F = Gx + \eta_1 \dot{x} \qquad (2.2)$$

where G and η_1 are the spring constant and viscosity coefficient respectively.

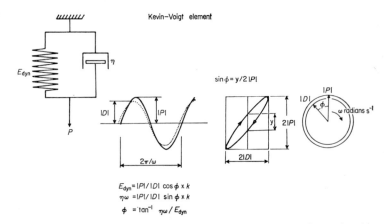

Kevin–Voigt element

$\sin\phi = y/2\,|P|$

$E_{dyn} = |P|/|D|\cos\phi \times k$

$\eta\omega = |P|/|D|\sin\phi \times k$

$\phi = \tan^{-1}\ \eta\omega / E_{dyn}$

Fig. 2. The Kelvin–Voigt element; a parallel arrangement of a spring (dynamic elastic modulus, E_{dyn}) and a dashpot (with a coefficient of viscosity η). A sinusoidal force with a magnitude $|P|$ causes a displacement of the magnitude $|D|$ which lags behind P by ϕ radians. ϕ may be evaluated from the hysteresis loop as shown or by substracting the phase of the D from P.

On solution of the equation one obtains for dynamic conditions:

$$G = \left|\frac{F}{x}\right| \cos \phi \qquad (2.3)$$

$$\eta_1 \omega = \left|\frac{F}{x}\right| \sin \phi \qquad (2.4)$$

$$\tan^{-1} \phi = \eta_1 \omega / G \qquad (2.5)$$

where $|F|$ and $|x|$ are the magnitudes of force and displacement respectively, ϕ the phase lag of displacement behind force and ω is the angular frequency. Thus the time-dependent properties of a material may be observed as stress relaxation, creep or hysteresis.

B. HYSTERESIS LOOP BEHAVIOUR OF VASCULAR TISSUE

Although stress relaxation, creep and hysteresis describe viscoelastic behaviour the former two relate to materials subjected to transient changes in wall stress. Hysteresis on the other hand is observed when a strip of tissue or intact vessel is subjected to cyclic stress changes.

Hysteresis has been extensively studied in arteries, veins and other tissues (see Remington, 1963; Alexander, 1963; Goto and Kimoto, 1966). Typical behaviour observed by Remington (1955) in a ring of aorta is shown in Fig. 3.

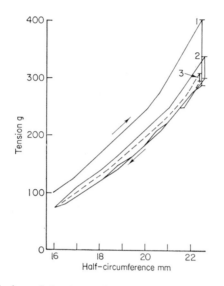

FIG. 3. Hysteresis loop behaviour of an aortic ring subjected to consecutive stretch and release cycles (1–3) which demonstrates the stability of the descending limb (release) and collapse of the loop at the expense of the ascending limb. (Redrawn from Remington, 1955.)

When a relaxed segment of artery is stretched and released cyclically the loop is wide at first, becoming narrower with successive cycles and finally becoming stable. Two or three cycles are sufficient in the case of the aorta while more are required with muscular arteries (Remington, 1963). The changes are greatest in the ascending limbs (Remington, 1963; Goto and Kimoto, 1966). The latter workers observed that formic acid digestion of the collagen fibres abolished the hysteresis loop whereas trypsin digestion of the elastin widened the loop. They concluded that the ascending limb was due to the properties of smooth muscle while the upper and lower parts of the descending loop were due to collagen and elastin respectively. Stability of the descending limb is also seen with veins (Alexander, 1963; Thron, 1968).

The existence of a loop in which the descending limb is stable and the ascending one is not, is a complex situation and clearly no combination of springs and dashpots will model this. However, Wezler and Schlüter (1953) have shown that for mesenteric arteries the descending limb of the loop is far from stable initially; with each successive cycle the curve creeps along the diameter axis. A model composed of two Kelvin–Voigt elements in series could mimic this behaviour. One dashpot would need to contain a non-Newtonian fluid; that is, one in which the viscosity was dependent on shear and on previous strain history. Such behaviour is exhibited by thixotropic materials (Bauer and Collins, 1967) which include many biological substances. The complex behaviour described by Remington and others may not be wholly relevant to the intact artery *in vivo* because the living artery is subjected to a steady stretch on which pulsations are superimposed. At no time in life is an artery unstressed. However, there are one of two observations which are relevant to the *in vivo* situation. First, Remington (1955) found that the width of the stable loop in the aorta increased with increased amplitude of stretch but at any amplitude it was independent of rate of stretch. Secondly vasoconstriction (adrenaline) and vasodilatation (sodium nitrite) had negligible influence on the width of the loop. These findings are particularly relevant to the factors influencing wall viscosity and will be discussed below.

C. STRESS RELAXATION AND CREEP OF VASCULAR TISSUE

It is clear from the work of Zatzman *et al.* (1954) and Speden (1960) that the decay of tension in an abruptly stressed arterial tissue is not exponential. Also no simple model of springs and dashpots will explain the observed time-dependent behaviour. In both these investigations non-linear relationships were obtained when the logarithm of pressure in the vessel or tension in the strip was plotted against time. On the other hand, when force was plotted against the logarithm of time the relationship was linear for about two log units. This behaviour is not unlike that of rubber which has been modelled by an array of many Maxwell elements with a wide and uniform distribution function of time constants (Tobolsky *et al.*, 1951). Such an arrangement has little physical reality in terms of the architecture or composition of vascular wall substance.

It seems certain that the stress relaxation of blood vessels occurs mainly in the smooth muscle. The umbilical artery, a particularly muscular vessel, shows greater stress relaxation than the carotid artery, an intermediate type (Zatzman *et al.*, 1954), but the time course of the relaxation of the two vessels is virtually identical. When the muscle in a blood vessel constricts the amount of stress relaxation increases (Leonard and Sarnoff, 1957; Wiederhielm, 1965a; Attinger, 1968). In the vena cava, constriction shifts the entire curve to higher pressures (Fig. 4) without altering the time course of the relaxation (Attinger, 1969).

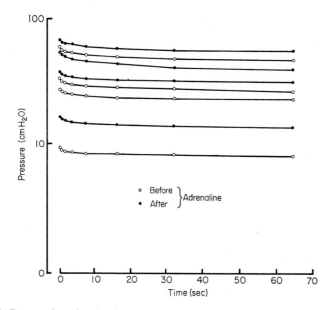

FIG. 4. Stress relaxation in the wall of a dog's jugular vein following the rapid injection of fluid. The effect of contraction of the venous smooth muscle is an increase in the resulting pressure without altering the time-course of stress relaxation. (Redrawn from Attinger, 1969.)

Mikami and Attinger (1968) derived an expression for the fall in pressure with time in arteries, veins and rubber tubes; this is

$$P = P_o^1 \exp{(-\alpha t)} - P_a \qquad (2.6)$$

where P = pressure in the vessel at any instant
P_o = initial pressure
P_a = asymptotic pressure
$P_o^1 = P_o - P_a$
α = damping coefficient.

This exponential relationship does not fit the entire time course of relaxation, the constants P_o, P_a and α being functions of the sampling times chosen. When the logarithm of the time constants was plotted against the logarithm of the sampling time a linear relationship was obtained and there was relatively little difference in the behaviour of either arteries, veins or rubber tubes. In view of the vast differences in these materials this finding is perhaps suggestive of some fundamental explanation for stress relaxation, perhaps more to do with the properties of macromolecules than the architecture of the wall.

The unreality inherent in the various combinations of viscoelastic elements used to explain the time-dependent behaviour of arterial tissue led Stacy (1957) to seek an alternative. The initial hypothesis was that the mechanical responses are due to transitions from the short to the long state of some elements having two possible states. Long elements would become short provided their potential energy was elevated sufficiently. Stressing the tissue favoured the short-to-long transition. Stacy derived an expression in which the decay of tension was determined by the ratio:

$$[K_1 + \exp(-xt)]/[K_2 - \exp(-xt)] \qquad (2.7)$$

where $x = K_s \exp(C_s T)$; K_1 and K_2 are determinable constants, K_s the reaction rate for short-to-long transformations and C_s is a constant describing the effect of tension on reaction rate. When K_s was 100 times greater than K_L (the reaction rate from long-to-short) the theoretical relationship fitted the observed data from carotid arteries very well. It follows that on the removal of the stress the relaxation process would not be repeated for several minutes. Excellent agreement with theory was obtained when the arterial tissue was re-stressed at variable time intervals after removal of the initial stress.

In studies on relaxed and constricted frog arterioles Wiederhielm (1965a) found that the creep occurred at a linear rate following a step rise in distending pressure. Since a linear increase in diameter occurred in the face of a rising wall stress (resulting from the law of Laplace and a diminishing wall thickness) it was concluded that viscosity must also have been incrsasing. This

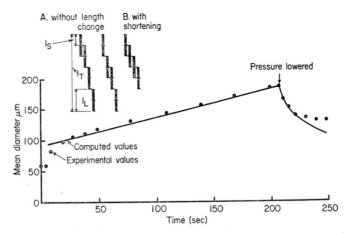

Fig. 5. Creep behaviour of a frog arteriole modelled using reaction-rate kinetics. The muscle is assumed to behave as a population of polymer chains which join to form either short- or long-length configurations (see text). (Redrawn from Wiederhielm, 1965a.)

finding underlines the difficulties which arise when classical concepts of stress, strain and viscosity are used to explain the mechanical behaviour of arteriolar walls. To avoid this Wiederhielm followed Stacy (1957) and used a model based on reaction rate kinetics to explain the time course of creep. The velocity of shortening in his model is given by the expression

$$V = (L_L - L_s)[K_s n_s - K_L(n_t - n_s) \exp(-C_s S)] \qquad (2.8)$$

where L_L and L_s are the lengths of the long and short elements; K_s and K_L are reaction rate constants for short-to-long and long-to-short transitions respectively, n_s and n_t are the numbers of short and the total number of elements respectively, C_s is a constant and S is the strain. The degree of agreement between theoretical and observed points using this model can be seen in Fig. 5. It is hoped that further investigations on time-dependent properties of vascular tissues will produce models which will not only explain the time-course of stress relaxation but also permit all constants to be determined experimentally.

D. THE USE OF THE KELVIN–VOIGT ELEMENT TO DESCRIBE THE DYNAMIC BEHAVIOUR OF THE ARTERIAL WALL

While arrays of springs and dashpots do not provide a satisfactory model of the transient response of vascular tissue to applied stress, a single spring and dashpot (Kelvin–Voigt) model leads to one useful way of separating elastic and viscous components at a single frequency. This approach was used by Dillon et al. (1944) to describe the viscoelastic properties of rubber and by Hardung (1953) to describe the elastic and viscous constants of arterial wall. He was then able to introduce these constants into mathematical models of the arterial system.

Consider a parallel arrangement of lumped elastic elements of modulus E_{dyn} and lumped viscous elements with a viscosity coefficient, η; (2.3) to (2.5) then become

$$E_{dyn} = \left(\left| \frac{P}{D} \right| \cos \phi \right) \times k \qquad (2.9)$$

$$\eta \omega = \left(\left| \frac{P}{D} \right| \sin \phi \right) \times k \qquad (2.10)$$

$$\tan^{-1} \phi = \eta \omega / E_{dyn} \qquad (2.11)$$

where k is $1 \cdot 5 \bar{r}_o . r_i^2 / (r_o^2 - r_i^2)$. It can be seen from these equations, when ϕ is small, that at a given mean pressure, the frequency behaviour of elasticity depends almost solely on that of $|P|/|D|$. For practical purposes the modulus E_{inc} in (1.1) equals E_{dyn} since ϕ has been shown to be small (Bergel, 1961b; Gow and Taylor, 1968).

Using an optical method of diameter measurement and sinusoidal pressure changes of ± 5 mmHg Bergel (1961b) found little frequency dependence of elastic (E_{dyn}) and viscous modulus ($\eta\omega$) in excised segments of dog aorta, carotid and femoral arteries at frequencies between 2 and 18 Hz. The importance of this investigation is that it provided values for dynamic elasticity (E_{dyn}) in the range of physiological pulsatile frequency components. Bergel (1961b) and Learoyd and Taylor (1966) confirmed the findings of Hardung (1953) and Kapal (1954) that the dynamic modulus of elasticity

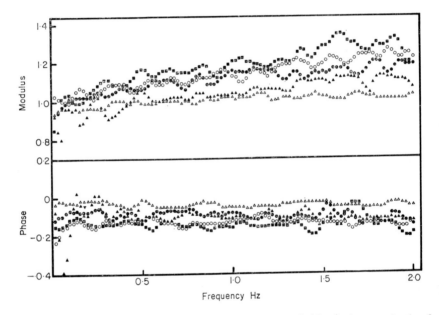

FIG. 6. Frequency behaviour of the elastic parameter, $|P|/|D_L|$, the magnitude of pressure to magnitude of "linearized" diameter, (labelled modulus) and viscous parameter, ϕ(labelled phase) between zero and 2 Hz. $\triangle$ Thoracic aorta; $\bullet$ Carotid artery; $\bigcirc$ Iliac artery; $\blacksquare$ Femoral artery; $\blacktriangle$ Abdominal aorta. (From Gow, 1969.)

was greater than the static. Gow (1969) demonstrated that this was also the case for arteries in the living dog. The significance of this finding relates to pulse wave velocity prediction; because the phase velocity is estimated from the high frequency components it is important that the dynamic elasticity be known at these frequencies. The frequency dependence of elasticity at very low frequencies up to 2 Hz (Fig. 6) was recently observed by Gow (1969) in living arteries using an electrical caliper (Gow, 1966) which records diameter pulsations faithfully without loading the vessel. It can be seen that the more muscular the artery the greater is the rise in dynamic stiffness over this frequency range, which is in agreement with the findings of Bergel (1961b) and Learoyd and Taylor (1966) for excised vessels.

The frequency behaviour of the linearized elastic parameter, $|P|/|D_L|$ (modulus) between zero and 16 Hz for several sites in the arterial tree is shown in Fig. 7. These data, along with measurements of phase lag of diameter

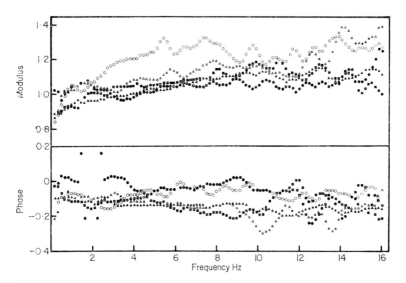

FIG. 7. Frequency behaviour of the elastic parameter, $|P|/|D_L|$, the magnitude of pressure to magnitude of "linearized" diameter, (labelled modulus) and viscous parameter, ϕ(labelled phase) between zero and 16 Hz. $\triangle$ Thoracic aorta; ● Carotid artery; ○ Iliac artery; ■ Femoral artery; ▲ Abdominal aorta. (From Gow, 1969.)

behind pressure, were obtained from spectral analysis (Taylor, 1966) of randomly varying pressure and diameter waves. The values of $|P|/|D|$ have been "normalized"† by a computer program which takes account of the non-linear relationship between P and D (Gow, 1969). The greatest increase in $|P|/|D_L|$ occurred in the femoral artery, the most muscular of those studied, confirming the work on excised vessels of Bergel (1961b) and of Learoyd and Taylor (1966). Between 2–16 Hz a steady increase in stiffness of 10 per cent was obtained for the descending thoracic aorta and of about 25 per cent for the abdominal aorta, iliac, femoral and carotid arteries.

† This program results in $|P|/|D_L|$, the ratio of the magnitude of pressure to linearized diameter magnitude. The result of this procedure is roughly equivalent to dividing all estimates of $|P|/|D|$ by its value at zero frequency, the latter being obtainable by back extrapolation of the plot.

The relative independence of ϕ on frequency in both frequency ranges (0–2 and 0–16 Hz) is interesting since it means that within this range the product $\eta\omega$ is independent of frequency and thus η is markedly frequency dependent. Shear-dependent viscosity is not uncommon in solutions containing polymers (Weltmann, 1960), such behaviour being known as pseudoplasticity. The relative constancy of ϕ explains the phenomenon (Remington, 1955; Gow, 1969) of a stable pressure-diameter hysteresis loop with a width that is independent of frequency.

Whether the contraction of vascular smooth muscle alters the viscous properties of arteries may depend on how viscosity is defined. It is significant, however, that similar values of ϕ have been obtained with excised arteries (Bergel, 1961b; Learoyd and Taylor, 1966; Gow, 1969) and with arteries measured *in vivo*. It has generally been assumed that there is a greater degree of muscular contraction in the living vessel *in situ* than in an excised vessel. If this is true, and there is no direct evidence either way, ϕ is unaltered by muscular contraction and hence the "time constant" (η/E_{dyn}, Ballou and Smith, 1949) will be the same for a given frequency in constricted and relaxed vessels. This finding is supported by Attinger (1969) who found similar time constants in relaxed and constricted veins.

The extent to which viscosity is influenced by wall strain is not certain. I found no evidence that ϕ was a function of mean pressure (Gow, 1969), but no experiments were done specifically to examine this proposition. If it is true that ϕ is independent of mean pressure then, because E_{dyn} increases with mean pressure, η must do likewise ($\eta/E_{dyn} = \tan \phi$). Therefore a rise in mean pressure which increases wall strain will also increase the effective wall viscosity (η). Wiederhielm (1965b) came to a similar conclusion from observations of creep in arterioles.

It is important to realize the limitations of a viscosity coefficient calculated in this way. The value is dependent on many other parameters and it is necessary that these be known and specified also. For the purpose of a quantitative description it is desirable to abstract the time-dependent behaviour into the simplest practical equation. While it can be seen that no single elastic or viscous parameter or group of such quantities will represent all behaviour, it has been found useful for certain applications, e.g. pulse wave propagation and related phenomena (Hardung, 1963). It appears that, at a given mean pressure, the motion of the artery wall can be satisfactorily derived from a knowledge of the frequency-dependent viscoelastic parameters $\Delta P/\Delta D$ and ϕ. Thus Taylor (1966a, b) using a randomly branched, viscoelastic tube as a model of the circulation was able to model the effects of wall viscosity on vascular input impedance and wave propagation by using the equation:

$$E = |E| \exp (i\phi) \qquad (2.12)$$

this, for any one frequency, being the behaviour of a Kelvin–Voigt model. In this example the frequency-dependence of ϕ was expressed empirically by

$$\phi = \phi_o[1 - \exp(-2\omega)] \tag{2.13}$$

which is a reasonable approximation to the experimental results.

In summary it can be said that there is good evidence to show that the stress relaxation of vascular tissues is a function of the smooth muscle content. However, the time dependent behaviour of vascular tissues is complex and not explicable in terms of simple linear viscoelastic models. Mathematical models based on reaction-rate kinetics predict the time course of relaxation well but employ constants which are difficult to determine experimentally. From a haemodynamic standpoint the time-dependent properties of arterial tissues can be quantified within the frequency domain by considering the wall to behave as a Kelvin–Voigt element at each frequency. By this means it has been possible to construct more realistic models relating pressure and flow in the arterial system.

3. The Effects of Contraction and Relaxation of Vascular Smooth Muscle on the Elasticity of Blood Vessels

In a recent and comprehensive review on vascular smooth muscle, Somlyo and Somlyo (1968) held to the thesis that vasoconstriction increases, and vaso-dilatation decreases, the elastic modulus of the vessel wall. However, the experimental evidence cited to support this conclusion came from a variety of vascular preparations under different experimental conditions. While there is much to be said for the controlled conditions under which a strip of blood vessel may be observed in an isolated organ bath, the conclusions reached are often difficult to apply to the intact vascular tree. Hence the haemodynamic consequences of nervous activity or circulating vasoactive substances are similarly difficult to predict in any quantitative sense. Despite technical difficulties and experimental limitations it is preferable that elasticity measurements be made on a length of intact vessel. The measurements should be made *in vivo* wherever possible and ideally, in a conscious animal. With these remarks in mind, the effects of vasoconstriction and dilatation on the elastic properties of individual sites in the vascular tree will now be considered.

A. aorta

Although arterial tissue is popular as a bioassay material for vasoactive drugs (Furchgott, 1955), Remington (1962) was unable to produce aortic constriction in the intact vessel *in vivo* either by local application of drugs or by electrical stimulation. Remington (1963) remarked that for an aortic strip to be effective as a bioassay material it was necessary that it was kept at minimum tensions. He found that aortic rings which had been soaked in adrenaline readily yielded to loads equivalent to those generated by physiological levels of arterial pressure, and following repeated stretches they behaved the same as relaxed rings. His conclusions stood in contrast to those of Wiggers and Wégria (1938) who, with an "aortograph", showed that following a brief episode of acute hypertension the mean diameter of the aorta in living dogs was reduced while the distensibility ($\Delta V/\Delta p$) was increased. The changes in the distensibility of the aorta were most likely due to changes in muscle tone. In one series of experiments the hypertension was induced by stimulation of the central ends of the divided vagi which presumably produced a large increase in sympathetic activity. In a second series adrenaline was infused. The cause of the aortic vasoconstriction in the experiments is obscure. It is possible that it resulted from increased sympathetic activity and adrenaline or as the result of a circulatory vasoconstrictor substance. However, the fact that large arteries exhibit myogenic properties (Furchgott and Bhadrakom, 1953; Lundholm and Mohme-Lundholm, 1966) suggests the possibility that the contraction was initiated by the increased wall stress which occurred during the hypertensive phase. (cf. the conclusions of Gerová and Gero (1962) from work on carotid sinus distensibility during acute hypertension.)

In contrast to the results of Wiggers and Wégria (1938), Barnett et al. (1961) found, using Mallos' (1962) electrical caliper, that $\Delta p/\Delta D_o$ was increased during acute, noradrenaline-induced hypertension. The fall in distensibility ($\Delta V/\Delta p$) in nine dogs was found to be 9–19 per cent (15 per cent average) but changes in mean diameter were, unfortunately, not reported. Although Peterson et al. (1960) concluded that noradrenaline given intravenously increased the elastic modulus (E_p) of the wall, no figures were given. Furthermore since E_p is a function of mean pressure (Bergel, 1961a) and because mean pressure does not appear to have been controlled, one is reluctant to accept their conclusion.

In a most comprehensive study of aortic distensibility Pieper and Paul (1969), found, at a given pressure, that haemorrhage resulted in aortic constriction (Mean 9·9 per cent, $0·02 < P < 0·05$); the change in the parameter $\Delta p/\Delta D_o$ however, was not significant. An elastic modulus was calculated from the expression $(dp/dr)(r_d^2/a_d)$ where dp/dr was taken from the slope of the pressure–inner radius relationship, r_d was the end diastolic radius and a_d the wall thickness at a radius r_d. This (incremental) modulus was diminished during haemorrhage-induced vasoconstriction.

B. PULMONARY ARTERY

The intravenous injection of noradrenaline into anaesthetized dogs reduced the radius of the pulmonary artery by 6·4 per cent of its value at the same mean distending pressure (Patel *et al.*, 1960); the ratio $\Delta r_o/\Delta p$ was decreased by 19 per cent. If these data are used to calculate an incremental modulus it is found (assuming $\gamma = 0.1$ or lower) that noradrenaline marginally reduces the elastic modulus but slightly increases the volume elasticity ($V\Delta p/\Delta V$) and hence the predicted wave velocity.

Different conclusions were reached by Bevan *et al.* (1964) who stressed the necessity of taking wall thickness into account when assessing elasticity changes. Although their pulmonary segments were not prestressed either circumferentially or longitudinally, the elastic moduli, computed as a function of both strain and calculated equivalent distending pressures, showed the constricted segment to have a lower elastic modulus than the control. Bevan *et al.* (1964) believed that the opposite conclusion reached by Patel *et al.* (1960) could be explained on the basis of different expressions used to calculate elastic moduli. However, the consistent rise in $\Delta p/\Delta r$ found by Patel *et al.* contrasts with variable or opposite changes in this parameter in the aorta (Pieper and Paul, 1969) and femoral artery (Gero and Gerová, 1969; Gow, 1970). While it is regrettable that no measurements of wall thickness were made in Patel's study the results, however, stand as the only measurements of pulmonary dynamic elastic properties made *in vivo*.

Bargainer (1967) found reasonable agreement between elastic modulus computed from measured phase velocities and that calculated from the expression, $c = c_o/(1-\sigma^2)^{\frac{1}{2}}$ (Womersley, 1957) where $c_o = (V\Delta p/\Delta V\rho)^{\frac{1}{2}}$; elasticity values were obtained from Patel *et al.* (1960) and Frasher and Sobin (1965). Following the infusion of serotonin the phase velocity (average of the apparent phase velocities measured at frequencies between 8–18 Hz) rose by 50 per cent, corresponding to an increase in volume elasticity of 125 per cent. Since volume elasticity increases with mean distending pressure, it is not known how much of this large increase in elasticity was due to this effect: it is always necessary to measure the phase velocity at comparable mean distending pressures before and during vasoconstriction if one is to ascertain the effects of smooth muscle contraction on wall elasticity.

C. CAROTID ARTERY

A recent investigation by Dobrin and Rovick (1969) on excised common carotid arteries of dogs has shown that the elastic modulus of a constricted vessel will be higher than that of a dilated one if the modulus is plotted as a function of strain, but lower if the modulus is plotted as a function of transmural pressure. They believe that this provides an explanation for the existing disagreement on the effects of constriction. However, their conclusions on strain-dependency rest on the rather arbitrary choice of the constricted vessel dimensions from which they defined "zero strain". Because

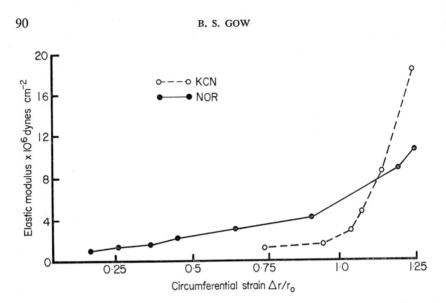

FIG. 8. The elastic modulus of an excised canine carotid artery plotted as a function of strain during constriction (NOR, ●————●) and dilatation (KCN, ○ – – – – ○). (Redrawn from Dobrin and Rovick, 1969.)

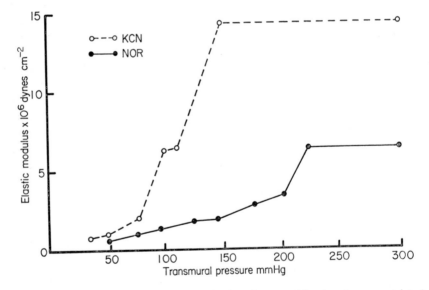

FIG. 9. The elastic modulus of an excised canine carotid artery in a constricted (●————●) and dilated (○ – – – – ○) state as in Figure 8, in this case plotted as a function of transmural pressure. (Redrawn from Dobrin and Rovick, 1969.)

the "unstressed" circumference of the constricted vessel is smaller than its relaxed counterpart it means that at low stresses comparable elastic moduli for constricted and dilated vessels can only be expected to occur at widely different strains. The outcome of the comparison would have been different had separate "zero strain" values been defined for the dilated and constricted vessel; the KCN curve (Fig. 8) would have been shifted along the strain axis to the left indicating, except at perhaps the lowest strains, that the constricted vessel has the lower modulus. When the elastic moduli for constricted and dilated vessels were plotted at the same mean pressures (Fig. 9) the conclusion was that vasoconstriction decreased the modulus of elasticity and vasodilatation increased it. This conclusion was also reached by Jaeger (1966) using intact vessels *in vitro* and Laszt (1968) who used strips of cow carotid artery.

D. MUSCULAR ARTERIES

In recent studies (Gow, 1969, 1970) the effects of vasoconstriction and dilatation on the elastic modulus and volume elasticity of the femoral artery were observed in anaesthetized dogs. This artery was chosen because of ease of access and also because being of intermediate structure it might provide representative behaviour of the arterial tree; that is, the large, elastic arteries would be less responsive to vasoactive substances while the converse can be assumed to apply to smaller and more muscular vessels.

Arterial diameter was measured using electrical calipers (Gow, 1966) modified to record large excursions in mean diameter. Details of the modified transducer are seen in Fig. 10. Because the legs of the caliper move in a circular locus the secondary of the differential transformer was wound on a former which was bent in the arc of a circle. By this means it was possible to achieve adequate linearity, sensitivity, lightness and low mechanical impedance.

The effect of topically applied acetylcholine (1 mg ml^{-1}) on the diameter of a femoral artery of a greyhound dog is seen in Fig. 11. The mean pressure was constant within ± 5 mmHg during the period of observation. After the peak dilatation had been reached noradrenaline ($0\cdot1 \text{ mg ml}^{-1}$) was applied. Dynamic incremental elastic moduli were calculated (1.1) and are shown at arbitrarily chosen points along the record. It can be seen that, at a constant distending pressure, the incremental elastic modulus was increased during vasodilatation and decreased during vasoconstriction. Acetylcholine increased the mean diameter by 9·4 per cent ($P < 0\cdot001$, $N = 7$) while noradrenaline decreased the diameter by 10·7 per cent ($P < 0\cdot001$, $N = 9$). The mean pressure for the group was approximately 140 mmHg. The maximum constriction was 19·2 per cent of the fully dilated diameter. (cf. 17·1 per

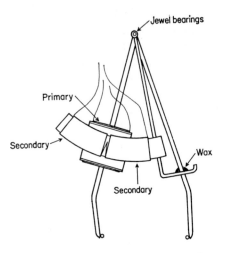

FIG. 10. Schematic diagram of electrical caliper used to record mean and pulsatile diameter changes of arteries *in vivo*. The coils were wound with 40 B and S enamel wire, the secondaries being each a single layer wound in opposite directions on a short piece of PVC catheter. The secondary former was bent around a circular mandrel and its shape stabilized by injecting acrylic resin along its lumen.

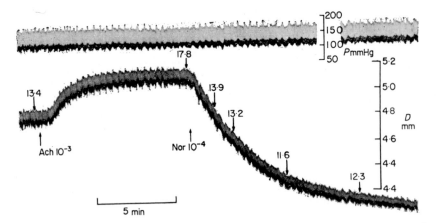

FIG. 11. The effects of a topical application of acetylcholine (ACH) and noradrenaline (NOR) on the diameter of a femoral artery in a living dog. The dynamic incremental elastic modulus (dynes $cm^{-2} \times 10^6$) is indicated at selected points along the diameter record. The upper trace is pressure. (From Gow, 1970 by courtesy of the publishers.)

cent for the excised carotid artery obtained by Dobrin and Rovick, 1969). However, it is slightly less than that obtained for the femoral artery by Gerová and Gero (1969) who, with a method similar to that used by Peterson *et al.* (1960), obtained 22 per cent dilatation following lumbar sympathetic trunk section, followed by a return to within 4 per cent of the control diameter within 15 minutes. When the distal end of the sympathetic trunk was then stimulated, a constriction of 13 per cent occurred which represents a range of 25 per cent relative to the dilated diameter. It has not, however, been established whether the transient dilatation which occurs on cutting the sympathetic trunk corresponds to a state of complete relaxation of the smooth muscle.

When calculations of incremental circumferential moduli of elasticity were made using measurements of $\Delta p/\Delta r_o$, $\bar{r}_o$ and wall thickness, Gow (1969) found that vasoconstriction reduced the elastic modulus of the dog femoral artery by 29 per cent and vasodilatation increased it by 46 per cent. Decreases in elasticity in constriction and increases in dilatation were to be expected from the fact that there was no statistically significant changes in $\Delta p/\Delta r_o$. When changes in volume elasticity were calculated from (1.3), dilatation produced an increase (mean 33 per cent, $0.01 < P < 0.02$) in six out of seven experiments while constriction produced slight decreases (mean 10.9 per cent, $0.02 < P < 0.05$) in eight out of nine experiments. The same general conclusions were reached in a single experiment when E_{inc} and $V\Delta p/\Delta V$ were calculated at an elevated mean blood pressure induced by noradrenaline infusion; acetylcholine and noradrenaline having previously been topically applied as before. Although Gerová and Gero (1969) did not calculate elasticity it is clear from their records (reproduced in Figs. 13 and 14) that $\Delta p/\Delta r_o$ showed little variation following constriction or dilatation as in my own experiments (Gow, 1970). Subsequently Gero and Gerová (1969), showed that $\bar{D}_o\Delta p/\Delta D_o$ ($= E_p$) was lower for a constricted femoral artery than that for the control. In view of the reduction in radius and the Laplace relationship it must be concluded, quite apart from any consideration of wall thickness changes, that vasoconstriction increased the extensibility of the wall and lowered its elastic modulus.

Hinke (1965) found that E_{inc} of the rat caudal artery at a mean pressure of 105 mmHg was reduced by 65 per cent during noradrenaline-induced vasoconstriction. When the mean pressure was 75 mmHg the incremental modulus was reduced by 76 per cent while at 40 mmHg the modulus was unchanged. Hinke interpreted the lack of change of E_{inc} and its low value at low pressures to mean that the smooth muscle was the sole stress-bearing component. Speden (1970) also found E_{inc} to be consistently lower in the constricted rabbit ear artery than when fully dilated (four observations *in vitro*).

E. VEINS

Unlike arteries veins are often partially collapsed, and the non-circular cross-section creates difficulty in calculating a modulus of elasticity from measurements of pressure and radius. The volume elasticity formula ($V\Delta p/\Delta V$) can be used, although from physiological stand-point, $\Delta p/\Delta V$ or its reciprocal is probably a more useful parameter when applied to the venous system since it is important to know the absolute changes in volume which correspond to given changes in pressure. As with arteries $\Delta p/\Delta V$ increases with increasing mean pressure. Thron (1968) found that $\Delta p/\Delta V$ changed during constriction and relaxation of the veins in the isolated perfused dog paw. Papaverine relaxed the smooth muscle and, as far as the ascending limb of the pressure volume relationship is concerned, decreased $\Delta p/\Delta V$ at all pressures, i.e. increased the extensibility of the wall. Noradrenaline increased $\Delta p/\Delta V$ below 30 mmHg and decreased it above this pressure. Similar results were obtained when the sciatic nerve was stimulated at 5–10 impulses s^{-1}. One would conclude from these experiments that vasoconstriction reduced the extensibility of the venous wall. Using venous strips, Leonard and Sarnoff (1957) found that the "strong" contraction of venous smooth muscle produced by aramine resulted in a decrease in the extensibility ($\Delta L/LF$), where ΔL, L and F are changes in length, unstressed length and force respectively. At tensions above 0·2 g the extensibility of normal and constricted strips was similar. It is not certain whether this tension is high or low compared to that normally found in the walls of these particular veins. Alexander (1967) found that the slope of the length–tension relationship was not markedly altered by contraction.

The incremental modulus of dog jugular vein, plotted as a function of outer radius, was higher when the vessel was in spasm than when relaxation was produced with xylocaine (Bergel, 1964). However, had this comparison been made by plotting modulus as a function of pressure the conclusion would have been similar to that for the carotid artery (Dobrin and Rovick, 1969), i.e. at a given pressure vasoconstriction decreases the elastic modulus.

F. ELASTIC PROPERTIES OF ARTERIOLES

In contrast to the numerous studies on large arteries and veins very few have been done on single vessels within the microcirculation largely because of the unavailability of suitable methods. Reference has already been made to the technical contributions of Wiederhielm (1965a) and Johnson and Greatbatch (1966). Johnson's (1968) observations highlight the importance of myogenic tone (Bayliss, 1902; Folkow, 1964; Johnson, 1964) by demonstrating that an increase in pressure at the arterial end of an arteriole was followed by a decrease in its diameter. Hence the concept of a viscoelastic tube which passively follows transmural pressure changes has limited application to vessels of this type.

The form of the pressure-radius relationship for a mesenteric arteriole in a cat is shown in Fig. 12 (Johnson, 1968). Below an arterial pressure of 50 mmHg the muscle is fully relaxed and the vessel exhibits the passive properties of a tube of relaxed muscle cells. Similaily, at very high pressure

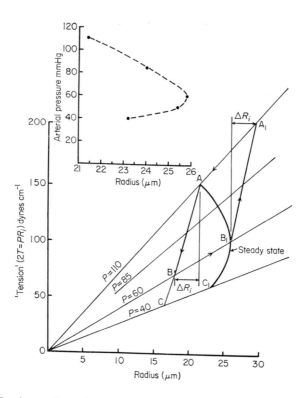

FIG. 12. Tension–radius relationship for a cat mesenteric arteriole. The inset is a pressure–radius plot using five points on the steady-state curve. (Redrawn from Johnson, 1968.)

the muscle cells are maximally contracted and the vessel again behaves as a passive tube. The tension–radius relationship in the mid-pressure region demonstrates what is known as autoregulation. It can be seen that a fall in arterial pressure from 110 to 60 mmHg results in a passive radius decrease from A to B. Subsequently the vessel dilates (time constant approximately 37 s) to B_1 on the steady-state relationship. With a return of pressure to

110 mmHg the radius increases initially but, as the result of muscular contraction, returns along OA_1 to A.

No measurements of elasticity or viscosity of the arteriolar wall were made by Johnson (1968) nor any measurements of wall thickness. However, the author has calculated incremental moduli for a relaxed and constricted vessel at an arterial pressure of 85 mmHg using his data. In the constricted case the passive relationship AB for a fall of 50 mmHg between 110 and 60 mmHg was used and in the relaxed state, the 50 mmHg change between 60 and 110 mmHg along A_1, B_1. A wall thickness to vessel inner diameter ratio of 1/30 (Van Citters et al., 1962) was assumed. The more constricted vessel (at 110 mmHg) was found to have an elastic modulus of $1 \cdot 90 \times 10^6$ dynes cm^{-2} which is notably less than that calculated for the same vessel in the more relaxed state ($5 \cdot 5 \times 10^6$). While undoubtedly there are errors in the incremental modulus calculated in this way these would not be expected to alter the conclusion.

A study of the elastic and viscous behaviour of frog arterioles (~ 150 μm diameter) was recently made by Wiederhielm (1965a, b). These vessels were larger than those studied by Johnson (1968) and showed no myogenic tone. The stress strain diagram plotted from pressure and diameter data was convex to the strain axis (like larger blood vessels). Accordingly, the Young's modulus was strain-dependent and markedly so when pressures outside the normal range were used. That vasoconstriction increases the Young's modulus of the arterial wall is not apparent from Wiederhielm's (1965a) data. While the wall of the constricted vessel was continuously creeping up to the point when the pressure was returned to zero, the diameter of the relaxed vessel stabilized rapidly (Fig. 5). The increase in diameter of the relaxed vessel was about 25 μm while that of the constricted vessel reached 100 μm and presumably would have increased further had the pressure step of 50 mmHg been maintained. In view of the greater extensibility of the constricted arterial wall one is led to the opposite conclusion that vasoconstriction decreases the elastic modulus of the wall of arterioles.

G. CONCLUSIONS

When vascular smooth muscle contracts, the diameter of a blood vessel falls and its wall thickness increases. In the majority of direct observations of vasoconstriction and dilatation the elasticity coefficient $\Delta p/\Delta r_o$ did not alter sufficiently to offset the effects of wall thickness changes on the calculated modulus. Therefore, at a constant distending pressure, vasodilators increase and vasoconstrictors decrease the elastic modulus of the wall.

The incremental modulus has been shown to predict pulse wave velocity fairly well in the aorta where changes in calibre resulting from vasomotor changes will in all probability be less than 10 per cent. It remains to be shown that the wave velocity falls in a constricted vessel and rises in a dilated one, and can in both instances be predicted with some degree of accuracy from this modulus.

4. VASOMOTOR CHANGES IN CONDUIT ARTERIES AND LARGE VEINS in vivo AND THEIR HAEMODYNAMIC CONSEQUENCES

A. CONDUIT ARTERIES

The only detailed information on the relationship of sympathetic outflow to the calibre of large arteries comes from the series of investigations made in anaesthetized dogs by Gero and Gerová in Czecho-Slovakia and from one or two preliminary experiments done in this laboratory. Their earlier experiments in dogs anaesthetized with thiopentone (Gerová and Gero, 1967) demonstrated convincingly that the vasoconstriction occurring in the femoral artery as the result of bilateral common carotid artery occlusion was of negligible physiological importance (3 per cent constriction of the outer diameter). When the carotid sinus receptors were stimulated by inflation of a balloon within it, the femoral artery dilated by 5 per cent (22 experiments). This clearly demonstrated the presence of maintained activity in the sympathetic nerves supplying the femoral arteries and presumably, other conduit arteries. The absence of a significant constrictor response to carotid artery occlusion has also been a consistent finding in the author's experiments. In two greyhounds the diameter of the femoral artery was monitored with an electrical caliper during bilateral common carotid artery occlusion. The mean pressure within the femoral artery was held constant during the pressor response by controlled clamping of the common iliac artery. Less than 1 per cent constriction occurred. Negligible constriction was also found in the common carotid artery held at a constant mean pressure during occlusion of the contralateral common carotid artery. The sheep common carotid was also unresponsive (< 1 per cent constriction) when pressure in the isolated, perfused, contralateral sinus was lowered to zero (Gow and Carney, unpublished observations). This artery, however, was highly reactive to direct electrical stimulation of its sympathetic supply; stimulation of the cephalic end of the divided ipsilateral sympathetic trunk (8 Hz, 5V and 15 ms duration) produced 25 per cent reduction in the outer diameter. This finding confirms that of Keatinge (1966) who reported decreases in sheep common carotid artery diameter ranging up to 40 per cent. One concludes from these observations that although the diameter of conduit arteries such as the femoral and carotid can, under certain experimental conditions, be reduced considerably, they are little influenced by the carotid sinus baroreceptors. Gerová and Gero (1969) have demonstrated the range of sympathetic control of the femoral artery in the dog (Figs. 13, 14).

Following division of the lumbar sympathetic trunk the femoral artery
dilated by 22 per cent above the resting diameter. The surprisingly rapid
and almost complete return to 4 per cent above control diameter within
15 min has important implications regarding myogenic tone, for it indicates

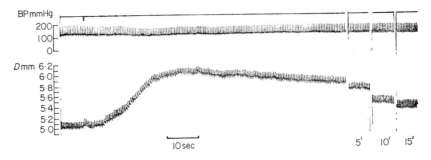

FIG. 13. Effect of section of the sympathetic trunk at the L3 to L4 level on blood
pressure (*BP*) and the diameter (*D*) of the femoral artery in a dog. (Reproduced
with permission from Gerová and Gero, 1969.)

that the calibre of conduit arteries can be maintained in the absence of
a sympathetic supply. These observations stand in contrast to the larger
concomitant changes in the microcirculation where Gerová and Gero (1969)
found that following lumbar sympathetic nerve section the femoral resistance

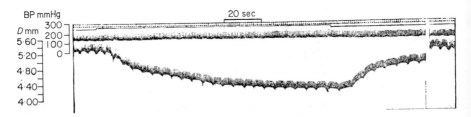

FIG. 14. Effect of stimulation of the sympathetic trunk at the L3 to L4 level on
blood pressure (*BP*) and diameter (*D*) of the femoral artery in a dog. Rectangular
stimulus pulses of 5 ms duration, amplitude 4·2V and frequency 15 Hz were used.
(Reproduced with permission from Gerová and Gero, 1969.)

vessels dilated by (calculated) 58 per cent; after 15 min these vessels had
only constricted back to 22 per cent above the control value.

Small active diameter changes in the aorta have been shown as the result
of changes in sympathetic activity. Gerová and Gero (1969a) showed that

the abdominal aorta of anaesthetized dogs constricted by 5·5 per cent following electrical stimulation of the second lumbar sympathetic ganglion. A constriction of 9·9 per cent in the thoracic aorta following a haemorrhage (Pieper and Paul, 1969) is higher than might have been expected from the above results, especially since the thoracic aorta contains relatively less smooth muscle. However, the reasons for the vasoconstriction on haemorrhage were not elucidated in this study. Several possibilities exist, one being the effects of circulating vasoactive substances. There is also the likelihood of an increased activity in the vasomotor nerves supplying the aorta. For instance it can be assumed that the stabilization of the carotid sinus pressure without a pulsatile component would have produced a state of increased sympathetic outflow. Apart from this, Bard (1963) has shown that spinal (i.e. reflexless) animals undergo vasoconstriction after haemorrhage. Further work must be done to show the range of active diameter changes along the entire length of the aorta. At present, it seems likely that active diameter reductions will be less than 10 per cent. If the results of Bevan et al. (1964) on the isolated nerve-pulmonary artery preparation at an (estimated) distending pressure of 15 mmHg can be extrapolated to the living animal it can be expected that intense sympathetic activity will cause about 13 per cent reduction in pulmonary artery diameter.

The above observations suggest for the most part that changes in vasomotor tone in conduit arteries are small. There are, however, situations where larger changes in conduit arteries might occur. Vascular spasm is a well-known phenomenon especially in the smaller arteries and veins. The changes in diameter in this situation are often enormous and stand in contrast to the smaller changes discussed above. Weckman (1960) induced marked constriction in rabbit arteries by stimulating the hypothalamus. Whether the same phenomenon can be evoked in selected arteries in dogs remains to be seen. However, the author has observed that when dissecting rabbit femoral arteries, spasm is a common occurrence, but this does not happen in greyhounds and probably not in other breeds. Similarly, sheep have a diminutive femoral artery rich in smooth muscle and quite unlike the large superficial vessel of the dog. Keatinge (1966) found the sheep's carotid artery could constrict by up to 40 per cent of its diameter. The author has never observed changes as large as this. All of this suggests that species differences are to be expected regarding reactivity of the conduit arteries to changes in physico-chemical environment and neural activity.

It may be concluded that we know very little about the normal variations in the conduit arteries. What the extent of vasomotor changes is in these arteries in such situations as shock, fright, rage, reactive hyperaemia, exercise etc. are questions awaiting answers. The long-term active variations in conduit artery diameter are also unknown. What is needed are devices for diameter measurement which can be chronically implanted into living animals and which do not produce sufficient disturbance in the artery and its local environment to invalidate the results. Until such techniques become available many of the above questions and others will remain unanswered.

B. VEINS

Unlike arteries the veins hold the bulk of the blood volume. Estimates by Wiedeman (1963) put 85 per cent of the blood in the veins and venous reservoirs. The haemodynamic consequences of venomotor changes will therefore be those of capacitance changes. Gero and Gerová (1968) observed active changes in the femoral vein in anaesthetized dogs on cutting and stimulating the lumbar sympathetic trunk. Following transection of the ipsilateral trunk the vein dilated by 22 per cent and returned to 10 per cent of the control value after 5–6 min. Stimulation at 15 impulses s^{-1} produced maximal contraction of 12·7 per cent. The behaviour of the vein was very similar to that of the artery. While peripheral veins are capable of forceful contractions, Gauer and Thron (1965) believe that the evidence suggests that the venous system behaves as a low pressure system with passive walls during disturbances in circulatory homeostasis. Provided that the subject is in a recumbent position large volumes of blood may be sequestered within the periphery without evidence of active venoconstriction (Wood and Eckstein, 1958). Similarly, Öberg (1967) found that active constriction of veins played little part in reducing the dimensions of the venous compartment when recumbent dogs were bled. Emptying of veins is a passive phenomenon (Thron and Scheppokat, 1958) if pressures are below 5–10 mmHg but results from active venoconstriction at higher pressures. Smooth muscle participates in venous emptying at higher pressures because of a favourable length–tension relationship (Speden, 1960; Sparks and Bohr, 1962) and is clearly advantageous in the mobilization of blood from the limbs when the animal is standing.

In experiments on conscious dogs Tafür and Guntheroth (1966) recorded active constriction of the superior vena cava in response to fright caused by a fire cracker explosion. Marked venoconstriction also occurs in the ischaemic pressure response (Guntheroth, 1969). In 26 per cent of Tafür and Guntheroth's experiments on exercising dogs simultaneous increases in venous pressure and decreases in diameter were recorded which clearly demonstrates active contraction and suggests that active venoconstriction may be an important prelude to the onset of exercise.

C. HAEMODYNAMIC CONSEQUENCES IN CONDUIT ARTERIES

Vasomotor changes in arteries will have two haemodynamic consequences, first, those arising from changes in cross-sectional area, second, those arising from changes in elastic and viscous moduli. On the basis of data published on the sympathetic control of conduit arteries (Gerová and Gero, 1969, 1969a) one can calculate the possible haemodynamic changes which might take place during a state of increased sympathetic activity. A 5·5 per cent constriction of the lumbar aorta reduces the cross-sectional area and volume per unit length by 13 per cent ($\gamma = 0.1$); a 13 per cent constriction of the femoral artery reduces its volume per unit length by 36 per cent. These volume reductions are of negligible significance since, in terms of the total vascular compartment, the volume changes only amount to 1 or 2 per cent. However, reductions in calibre of the conduit vessels will increase the resistance to blood flow. A 9·4 per cent increase and a 10·7 per cent decrease in femoral diameter (Gow, 1970) at the fundamental frequency of 2 Hz, leads to values of α, of 6 and 4·5. On the basis of Womersley's (1955) calculations the ratio of maximum oscillatory flow to steady flow at these values of α is 0·26 and 0·16 respectively (at frequencies corresponding to higher harmonics α is higher and the differences in these ratios are less). It is clear that in a situation where sympathetic activity was sufficient to cause a 10 per cent constriction of the aorta and its branches, there would also be greater percentage constriction in the microcirculation, unless, of course, there is some differential sympathetic outflow to the conduits as opposed to their terminal ramifications. Hence it is reasonable to conclude that any changes in resistance within the conduit arteries will be trivial compared to those occurring in the microcirculation.

Changes in elasticity will alter the wave velocity and hence the characteristic impedance (Z_o) in proportion to $(V\Delta p/\Delta V)^{\frac{1}{2}}$. However Z_o is inversely proportional to D_i^2 so that following any vasomotor change Z_o will be expected to be altered in proportion to $(V\Delta p/\Delta V)^{\frac{1}{2}}/D_i^2$. Using the changes in $V\Delta p/\Delta V$ and D_i in the dog femoral artery reported by Gow (1970) it was found that following dilatation the increases in Z_o due to $V\Delta p/\Delta V$ increases were, on the average, offset by the increases in cross-sectional area (1·4 per cent mean decrease in Z_o, range 30·8 per cent increase to 25 per cent decrease, $N = 7$). In the constricted artery, however, the reduction in cross-sectional area was incompletely offset by the changes in $(V dp/dV)^{\frac{1}{2}}$ and hence impedance was increased (mean 31 per cent, range 7 to 58 per cent, $N = 9$). Whether these changes are representative of all the major arterial segments has yet to be determined. Pieper and Paul (1969) found no consistent change in the predicted wave velocity with aortic constriction. In two out of four experiments predicted wave velocity increased by approximately 5 and 10 per cent while in the others it fell by about 5 and 7 per cent. In the remainder of experiments in which either the carotid sinus pressure was stabilized or the vagi were cut, the predicted wave velocity showed negligible changes in most instances, the maximum change being a decrease of about 8 per cent.

On the basis of the constancy of the predicted wave velocity these workers concluded that wave velocity is held constant despite the active constriction and thus helps to maintain a constant characteristic impedance. However, in view of the small changes in elasticity and the significant reduction in cross-sectional area the characteristic impedance will be increased following vasoconstriction.

The above calculations suggest minor haemodynamic consequences in dogs as the result of vasoconstriction or vasodilatation in the large arteries since it is unlikely that the changes would occur independently of those in the microcirculation. Furthermore the effects of these changes on the input impedance of the circulation and on pulsatile cardiac work would have to be thought minimal when considering the moderate changes in impedance which occur as the result of gross procedures such as total occlusion of the descending aorta or the brachiocephalic trunk and subclavian arteries (O'Rourke and Taylor, 1967). This poses the question: what is the function of vascular smooth muscle in conduit arteries? The aorta and pulmonary artery particularly have the important function of accommodating the ventricular ejection and buffering the pressure rise (Windkessel). From a teleological standpoint there seems little advantage in having contractile cells in the proximal aorta. However, since the smooth muscle cell is the only cell type in the aortic media (Pease and Paule, 1960) its role in laying down elastic and collagen fibres would seem the more important. As the conduit arteries become smaller and the relative smooth muscle content rises the contribution of these conduits to total resistance progressively increases, although this is always small compared with that of the arterioles.

Finally one should not forget the important role of smooth muscle con-traction of conduit arteries in haemostasis (Zucker, 1947). When an artery or even its branches are injured or severed, spasm of the smooth muscle occurs. This strongly contracted state in larger vessels would seem to be greater than any response elicitable by sympathetic stimulation. Whether or not spasm is qualitatively different from "normal" vasoconstriction awaits further investigation.

5. SUMMARY AND PROBLEMS FOR FUTURE STUDY

The structure and elastic properties of blood vessels have been reviewed with reference to the influence exerted by vascular smooth muscle. From the relation between pressure and volume one can conclude that arteries and veins in general behave as passive viscoelastic tubes; the contribution of myogenic tone to the determination of calibre in these vessels remains obscure. Arterioles with autoregulatory properties behave as passive viscoelastic tubes at extremes of pressure, but in the physiological pressure range, respond to an increase of pressure by decreasing their diameter.

The inadequacy of linear viscoelastic elements in explaining the time- and frequency-dependent properties was emphasized. Notwithstanding this, the Kelvin–Voigt element was shown to be useful in quantitating the motion of the arterial wall at a given frequency and blood pressure. On the other hand the use of reaction-rate kinetics was shown to provide a plausible explanation for the time-dependent mechanical properties of blood vessels. This approach, however, did not allow the interaction of muscle and passive elastic elements to be evaluated.

The incremental modulus of the intact vascular wall is decreased during vasoconstriction and increased during vasodilatation at any given mean distending pressure. Although the use of this modulus gives a satisfactory prediction of the foot-to-foot velocity under control conditions it has not yet been established whether this modulus also predicts wave velocity in a vasoconstricted and in a vasodilated vessel.

While there is now quantitative data on the amount of active constriction of conduit arteries in dogs there is very little information for other species; comparable measurements for veins are also sadly lacking. For the femoral artery in the dog, maximal vasoconstriction results in a reduction in calibre of about 10–15 per cent. The haemodynamic consequences of these changes in calibre are small if compared with expected concomittant changes in the microcirculation; changes in the aorta probably rarely exceed 5 per cent and since the elastic properties of the excised aorta are similar to that *in vivo*, it is concluded that contraction of vascular smooth muscle in the aorta of the dog has little haemodynamic consequence. Hence the role of vascular smooth muscle cells in the large vessels is primarily one of laying down the fibrous proteins and maintaining the integrity of the wall. In large veins, however, there is evidence to suggest that vascular smooth muscle contraction with resulting decreases in venous capacity, provides an important mechanism for rapidly adjusting the venous return.

From the preceding review several problems stand out as worthy of future study.

1. There is a need to improve current models of the arterial wall giving attention to the structural arrangement of collagen, elastin and smooth muscle. Future models will be expected to explain quantitatively changes in wall extensibility following an active shortening or lengthening of the muscle component.
2. Further work is required to provide adequate explanations for the time-dependent properties of vascular tissues.
3. An elasticity modulus is required which not only predicts the phase velocity under control conditions but also when the artery is in a state of constriction and dilatation.

4. New techniques are required to provide a continuous monitor of vascular dimensions in conscious animals thus allowing the precise measurement of the normal physiological variations in vascular calibre and viscoelastic properties. Such implanted devices would have to be rigorously tested to eliminate the possibility of serious interference to the vessel and its environment.

5. The relationship of myogenic tone to the maintenance of vascular calibre is an interesting but largely unanswered problem; for example the mechanisms which almost completely restore femoral artery diameter following lumbar sympathectomy are at present a matter for speculation.

ACKNOWLEDGEMENT

The author gladly acknowledges the able technical assistance of Mrs. Sandra Elliott and Mr. Ted Foster in the preparation of the figures.

REFERENCES

Abrahamson, D. I. (1962). "Blood Vessels and Lymphatics," Academic Press, London and New York.

Alexander, R. S. (1963). The peripheral venous system. In "Handbook of Physiology" (W. F. Hamilton, ed.), Vol. 2, pp. 1075–1098, American Physiology Society, Washington, D.C.

Alexander, R. S. (1967). Contractile mechanics of venous smooth muscle. Am. J. Physiol. 212, 852–858.

Attinger, E. O. (1963). Pressure transmission in pulmonary arteries related to frequency and geometry. Circulation Res. 12, 623–641.

Attinger, E. O. (1969). Wall properties of veins. IEEE Transactions on Bio-Med. Eng. BME–16, 253–261.

Attinger, E. O., Sugawara, H., Navarro, A., Riccetto, A. and Martin, R. (1966). Pressure-flow relations in dog arteries. Circulation Res. 19, 230–246.

Attinger, F. M. L. (1968). Two dimensional in vitro studies of femoral arterial walls of the dog. Circulation Res. 22, 829–840.

Bader, H. (1963). The anatomy and physiology of the vascular wall. In "Handbook of Physiology" (W. F. Hamilton, ed.), Vol. 2, pp. 865–889, American Physiology Society, Washington, D.C.

Ballou, J. W. and Smith, J. (1949). Dynamic measurements of polymer physical properties. J. Appl. Phys. 20, 493–502.

Bard, P. (1963). Central nervous control of vascular flow. In "The Peripheral Blood Vessels" (J. L. Orbison and D. E. Smith, eds.), pp. 106–133, Williams and Wilkins, Baltimore.

Bargainer, J. D. (1967). Pulse wave velocity in the main pulmonary artery of the dog. Circulation Res. 20, 630–637.

Barnett, G. O., Mallos, A. J. and Shapiro, A. (1961). Relationship of aortic pressure and diameter in the dog. J. Appl. Physiol. 16, 545–548.

Bauer, W. H. and Collins, E. A. (1967). Thixotropy and dilatancy. *In* "Rheology Theory and Applications" (F. R. Eirich, ed.), Vol. 4, pp. 423–459, Academic Press, New York and London.

Bayliss, W. M. (1902). On the local reactions of the arterial wall to changes of internal pressure. *J. Physiol.* **28**, 220–231.

Benninghoff, A. (1927). Über die Beziehungen zwischen elastischem Gerüst und glatter Muskulatur in der Arterienwand und ihre funktionelle Bedeutung. *Z. Zellforsch. Mikrosk. Anat.* **6**, 348–396.

Benninghoff, A. (1930). Blutgefässe und Herz. *In* "Handbuch der Mikroskopischen Anatomie des Menschen" (W. von Mollendörff, ed.), Vol. VI, Part 1, Springer, Berlin.

Bergel, D. H. (1960). The viscoelastic properties of the arterial wall. Ph.D. Thesis, University of London.

Bergel, D. H. (1961a). The static elastic properties of the arterial wall. *J. Physiol.* **156**, 445–457.

Bergel, D. H. (1961b). The dynamic elastic properties of the arterial wall. *J. Physiol.* **156**, 458–468.

Bergel, D. H. (1964). Arterial viscoelasticity. *In* "Pulsatile Blood Flow" (E. O. Attinger, ed.), pp. 275–292, McGraw-Hill, New York.

Bergel, D. H. (1966). Stress-strain properties of blood vessels. *Lab. Pract.* **15**, 77–81.

Bergel, D. H. and Milnor, W. R. (1965). Pulmonary vascular impedance in the dog. *Circulation Res.* **16**, 401–415.

Bevan, J. A., Johnson, R. C. and Verity, M. A. (1964). Changes in elasticity of pulmonary reflexogenic area with sympathetic activity. *Am. J. Physiol.* **206**, 36–42.

Bramwell, J. C. and Hill, A. V. (1922). The velocity of the pulse wave in man. *Proc. R. Soc. B.* **93**, 298–306.

Brenner, O. (1935). The pathology of vessels in the pulmonary circulation. *Arch. Intern. Med.* **56**, 211–237.

Burton, A. C. (1954). Relation of structure to function of the tissue of the wall of blood vessels. *Physiol. Rev.* **34**, 619–642.

Carew, T. E., Vaishnav, R. N. and Patel, D. J. (1968). Compressibility of the arterial wall. *Circulation Res.* **23**, 61–68.

Cleary, E. G. (1963). A correlative and comparative study of the non-uniform arterial wall. M.D. Thesis, University of Sydney.

Dillon, J. H., Prettyman, I. B. and Hall, G. L. (1944). Hysteretic and elastic properties of rubber-like materials under dynamic shear stresses. *J. Appl. Phys.* **15**, 309–323.

Dobrin, P. B. and Doyle, J. M. (1970). Vascular smooth muscle and the anisotropy of dog carotid artery. *Circulation Res.* **27**, 105–119.

Dobrin, P. B. and Rovick, A. A. (1969). Influence of vascular smooth muscle on contractile mechanics and elasticity of arteries. *Am. J. Physiol.* **217**, 1644–1651.

Folkow, B. (1964). Description of the myogenic hypothesis. *Circulation Res.* **15**, Suppl. I, 279–287.

Frasher, W. G., Jr. and Sobin, S. S. (1965). Pressure-volume response of isolated living main pulmonary artery in dogs. *J. Appl. Physiol.* **20**, 675–682.

Furchgott, R. F. (1955). The pharmacology of vascular smooth muscle. *Pharmac. Rev.* **7**, 183–265.

Furchgott, R. F. and Bhadrakom, S. (1953). Reactions of strips of rabbit aorta to epinephrine, isopropylarterenol, sodium nitrite, and other drugs. *J. Pharmacol. Exp. Ther.* **108**, 129–143.

Fung, Y. C. (1966). Theoretical considerations of the elasticity of red cells and small blood vessels. *Fed. Proc. Fed. Am. Soc.* **25**, 1761–1772.

Gauer, O. H. and Thron, H. L. (1965). Postural changes in the circulation. In "Handbook of Physiology" (W. F. Hamilton, ed.), Vol. 3, pp. 2409–2439, American Physiology Society, Washington, D.C.

Gero, J. and Gerová, M. (1968). Sympathetic regulation of collecting vein. *Experientia* **24**, 811–812.

Gero, J. and Gerová, M. (1969). Sympathetic regulation of arterial distensibility. *Physiologica bohemoslov.* **18**, 480–481.

Gerová, M. and Gero, J. (1962). Dynamics of carotid sinus elasticity during pressor reaction. *Circulation Res.* **11**, 1010–1020.

Gerová, M. and Gero, J. (1967). Reflex regulation of smooth muscle tone of conduit vessel. *Angiologica* **4**, 348–358.

Gerová, M. and Gero, J. (1969). Range of the sympathetic control of the dog femoral artery. *Circulation Res.* **24**, 349–359.

Gerová, M. and Gero, J. (1969a). Sympathetic control of the lumbar aorta. *Physiol. Bohemoslov.* **18**, 481–482.

Goto, M. and Kimoto, Y. (1966). Hysteresis and stress relaxation of the blood vessels studied by a Universal Tensile Testing Instrument. *Jap. J. Physiol.* **15**, 169–184.

Gow, B. S. (1966). An electrical caliper for measurement of pulsatile arterial diameter changes *in vivo. J. Appl. Physiol.* **21**, 1122–1126.

Gow, B. S. (1969). A study of the viscoelastic behaviour of systemic arteries in the living dog. Ph.D. Thesis, University of Sydney.

Gow, B. S. (1970). Viscoelastic properties of conduit arteries. *Circulation Res.* **26** and **27**, Suppl. II, 113–122.

Gow, B. S. and Taylor, M. G. (1968). Measurement of viscoelastic properties of arteries in the living dog. *Circulation Res.* **23**, 111–122.

Guntheroth, W. G. (1969). *In vivo* measurement of dimensions of veins with implications regarding control of venous return. *IEEE Transactions on Biomed. Eng.* **BME–16**, 247–253.

Ham, A. W. and Leeson, T. S. (1961). "Histology", 4th Ed., Lippincott Co., Philadelphia.

Hardung, V. (1953). Vergleichende Messungen der dynamischen Elastizität und Viskosität von Blutgefässen, Kautschuk und synthetischen Elastomeren. *Helv. Physiol. Pharmacol. Acta* **11**, 194–211.

Hardung, V. (1963). Propagation of pulse waves in visco-elastic tubings. In "Handbook of Physiology" (W. F. Hamilton, ed.), Vol. 2, pp. 107–135, American Physiology Society, Washington, D.C.

Hardung, V. (1964). Die Bedeutung der Anisotropie und Inhomogenität bei der Bestimmung der Elastizität der Blutgefässe II. *Angiologica* **1**, 185–196.

Harkness, M. L. R., Harkness, R. D. and McDonald, D. A. (1957). The collagen and elastin content of the arterial wall in the dog. *Proc. R. Soc. B.* **146**, 541–551.

Harris, P. and Heath, D. (1962). "The Human Pulmonary Circulation: Its Form and Function in Health and Disease," Livingstone, London.

Hinke, J. A. (1965). *In vitro* demonstration of vascular hyper-responsiveness in experimental hypertension. *Circulation Res.* **17**, 359–371.

Horeman, H. W. and Noordergraaf, A. (1958). Numerical evaluation of volume pulses in man. I. The basic Formula. *Phys. Med. Biol.* **3**, 51–58.

Jaeger, M. (1966). L'élasticité des artères et son influence sur leur irrigation. *Helv. Physiol. Pharmacol. Acta* **17**, Suppl. XVII, 1–128.

Johnson, P. C. (1964). Origin, localization and homeostatic significance of autoregulation in the intestine. *Circulation Res.* **15**, Suppl. I, 225–232.

Johnson, P. C. (1968). Autoregulatory responses of cat mesenteric arterioles measured *in vivo*. *Circulation Res.* **22**, 199–212.

Johnson, P. C. (1969). Haemodynamics. *Ann. Rev. Physiol.* **31**, 331–352.

Johnson, P. C. and Greatbatch, W. H., Jr. (1966). The angiometer: A flying spot microscope for measurement of blood vessel diameter. *Methods Med. Res.* **11**, 220–227.

Kapal, E. (1954). Die elastischen Eigenschaften der Aortenwand sowie des elastischen kollagenen Bindegewebes bei frequenten zyclishen Beanspruchengen. *Z. Biol.* **107**, 347–404.

Keatinge, W. R. (1966). Electrical and mechanical response of arteries to stimulation of sympathetic nerves. *J. Physiol.* **185**, 701–715.

King, A. L. (1957). Some studies in tissue elasticity. *In* "Tissue Elasticity" (J. W. Remington, ed.), American Physiology Society, Washington, D.C.

Krafka, J. (1939). Comparative studies of the histo-physics of the aorta. *Am. J. Physiol.* **125**, 1–14.

Krafka, J. (1940). Changes in the elasticity of the aorta with age. *Archs Path.* **29**, 303–309.

Lambossy, P. and Müller, A. (1954). Vitesse des ondes dans les tubes. Influence de l'anistropie de la paroi. *Helv. Physiol. Pharmacol. Acta* **12**, 217–229.

Laszt, L. (1968). Untersuchungen über die elastischen Eigenschaften der Blutgefässe be im Ruhe-und im Kontraktionszustand. *Angiologica* **5**, 14–27.

Lawton, R. W. (1954). The thermoelastic behaviour of isolated aortic strips of the dog. *Circulation Res.* **2**, 344–353.

Learoyd, B. M. and Taylor, M. G. (1966). Alterations with age in the viscoelastic properties of human arterial walls. *Circulation Res.* **18**, 287–292.

Lee, J. S., Frasher, W. G. and Fung, Y. C. (1968). Comparison of elasticity of an artery *in vivo* and in excision. *J. Appl. Physiol.* **25**, 799–801.

Leonard, E. and Sarnoff, S. J. (1957). Effect of aramine-induced smooth muscle contraction on length–tension diagrams of venous strips. *Circulation Res.* **5**, 169–174.

Luisada, A. A. (1961). "Development and Structure of the Cardiovascular System", McGraw-Hill, New York.

Lundholm, L. and Mohme-Lundholm, E. (1966). Length at inactivated contractile elements, length-tension diagram, active state and tone of vascular smooth muscle. *Acta Physiol. Scand.* **68**, 347–359.

Mallos, A. J. (1962). An electrical calliper for continuous measurement of relative displacement. *J. Appl. Physiol.* **17**, 131–134.

McDonald, D. A. (1960). "Blood Flow in Arteries", Arnold, London.

McDonald, D. A. (1968). Haemodynamics. *Ann. Rev. Physiol.* **30**, 525–556.

Meyer, W. W. (1958). Die Lebenswandlung der Struktur von Arterien und Venen. *Verh. Deut. Ges. Kreislaufforsch.* **24**, 13–40.

Mikami, T. and Attinger, E. O. (1968). Stress relaxation of blood vessel walls. *Angiologica* **5**, 281–292.

Moreno, A. H., Katz, A. I., Gold, L. D. and Reddy, M. (1970). Mechanics of distension of dog veins and other very thin walled tubular structures. *Circulation Res.* **27**, 1069–1080.

Morris, M. J. (1965). Pressure and flow in the pulmonary vasculature of the dog. B.Sc. (Med). Thesis, University of Sydney.

Öberg, B. (1967). The relationship between active constriction and passive recoil of the veins at various distending pressures. *Acta Physiol. Scand.* **71**, 233–247.

O'Rourke, M. F. (1967). Steady and pulsatile energy losses in the systemic circulation under normal conditions and in simulated arterial disease. *Cardiovascular Res.* **1**, 312–326.

O'Rourke, M. F. and Taylor, M. G. (1967). Input impedance of the systemic circulation. *Circulation Res.* **20**, 365–380.

Patel, D. J., de Freitas, F. M., Greenfield, J. C., Jr. and Fry, D. L. (1963). Relationship of radius to pressure along the aorta in living dogs. *J. Appl. Physiol.* **18**, 1111–1117.

Patel, D. J. and Fry, D. L. (1969). The elastic symmetry of arterial segments in dogs. *Circulation Res.* **24**, 1–8.

Patel, D. J., Janicki, J. S. and Carew, T. E. (1969). Static anisotropic elastic properties of the aorta in living dogs. *Circulation Res.* **25**, 765–779.

Patel, D. J., Mallos, A. J. and Fry, D. L. (1961). Aortic mechanics in the living dog. *J. Appl. Physiol.* **16**, 293–299.

Patel, D. J., Schilder, D. P. and Mallos, A. J. (1960). Mechanical properties and dimensions of the major pulmonary arteries. *J. Appl. Physiol.* **15**, 92–96.

Pease, D. C. and Paule, W. J. (1960). Electron microscopy of elastic arteries: the thoracic aorta of the rat. *J. Ultrastruct. Res.* **3**, 469–483.

Peterson, L. H., Jensen, R. E. and Parnell, J. (1960). Mechanical properties of arteries *in vivo*. *Circulation Res.* **8**, 622–639.

Pieper, H. P. and Paul, L. T. (1968). Catheter-tip gauge for measuring blood flow velocity and vessel diameter in dogs. *J. Appl. Physiol.* **24**, 259–261.

Pieper, H. P. and Paul, L. T. (1969). Responses of aortic smooth muscle studied in intact dogs. *Am. J. Physiol.* **217**, 154–160.

Pürschel, S., Reichel, H. and Vonderlage, M. (1969). Vergleichende Untersuchungen zur statischen und dynamischen Wanddehnbarkeit von Vena cava und Aorta des Kaninchens. *Pflügers Arch.* **306**, 232–246.

Remington, J. W. (1955). Hysteresis loop behaviour of the aorta and other extensible tissues. *Am. J. Physiol.* **180**, 83–95.

Remington, J. W. (1957). Extensibility and hysteresis phenomena in smooth muscle tissues. *In* "Tissue Elasticity" (J. W. Remington, ed.), pp. 138–153, American Physiology Society, Washington, D.C.

Remington, J. W. (1962). Pressure-diameter relations of the *in vivo* aorta. *Am. J. Physiol.* **203**, 440–448.

Remington, J. W. (1963). The physiology of the aorta and major arteries. *In* "Handbook of Physiology" (W. F. Hamilton, ed.), Vol. 2, pp. 799–838, American Physiology Society, Washington, D.C.

Reuterwall, O. P. (1921). Über die Elastizität der Gefässwände und die Methoden ihrer näheren Prüfung. *Acta Med Scand.*, Suppl. 2, 1–175.

Roach, M. R. and Burton, A. C. (1957). The reason for the shape of the distensibility curves of arteries. *Can. J. Biochem. Physiol.* **35**, 681–690.

Roy, C. S. (1880). The elastic properties of the arterial wall. *J. Physiol.* **3**, 125–162.

Sinn, W. (1956). Die Elastizität der Arterien und ihre Bedeutung für die Dynamik des Arteriellen Systems. *Akad. Wiss. Lit.* **11**, 647–832.

Somlyo, A. P. and Somlyo, A. V. (1968). Vascular smooth muscle. I. Normal structure, pathology, biochemistry and biophysics. *Pharm. Rev.* **20**, 197–272.

Sparks, H. V., Jr. and Bohr, D. F. (1962). Effect of stretch on passive tension and contractility of isolated vascular smooth muscle. *Am. J. Physiol.* **202**, 835–840.

Speden, R. (1960). The effect of initial strip length on the noradrenaline-induced isometric contraction of arterial strips. *J. Physiol.* **154**, 15–25.

Speden, R. (1970). Personal communication.

Stacy, R. W. (1957). Reaction rate kinetics and some tissue mechanical properties. *In* "Tissue Elasticity" (R. W. Remington, ed.), pp. 131–137, American Physiology Society, Washington, D.C.

Stacy, R. W., Williams, D. T., Worden, R. E. and McMorris, R. O. (1955). "Essentials of Biological and Medical Physics", McGraw-Hill, New York.

Tafür, E. and Guntheroth, W. G. (1966). Simultaneous pressure, flow and diameter of the vena cava with fright and exercise. *Circulation Res.* **19**, 42–50.

Taylor, M. G. (1964). Wave travel in arteries and the design of the cardiovascular system. *In* "Pulsatile Blood Flow" (E. O. Attinger, ed.), pp. 343–372, McGraw-Hill, New York.

Taylor, M. G. (1966). Use of random excitation and spectral analysis in the study of frequency-dependent parameters of the cardiovascular system. *Circulation Res.* **18**, 585–595.

Taylor, M. G. (1966a). The input impedance of an assembly of randomly branching elastic tubes. *Biophys. J.* **6**, 29–51.

Taylor, M. G. (1966b). Wave transmission through an assembly of randomly branching elastic tubes. *Biophys. J.* **6**, 697–716.

Taylor, M. G. (1967). The elastic properties of arteries in relation to the physiological functions of the arterial system. *Gastroenterology* **52**, 358–363.

Thron, H. L. (1967). Das Verhalten peripherer Blutgefässe *in vivo* bei passiven und aktiven Weitenänderungen. *Arch. Kreislaufforsch.* **52**, 1–63.

Thron, H. L. (1968). The interrelation between active and passive diameter changes in resistance and capacitance vessels. *In* "Circulation in Skeletal Muscle" (O. Hudlická, ed.), pp. 295–314, Pergamon Press, Oxford.

Thron, H. L. and Scheppokat, K. D. (1958). Tonusänderungen peripherer kapazitiver Gefässe. *Verh. Deut. Ges. Kreislaufforsch.* **24**, 333–338.

Tickner, E. G. and Sacks, A. H. (1964). Theoretical and experimental study of the elastic behaviour of the human brachial and other human and canine arteries. *Vidya Rep.* 162, Itek Corporation, California.

Tobolsky, A. V., Dunell, B. A. and Andrews, R. D. (1951). Stress relaxation and dynamic properties of polymers. *Text. Res. J.* **21**, 404–411.

Van Citters, R. L., Wagner, B. M. and Rushmer, R. F. (1962). Architecture of small arteries during vasoconstriction. *Circulation Res.* **10**, 668–675.

Weckman, N. (1960). Local constriction and spasm of large arteries elicited by hypothalamic stimulation. *Experientia* **16**, 34–36.

Weltmann, R. (1960). Rheology of pastes and paints. *In* "Rheology Theory and Applications" (F. R. Eirich, ed.), Vol. 3, pp. 189–248, Academic Press, New York and London.

Wezler, K. and Schlüter, F. (1953). Cited by Bader (1963).

Wezler, K. and Sinn, W. (1953). "Das Strömungsgesetz des Blutkreislaufes", (cited by McDonald, 1960), Edns. Cantor, Aulendorf, Württ, W. Germany.

Wiederhielm, C. A. (1965a). Distensibility characteristics of small blood vessels. *Fed. Proc.* **24**, 1075–1084.

Wiederhielm, C. A. (1965b). Viscoelastic properties of relaxed and constricted arteriolar walls. *Bibl. Anat.* **7**, 346–352.

Wiedeman, M. P. (1963). Dimensions of blood vessels from distributing artery to collecting vein. *Circulation Res.* **12**, 375–378.

Wiggers, C. J. and Wégria, R. (1938). Active changes in the size and distensibility of the aorta during acute hypertension. *Am. J. Physiol.* **124**, 603–611.

Wolinsky, H. and Glagov, S. (1964). Structural basis for the static mechanical properties of the aortic media. *Circulation Res.* **14**, 400–413.

Wolinsky, H. and Glagov, S. (1967). A lamellar unit of aortic medial structure and function in mammals. *Circulation Res.* **20**, 99–111.

Womersley, J. R. (1955). Oscillatory motion of a viscous liquid in a thin-walled elastic tube. I. The linear approximation for long waves. *Phil. Mag.* **46**, 199–221.

Womersley, J. R. (1957). Oscillatory flow in arteries: the constrained elastic tube as a model of arterial flow and pulse transmission. *Phys. Med. Biol.* **2**, 178–187.

Wood, J. E. and Eckstein, J. W. (1958). A tandem forearm plethysmograph for study of acute responses of the peripheral veins of man: The effect of environmental and local temperature change and the effect of pooling blood in the extremities. *J. Clin. Invest.* **37**, 41–50.

Zatzman, M., Stacy, R. W., Randall, J. and Eberstein, A. (1954). Time course of stress relaxation in isolated arterial segments. *Am. J. Physiol.* **177**, 299–302.

Zucker, M. B. (1947). Platelet agglutination and vasoconstriction as factors in spontaneous haemostasis in normal, thrombocytopenic, heparinized and hypoprothrombinaemic rats. *Am. J. Physiol.* **148**, 275–288.

Chapter 13

Poststenotic Dilatation in Arteries†

MARGOT R. ROACH

*Departments of Biophysics and Medicine, University of Western
Ontario, London, Ontario, Canada*

1. INTRODUCTION

Poststenotic dilatation (PSD) implies that arteries enlarge in the low pressure region distal to a stenosis, rather than in the higher pressure region proximally. Radiologically the PSD is often easier to see than the stenosis. Although the exact incidence of PSD is unknown, it has been reported with virtually all types of stenosis: congenital and acquired, intrinsic and extrinsic.

The incidence of PSD with various lesions is hard to determine because few authors write on it specifically. However, about 50–60 per cent of patients with coarctation have it (Wood, 1956; Skandalakis *et al.*, 1960; Zaroff *et al.*, 1959). Age may be a factor as Kjellberg *et al.*, (1955) found a PSD in all of their 40 patients over age seven with a coarctation, but in only three out of ten younger patients with this lesion. Distal mycotic aneurysms also occur, and about 50 per cent of them rupture (Kieffer *et al.*, 1961).

† Supported by grants from the Ontario Heart Foundation and the Medical Research Council of Canada, and by a Scholarship from the Medical Research Council (1967–70).

Pulmonary valve stenosis is almost always associated with a PSD unless the stenosis is severe while pulmonary infundibular stenosis is rarely associated with it (Wood, 1956; Kjellberg *et al.*, 1955; Kincaid, 1960; Keith *et al.*, 1958), and Kincaid (1960) suggests it may be the only abnormality with mild pulmonary stenosis. Brock (1952), however, feels that all cases of infundibular stenosis are associated with both a PSD and a valvular stenoses.

Aortic valvular stenosis, either congenital or acquired, is usually associated with a PSD (Wood, 1956; Jarchow and Kincaid, 1961; Rochoff and Austen, 1963; Kiloh, 1950; Morrow *et al.*, 1959). Most authors (Morrow *et al.*, 1959; Castellanos and Hernandez, 1967) state PSD is rare with subvalvular and supravalvular stenoses, but Weintraub *et al.*, (1964) feel PSD is common with subvalvular stenoses.

Stenoses in the pulmonary arteries (Arvidsson *et al.*, 1955), renal arteries (Kincaid and Davis, 1961) and limb and neck arteries (DeBakey *et al.*, 1961) are often associated with a PSD, and in fact the PSD may be easier to see radiologically than the stenosis.

External compression of the subclavian artery by a cervical rib (Halsted, 1916) or other thoracic inlet anomalies (Eden, 1939) or of the popliteal artery by a tendon or ligament (Gedge *et al.*, 1961) can also produce a PSD.

Thus, almost any type of stenosis, whether valvular or peripheral, can create a PSD. However, short stenoses seem more likely to do so than longer ones. The reason will be discussed later.

2. Theories on the Ætiology of Poststenotic Dilatation

Early theories were based on the ætiology of subclavian aneurysms distal to cervical ribs and included damage to the vasa vasorum and stimulation of the nerva vasorum (Halsted, 1916). They obviously cannot explain PSD associated with intrinsic lesions.

Later theories have been based on the observation that flow distortions were produced by the stenosis, and probably were related to the development of the PSD. These include turbulence (Halsted, 1916; Holman, 1954a,b; Roach, 1963a,b), vortex formation (Bruns *et al.*, 1959) and cavitation (Robicsek *et al.*, 1958; Rodbard *et al.*, 1967). These flow distortions may cause structural fatigue in the wall, or alter the distending pressure, or the drag force and so lead to a PSD.

3. Experimental Production of Poststenotic Dilatation

A. *IN VIVO*

Although Luigi Porta (1845) published a picture of PSD in the abdominal aorta of a dog in 1845, little experimental work was done until Halsted (1909) roused interest in the subject early in the twentieth century. Pressure necrosis with rupture was common (Reid, 1916, 1924; Halsted, 1909) and discouraged most workers. However, once Reid (1924) showed that the abdominal aorta was less likely to rupture than the thoracic aorta, Halsted (1916) was able to do a series of experiments on the abdominal aorta of dogs with metal bands which led him to conclude that PSD would occur in the circumscribed area distal to a stenosis (65–75 per cent) which created whirlpools. He did not say how the whirlpools generated the PSD. Halsted (1918) also reported one remarkable clinical study of a 50-year-old woman who developed a large aneurysm of the right common carotid artery four years after he banded her innominate artery as treatment for a large aneurysm of the right subclavian artery. Here, too, turbulence was produced by the band.

Holman and his colleagues (Holman, 1954a,b; 1955; Holman and Peniston, 1955) studied PSD in rubber tubes, and by banding the thoracic aorta of newborn puppies. They concluded that turbulence produced the PSD by increasing the side pressure on the wall and so causing structural fatigue. In dogs, the PSD took several months to develop, while in rubber tubes it occurred after several days.

Rodbard et al. (1967) did similar experiments on chicks aged 11–15 weeks and sacrificed them after 1–28 days. They concluded that the incidence of PSD increased with time, and was not affected by an atherogenic diet. They suggested that drag forces produced by the flow alterations were important, and might alter the lumen by initiating local relaxation of arterial smooth muscle. They did not assess drag using Fry's method (1969).

Kline et al. (1962) felt the newborn pig was the ideal experimental animal because of its size and rapid growth. They produced stenosis in (i) the pulmonary artery, (ii) the ascending aorta, and (iii) the postductal aorta, and concluded after angiographic studies that turbulence caused the PSD, probably because of shattering of the jet on the vessel wall over a period of 4–5 months.

Aars (1963, 1968) constricted the aorta of rabbits with a tapered nylon ring and concluded angiographically that a PSD could develop in a few days if turbulence was present, and observed that the dilatation could extend into the branches in contrast to other authors who felt it stopped at bifurcations. He found with strip experiments that there appeared to be no alteration in arterial elasticity so could not explain why the dilatation occurred.

We (Roach, 1963a) produced three degrees of stenosis in the femoral and carotid arteries of adult dogs with a nylon taffeta band. Only the moderate stenoses which produced distal turbulence† as indicated by a thrill and bruit

---

† We have defined "turbulence" as a flow distortion sufficient to produce a thrill and bruit (with a wide frequency spectrum), and with apparently random mixing of injected dye. Other authors may use other definitions (see glossary and text) and some feel flow-generated turbulence is different from pipe-generated turbulence. This point is discussed further on page 126.

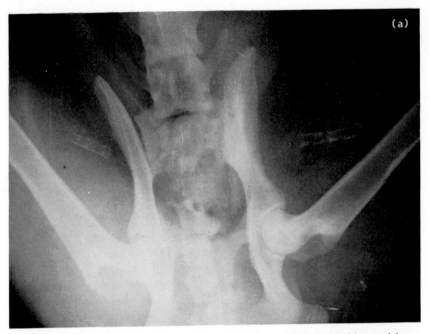

FIG. 1. (a) X-Ray of anaesthetized dog in supine position with hips and knees flexed to show femoral arteries painted with thorium dioxide. The stenosis is obvious on the right of the diagram.

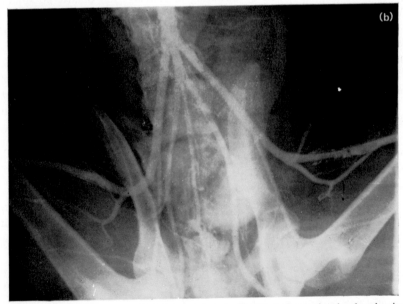

FIG. 1. (b) Arteriogram of the same dog to illustrate how closely the thorium dioxide outlines the artery. A small **PSD** is obvious on the right.

caused a PSD, but all of them did. Minimal stenoses with no distal turbulence and severe stenoses with no turbulence but a marked decrease in distal
pulsation did not cause a PSD, indicating turbulence was the causative agent.
The arteries were painted with a thick paste of thorium dioxide, a radio-
opaque powder taken up by reticulo-endothelial cells in the adventitia, and
so daily roentgenograms (Fig. 1) were able to be made to study the time
course of the development of PSD. Figure 2 shows mean curves for the three
types of stenosis, and indicates that the dilatation developed over the first

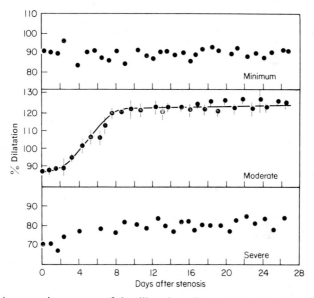

Fig. 2. Average time course of the dilatation after creation of a stenosis on day 0.
The top panel is the mean of seven arteries with minimal stenoses, the middle panel
the mean ± standard error of forty arteries with moderate stenoses, and the bottom
the mean of four arteries with severe stenoses. The variations are due both to
differences in position of the dogs, and different arteries in each group (Roach,
1963a). In this, and all subsequent figures, per cent dilatation was used to express the
ratio of distal to proximal diameter times 100.

ten days after banding, and then remained stable for periods up to ten
months. The long-term time course was predictable, but the immediate
response was variable (Fig. 3) for some undetermined reason which may be
related to muscle activity. It was shown that the thorium did not alter the
elastic properties of the arteries over the ten month period, although it is
known to cause fibrosis after 10–20 years (Amory and Bunch, 1948). We did
find considerable perivascular fibrosis if much powder was spilled around
the artery.

6*

While most authors (above) seem to feel that the flow distortion produced by the stenosis is turbulence, others have questioned this conclusion. Bruns (1959) argued strongly that turbulence is completely random and so cannot create enough energy to produce a murmur. He suggested that vortex formation (a Karman trail) was the most likely cause of murmurs. Unfortunately

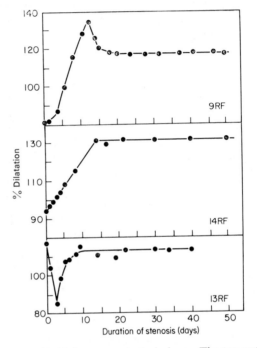

FIG. 3. Three types of initial response to turbulence. The top pattern occurred in six dogs, the middle in thirty-two, and the bottom in three arteries. The reason for the difference is obscure. Adapted from Roach (1963a).

the engineering literature to which he referred is for a weir rather than an orifice. Vortex formation probably does cause the musical murmur of calcific aortic stenosis, but musical murmurs (typical of Karman trails) are rare. However, Bruns et al. (1959), after vibrating rubber tubes, postulated that this was the cause of PSD.

Another group (Robicsek et al., 1958; Rodbard et al., 1967) feel cavitation is the most likely cause of murmurs and hence of PSD. They have demonstrated bubble formation in water flowing in glass tubes, but have not done so with blood. Harvey (1950) states that cavitation is rare in blood, and that several atmospheres of negative pressure are needed to create it. The sound produced is a high-pitched hiss (10 000–20 000 Hz) very unlike most murmurs.

Since the size of an artery is produced by a combination of the intraluminal pressure and the elastic properties of the wall, presumably the pressure must increase, or the vessel wall weaken to create a PSD. While Holman (1954a,b) suggested that turbulence increased the side pressure, all other authors agree

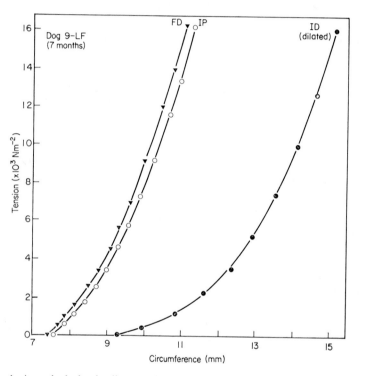

FIG. 4. A typical elastic diagram from an artery with a PSD present for seven months. The proximal (IP) and far distal (FD) segments have similar tension–length curves, but the dilated segment (ID) not only has a bigger initial circumference, it also distends more for each increment of tension.

that the pressure is unchanged or decreased by a stenosis (DeVries and van den Berg, 1958). Thus there must be some alteration in the vessel wall (Halsted, 1916; Holman, 1954a,b). The author (Roach, 1963b) showed that the dilated artery was more distensible than normal by doing pressure-volume curves on the proximal and distal segments using the method of Roach and Burton (1957). Figure 4 shows that the dilated segment of artery has a bigger initial circumference, and that the circumference increases more than that of the proximal segment with each increment of tension (or pressure). Figure 5 shows comparable curves of tension vs strain. It is obvious that the dilated segment is more distensible than those on either side of it. Using the results of previous digestion studies (Roach and Burton, 1957)

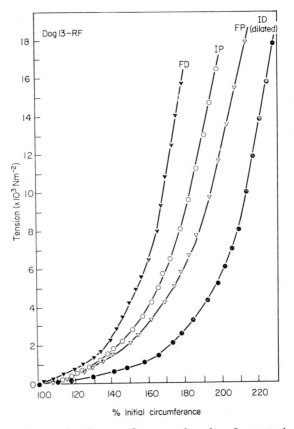

Fig. 5. A tension–strain diagram from another dog. In controls, the arterial segments became progressively less distensible toward the periphery. Here the dilated segment immediately distal to the stenosis (ID) is most distensible while the segment distal (FD) and proximal (IP) to it are less distensible. FP is most proximal of all.

which showed that the initial part of the tension–length curve was due to elastin, and the final part to collagen, it was concluded (Roach, 1963b) that the major change produced by the turbulence was in the elastin and probably in the "links" holding the collagen fibres together. This is shown by the p-values in Table 1.

TABLE 1

	Turbulence—No Turbulence			Distal—Proximal	
	Percentage dilatation	Distal	Proximal	Turbulence	No Turbulence
Initial elastance (elastin)	<0·01	<0·01	<0·1	<0·01 (negative)	<0·01 (positive)
Final elastance (collagen)	<0·9	<0·4	<0·9	<0·7	<0·5
Physiol. elastance (at 100 mmHg)	<0·01	<0·2	<0·4	<0·1	<0·6
Percentage stretch all collagen ("links")	<0·01	<0·2	<0·4	<0·2	<0·4

NOTE: p values are used to compare the effect of turbulence on the elastic properties of the carotid and femoral arteries of dog. The only significant values ($p<0·01$) are in the initial elastance (elastin), physiological elastance and the percentage stretch at all collagen which indicates something about the "links" between collagen fibres. The change is more marked distally. For details, see Roach (1963b).

In the left-hand part of the table the arteries were divided into two groups: with turbulence produced by the stenosis and with no turbulence. The various parameters of elasticity were then compared in the distal and proximal segments and with percentage dilatation. The only significant alteration ($p<0·01$) in the distal and proximal values was for the initial elastance of the distal segments, implying that the turbulence altered this part of the artery. Using percentage dilatation which decreased the deviation due to different diameters, all parameters except the final elastance were altered by the turbulence.

In the right-hand part of the table the distal and proximal segments of each artery were compared after they had been divided into two groups: with turbulence and with no turbulence. Here the only significant difference was in the initial elastance where the distal segment of the arteries with turbulence was more distensible than the proximal segment, while the converse was true without turbulence.

Thus we can conclude that a PSD will develop if the stenosis produces a flow distortion, probably turbulence, and that this alters the vessel wall in some undetermined way so that it becomes more distensible. The elastin and intercollagen "links" seem most prone to be altered.

B. ISOLATED PERFUSED ARTERIES

Roach and Harvey (1964) developed an apparatus to study the rate of dilatation in isolated perfused iliac arteries. Essentially this consisted of a constant pressure reservoir containing saline connected to a double-chambered brass plethysmograph with a plastic top. The two chambers were separated by a small hole into which plastic stenoses of different sizes could be fitted. Volume changes in the plethysmograph were measured with fine capillary tubing, and indicated either leakage of fluid through the artery wall, or a change in size of the artery. Blue dye was used to detect leaks, but some

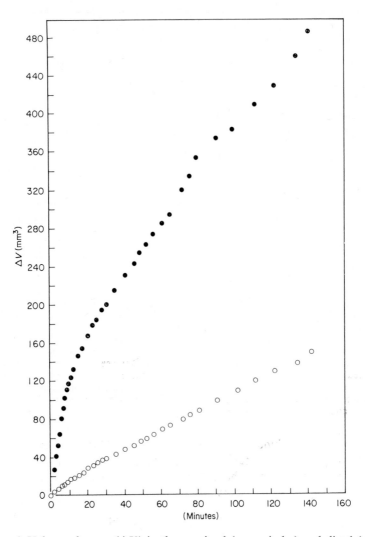

FIG. 6. Volume changes (ΔV) in the proximal (open circles) and distal (closed circles) chambers of the plethysmograph are plotted against time for the iliac artery of a 55-year-old man. Turbulence was present distally, and it is obvious that the volume change is much more marked in the distal chamber. The true dilatation (which compared well with calliper measurements) was found by subtracting one curve from the other. For details see Roach and Harvey (1964).

filtration occurred so that the curves from the two segments had to be sub-tracted to determine the volume change due to dilatation. Figure 6, a typical result, shows that the distal segment dilated rapidly over the first 20–30 minutes and then more slowly. All arteries where the stenosis created distal turbulence (a thrill and bruit) dilated, but none of the others did. The volume change in the plethysmograph was always greater than the amount of dilatation measured with callipers. Since no dye left the lumen, we concluded that this must have been filtration. Figure 7 illustrates that this filtration

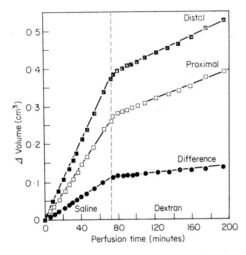

FIG. 7. A similar experiment to that in Fig. 6, but at 70 min the saline perfusate was switched to dextran. The volume changes/unit time in each chamber decreased, suggesting that at least some of the change was due to filtration of fluid through the wall. The viscosity of dextran was high enough that turbulence did not occur, and the dilatation which had been developing stopped.

decreased if dextran rather than saline was used as a perfusate. However, the viscosity of dextran was so high that turbulence could not be produced with it.

After 4–72 h the elastic properties of the proximal and distal segments of all arteries were measured as described above. Figure 8 is typical and illus-trates that if no turbulence was present the elastic properties of the proximal and distal segments were similar, but if turbulence had been present, the distal segment was always more distensible than the proximal one. It is obvious from Fig. 8 that the change is in the initial part of the curve, and the final slope is unaltered. Thus, *in vitro* as *in vivo*, turbulence appears to alter the elastin more than the collagen.

The degree of dilatation was small. Grade 3–4/6 murmurs caused 10–15 per cent dilatation after three days, and Grade 5–6/6 murmurs produced

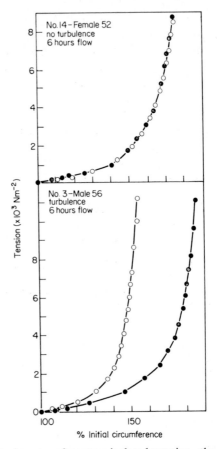

FIG. 8. Tension–strain curves from two isolated arteries—the top with a minimum stenosis and no turbulence, and the bottom with distal turbulence. The open circles in each case are from the proximal segment, and the closed circles from the distal one. The distal segment was always more distensible than the proximal one if turbulence was present.

24–31 per cent dilatation. The murmurs were graded from 0 to 6 on the basis of the standard clinical method, i.e.

Grade 0—no murmur at any time.

Grade 1—a faint murmur, made definite by exercise.

Grade 2—a soft murmur, audible to most observers.

Grade 3—audible to all.

Grade 4—questionable thrill with a loud murmur.

Grade 5—definite thrill and loud murmur.

Grade 6—audible without a stethoscope.

Our plethysmographic method could detect very small volume changes (0·005 cm³) which may explain why dilatation was more readily detected than by Foreman and Hutchison (1970) who tried to measure the changes with a travelling microscope. Since the dilatation was not always uniform, and the curvature caused problems with parallax we felt the travelling microscope was less accurate than the plethysmograph. In addition, Foreman and Hutchison do not comment on the intensity of the murmur generated by their stenoses, so the experiments may not be comparable.

C. VIBRATION OF ISOLATED ARTERIES

Since there appeared to be some relation between vibration of the arterial wall produced by turbulence and the development of a PSD, it was decided to study the effect of vibrations alone on the arterial wall. Initially the author did a few very crude experiments (Roach, 1963b) where an isolated iliac artery was placed over the vibrating rod of a cocktail shaker for several hours. In all cases, the vibrated artery was more distensible than comparable controls.

Roach and Melech (1971) then attempted to determine if the frequency of the vibration altered the response of the arterial wall. Isolated, non-distended, human iliac arteries were vibrated by connecting a modified phonocatheter

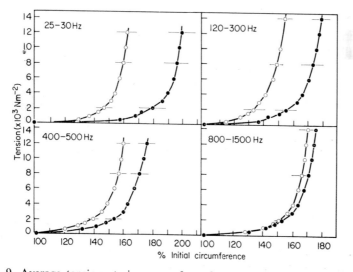

FIG. 9. Average tension–strain curves from four sets of arteries vibrated with sound played through a phonocatheter inside the artery. In all cases the open circles are before vibration and the closed circles after. The lines show one standard error of the mean. The low frequencies are most effective for altering the distensibility, and frequencies >800 Hz have no effect.

M. R. ROACH

to a sound generator. The low frequencies were more effective than the high ones in altering the elastic properties of the artery. As Fig. 9 shows, while there was considerable scatter, frequencies of 25–30 Hz caused the greatest alterations, and frequencies of 800–1500 Hz virtually no change. In general, any frequency under 400 Hz seemed to cause some increase in distensibility compared to the control.

Boughner and Roach (1970) vibrated isolated human iliac arteries held at approximately *in vivo* length in a plethysmograph, and distended with 100 mmHg pressure (Fig. 10). The artery was connected to a sound generator

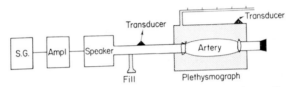

Fig. 10. Apparatus used by Boughner and Roach (1970) to vibrate distended isolated human iliac arteries. A Heathkit 1G-18 sound generator (SG) was connected to an amplifier (AMPL) and used to drive a Fanon HOA-5A-8, 15W, 8 Ω loud-speaker. This transmitted vibrations to the artery which could be monitored with the transducers as illustrated. Volume changes in the artery were measured with the plethysmograph.

by means of a loud-speaker, and volume changes produced in the artery measured at intervals of several hours. Transducers in the inlet tube and in the wall of the plethysmograph indicated that all frequencies were transmitted equally well through the arterial wall with no evidence of resonant peaks. Table 2 summarizes the results—young arteries dilated with low frequencies, and older arteries with higher frequencies; the effective range was quite narrow, and was significantly different for the young and old arteries

TABLE 2

Dilatation of vibrated arteries

| Frequency of vibration | Number dilated/total number vibrated | | |
	16–44 years	45–59 years	60–77 years
30–100 Hz	5 / 6	2 / 7	1 / 6
100–200 Hz	1 / 3	4 / 5	0 / 5
200–300 Hz	0 / 4	1 / 7	7 / 8

NOTE: The effect of the frequency of vibration on the presence or absence of dilatation in distended isolated human iliac arteries exposed to sonic vibrations as shown in Fig. 10. Young arteries (16–44 years) dilated with low frequencies (30–100 Hz) and old arteries (60–77 years) with higher frequencies.

$(p<0\cdot01)$. Since arteries get progressively stiffer with age (Roach and Burton, 1959), this difference in response is not surprising. In all cases where effective frequencies were used, the arteries dilated at the rate of $1\cdot2-2\cdot7$ per cent per day (Fig. 11), and the changes in the elastic diagram (Fig. 12) were comparable to those described above with turbulence.

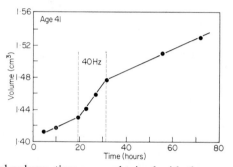

Fig. 11. A typical volume–time curve obtained with the apparatus described in Fig. 10. The pressure caused creep which had to be subtracted to assess the degree of dilatation. However, with the appropriate frequencies the artery dilated more rapidly—seen with 40 Hz.

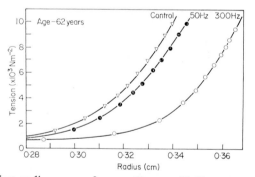

Fig. 12. Tension–radius curve from a 62-year-old iliac artery. No dilatation occurred with 50 Hz and the curve is not significantly altered. Dilatation did occur with 300 Hz and was associated with a marked increase in distensibility, mainly due to alterations in the initial part of the curve.

These results would suggest that the major frequency components of a murmur probably determine whether or not a PSD will develop. Boughner and Roach (1970) found this was true in eight patients with aortic valve stenosis. In all cases the presence or absence of a PSD was correlated with the presence or absence of the frequencies found to dilate iliac arteries of that age. We have no evidence that these frequency responses are similar for all types of arteries.

4. HISTOLOGICAL STUDIES OF POSTSTENOTIC DILATATION

Pathologically a dilatation shows no gross histological change, while an aneurysm contains obviously fragmented elastin. There is no general agreement on what changes are associated with a PSD.

A number of authors have studied aortas proximal and distal to coarctations. All agree that the most marked changes are in the region of the coarctation. Reifenstein *et al.* (1947) and Clagett *et al.* (1954) found few medial changes distally in over 100 cases reviewed unless an aneurysm was present. Martin *et al.* (1956) agreed but felt a jet lesion could develop with fibrous thickening and elastin fragmentation, and Frederiksen and Poulsen (1961) suggested the jet might even cause an aortitis. Heath and Edwards (1959) felt there was more elastin proximal to a coarctation than distal to it. Dunnill (1959) agreed, but suggested mucopolysaccharide accumulated proximally as well, and was often a precursor of atherosclerosis which was always present proximally if the diastolic pressure exceeded 100 mmHg.

Robicsek (1955) found elastin fragmentation in the dilated pulmonary artery beyond a pulmonary valve stenosis, and van Buchem (1956) showed similar changes with idiopathic dilatation. The changes with a pulmonary artery coarctation have not been studied.

Experimentally, Reid (1916) found atrophy of both muscle and elastin distal to metal bands placed on the aorta of dogs. Jensen and Svane (1967) concluded that the major change was a proximal medial thickening due to accumulation of acid mucopolysaccharides. No assessment has been made of how the degree of stenosis affects the histological changes, or if there are changes at the electron microscopic level. Haust *et al.* (1972) are now attempting to obtain this information.

5. EFFECT OF STENOSIS GEOMETRY ON THE DEVELOPMENT AND SIZE OF A POSTSTENOTIC DILATATION

Since the clinical literature suggests that short stenoses are more apt to create a PSD than long ones, we would predict that the geometry of the stenosis determines, at least in part, whether a PSD will develop, and perhaps determine its size. While the engineering literature contains many references to weirs and orifices (Dryden *et al.*, 1956), it contains little on stenoses of finite length, and virtually nothing on pulsatile flow.

Reynolds (1883) was the first to describe a method for quantitatively predicting when flow would change from laminar to turbulent in a long straight tube. He showed that four parameters were important—the diameter of the tube (d), and the velocity (v), density (ρ) and viscosity (η) of the fluid. He determined experimentally that if $\rho . v . d / \eta$ exceeded 2000, turbulence would develop. This number is now known as the Reynolds' number, and the value of it where turbulence develops is called the critical Reynolds' number, or Re_c. Coulter and Pappenheimer (1949) repeated the same experiments with blood, and found a similar value for Re_c. Unfortunately they used radius rather than diameter and found an Re_c of just under 1000. Since Reynolds used diameter in the original description we will adhere to this. While Reynolds stressed the importance of a "long, straight tube far from the inlet", the value of 2000 has been widely, and unjustly, applied to the circulation and there are many statements in the biological literature that turbulence cannot occur in the cardiovascular system because the Re is <2000. Stehbens (1959) was one of the first to point out that this thinking was erroneous for bifurcations, and Ferguson and Roach (see chapter 14) have since shown that the angle of the bifurcation determines the Re_c. Stenoses are even more likely to lower the Re_c than bifurcations.

Harvey and the author (unpublished) did a few experiments to determine the relative importance of the diameter and length of a plastic stenosis on the Re_c in Tygon tubes. A constant pressure reservoir fed from the taps was used, and the flow controlled by creating a peripheral resistance with a variable array of capillary tubes arranged in parallel. The flow rate was varied by 5 ml/min steps from 5 to 2500 ml/min and measured to within ± 0.5 ml s^{-1} by arranging a series of electrodes vertically up a calibrated cylinder so that changes in fluid level triggered the timer on and off. Evans blue dye was injected proximal to the stenosis and the onset of turbulence noted visually. Table 3 illustrates that a two-fold change in diameter had a

TABLE 3

Critical Reynolds numbers for stenoses in 9·52 mm tube

Stenosis Width × length	Re_c Proximal	Re_c Distal	Re_c in stenosis (when distal turbulence)
2·38 × 2·5 mm	1799	88	354
4·76 × 2·5 mm	1827	376	752
4·76 × 20 mm	1821	423	846

NOTE: The critical Reynolds Number, Re_c, is shown for three plastic stenoses in Tygon tubes. Tight stenoses, especially if short, produce the most flow distortion and the lowest Re_c.

far greater effect on lowering the Re_c than an eight-fold change in length. Moreover, it is apparent that this Re is readily generated in the circulation so it is not surprising that stenoses do create turbulence.

Unfortunately there is still no way to quantitate turbulence (Corrsin, 1961; McDonald, 1960, pp. 69–77; Powell, 1958), so we cannot assess how much turbulence different types of stenosis produce. However, it is unlikely that the stenosis will create turbulence for more than a short distance, i.e. not beyond the "inlet".† McDonald (1960, pp. 47–48) states that the inlet length, $x = 0.057.r.Re$ for laminar flow, and is $1.386 \times r \times (Re)^{\frac{1}{4}}$ for turbulent flow where r = radius. He predicts that the former would include the whole length of the aorta, and the latter the proximal half of the aorta. The effect of pulsatile flow on these values has not been determined.

Heart valves are common sites for stenosis (congenital or rheumatic). Goldstein (1938) states that for a projection of height ε in a tube of radius r, the flow will remain laminar if $\varepsilon/r < 4/(Re)^{\frac{1}{2}}$. Gorlin and his colleagues (Gorlin and Gorlin, 1951; Gorlin et al., 1951; Gorlin et al., 1955) have

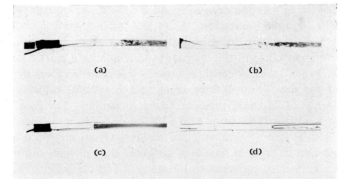

FIG. 13. Examples of flow distortion produced by plastic stenoses in Tygon tubes. The upper right-hand panel (b) shows a long stenosis, and the others short stenoses. Flow is from left to right. The jet is obvious in the top two (a), (b) with turbulence downstream but not in the stenosis. In the lower left-hand panel (c) the turbulence has extended back to the stenosis. In the lower right-hand panel (d) dye is injected distally with a fine bent tube. The flow has become laminar (same flow as (c)) indicating that turbulence is limited to the "inlet", rather than being propagated downstream.

provided formulas for calculating valve areas based on measurements of cardiac output and pressure gradient, but do not say how these are related to turbulence.

A number of authors have studied the effects of experimental stenoses in peripheral arteries. All of these (Mann et al., 1938; May et al., 1963; May et al., 1963; Vonruden et al., 1964; Killen and Oh, 1968; Kindt and Youmans, 1969) found that the diameter of the stenosis was far more important than the length in producing alterations in pressure gradient and flow, and that

† Throughout this chapter "inlet length" refers to the zone beyond the stenosis where the flow profile is distorted. The end of this zone is defined as the downstream point where the parabolic flow profile reappears. (See Goldstein, 1938, p. 139).

stenoses had to reach 60–70 per cent before they produced any significant effect. Gupta and Wiggers (1951) and Spencer, *et al.* (1958) found a systolic murmur appeared with a stenosis of 50–60 per cent and then became longer and extended through diastole for an 80 per cent stenosis, but disappeared with very severe stenoses. These authors did not state how far distal to the stenosis the murmur was propagated.

Since there was so little information on the inlet length with different types of stenoses, Stockley and Roach modified the method used by Roach and Harvey (1964) to determine the inlet length. All experiments were done with $Re \approx 700$. Dye was injected proximal to the stenosis to determine the distance downstream that the jet broke up to flow both proximally and

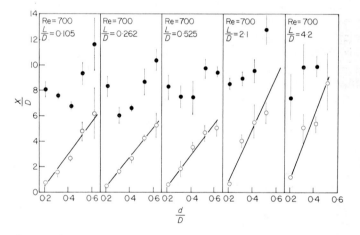

FIG. 14. Data from model experiments. D = tube diameter, d = stenosis diameter, L = stenosis length, and X = distance from stenosis. All parameters are expressed as tube diameters. The open circles show the length of the jet ($\pm$ S.E.M.) and the closed circles show where the flow becomes laminar again ($\pm$ S.E.M.).

distally (Fig. 13), and was injected from the distal end with a fine curved tube to determine where the stream again became laminar (Fig. 13). These two distances are plotted for different diameters and lengths of stenosis in Fig. 14. The jet moved closer to the stenosis as the diameter decreased, and was slightly altered by the length of the stenosis. The inlet length was more variable, but was probably roughly inversely proportional to the diameter of the stenosis. Comparable experiments are now under way for pulsatile flow. While Harvey and Roach also did some preliminary sound measurements with a phonocatheter, these did not produce any significant results. They are still not able to predict exactly how the geometry of the stenosis determines flow in the inlet.

6. FACTORS WHICH AFFECT THE SIZE OF THE POSTSTENOTIC DILATATION

The size of any artery, or part of an artery, is determined by the intraluminal pressure and the elastic properties of the wall. Since most stenoses
which create significant murmurs are severe enough to cause a pressure
gradient, it is not surprising that no correlation has been found between the
degree of stenosis and the size of the PSD either with aortic (Jarchow and
Kincaid, 1961; Castellanos and Hernandez, 1967) or pulmonary (van Buchem,
1956; Rudhe *et al.*, 1962; D'Cruz *et al.*, 1964) valve stenoses. Roach (1963b)
found that the degree of dilatation was not related either to the degree of
stenosis or to the change in elastance in the femoral and carotid arteries of dogs.

With the hope that the factors which determined the inlet length might be
less complicated than those which determined the magnitude of turbulence
and the pressure drop, Roach and MacDonald (1970) measured the length
and diameter of the PSD in arteriograms from patients with renal artery
stenosis. While there was no correlation between the diameter of the PSD and
the stenosis size, there was a highly significant inverse correlation of the
length of the PSD with the diameter of the stenoses (Fig. 15). Thus a long
PSD implies a tight stenosis and a short PSD implies a less severe stenosis.

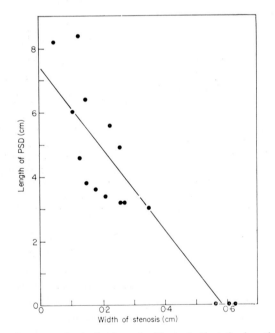

FIG. 15. Data from renal arteriograms to illustrate that the length of the PSD is
inversely related to the width of the stenosis. The correlation coefficient is −0·88.
The three points with no PSD show the normal diameter of the renal artery.

Since it is so difficult to quantitate turbulence, it is difficult to predict how the frequency spectrum of the murmur, the age of the patient, and the pressure drop produced all work together to determine the diameter of the artery in the region of the PSD. The active tension in the wall produced by the muscle (Burton, 1954) may also play a role as Rodbard *et al.* (1967) suggest. Whether resonance is a factor as Foreman and Hutchison (1970) imply

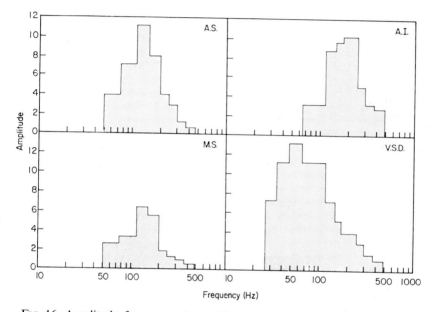

FIG. 16. Amplitude–frequency plots of four types of murmurs—aortic stenosis (AS), aortic insufficiency (AI), mitral stenosis (MS), and a ventricular septal defect (VSD). Each murmur is from a single patient with a pure lesion of the type specified. All recordings were made externally with a microphone with a flat frequency response. The amplitudes are consistent in any one panel, but not between panels. All murmurs have a wide frequency spectrum and appear very similar. The intensity scale is arbitrary and linear.

remains to be determined. Boughner has analysed the frequency spectrum of a variety of murmurs recorded from the anterior chest wall. The frequency spectrum is remarkably similar for all types of murmurs studied (Fig. 16) and no sharp resonant peaks were seen. The absolute amplitude has not been determined as yet. However, we have compared the frequency spectra of the same murmur recorded with an intracardiac phono-catheter and the above chest wall recording. Figure 17 indicates that the high frequencies appear to be damped out more than the low ones in passing through the various tissues between the arterial lumen and the chest wall.

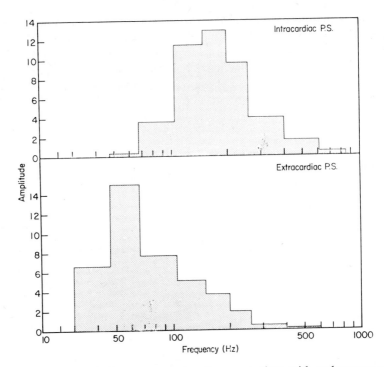

Fig. 17. Amplitude-frequency spectra from a patient with pulmonary valve stenosis recorded with an intracardiac phonocatheter in the pulmonary trunk (top panel) and with a chest microphone (bottom panel). The high frequencies are attenuated most. Amplitudes are arbitrary.

Workers are now trying to determine quantitatively if this attenuation occurs in the lung or elsewhere. Animal experiments will be required to answer this, and to say if the energy lost in the arterial wall is sufficient to cause the changes in distensibility that are observed.

7. REVERSIBILITY OF THE DILATATION

With modern advances in cardiac surgery, it is important to know if the dilatation will increase (due to a pressure increase) or decrease (due to decrease in turbulence) when the stenosis is corrected. There are at least three reports (Imler *et al.*, 1951; Steinberg, 1957; and MacFee, 1940) of a subclavian artery aneurysm disappearing after removal of a cervical rib. Roach (1963a) reported previously that a femoral artery dilatation in a dog femoral disappeared when the dog became pregnant, presumably because the femoral flow decreased as the uterine flow increased (Fig. 18). However, this dilatation had been present for only a few days so the situation was not analogous to the chronic one seen clinically. Since the degree of dilatation did not alter in the stenosed carotid arteries of the same dog, we presume that alterations in cardiac output, hormone levels, etc. are not involved.

Roach (1971) studied the effect of band removal on the PSD created in the femoral arteries of dogs. In all cases the PSD disappeared within 24 hours of when the murmur disappeared even if the PSD had been present for six months. In six dogs, the bands were removed on the X-ray table and films taken at $\frac{1}{2}$–1 h intervals. In all cases where the murmur disappeared the PSD

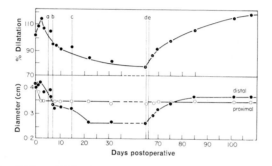

Fig. 18. Reversibility of PSD in the femoral artery of a pregnant dog, with recurrence of the PSD after delivery. The top panel shows the dilatation against time; the bottom the proximal (open circles) and distal (closed circles) diameters after a stenosis with a loud murmur was produced on day 0. At "a" the murmur was faint and the PSD decreasing, at "b" the murmur was gone. At "c" it was apparent the dog was pregnant and we suspected that the increased uterine flow had decreased the femoral flow. At "d" seven pups were delivered, and by the next day "e" the murmur had returned and the PSD developed as before. Adapted from Roach (1963a).

was completely gone in 6–8 hours (Fig. 19), and the altered elastic properties previously seen in the dilated segment had disappeared. The mechanism for this rapid reversion is obscure. It is much too fast to be produced by laying down new connective tissue since both elastin (Slack, 1954) and collagen (Kao et al., 1961) have very long turnover times. It is too slow to be due to changes in muscle tone, but probably could be due to alterations in cross-linking. Collagen cross-linking can be altered by ultrasonic vibrations (Harding, 1965), but comparable studies on elastin are not available (Banga, 1966).

Clinical studies on the reversibility of PSD are in progress, but are harder to assess as the dilated segment is often incised or extensively manipulated during the surgery.

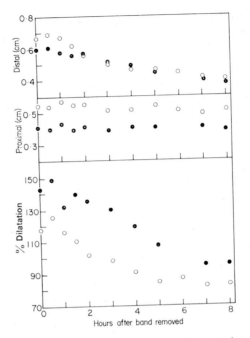

FIG. 19. Curves from two arteries with large dilatations to show how rapidly the dilatation disappeared after the band was removed. The solid dots are from an artery with a PSD present for seven months, the open dots from one present for three weeks. Both disappeared within 6–8 hours.

8. SUMMARY

Poststenotic dilatation of arteries *in vivo* and *in vitro* appears to be produced by physical forces created by alterations in flow produced by the stenosis. Turbulence (indicated by a murmur) is the *sine qua non* for its development, and appears to cause vibration of the arterial wall as well as of the blood. This vibration usually has a wide frequency spectrum (30–500 Hz), but only certain frequencies are able to make the artery more distensible. While there is suggestive evidence that resonance may be involved, the evidence is not conclusive. Elastin is more susceptible to these vibrations than collagen, and is the wall component which appears to be altered both dynamically and histologically.

The factors which affect the size of the PSD are complex, but our work suggests that the length rather than the diameter of the PSD may be the most sensitive indicator of stenosis geometry.

The dilatation is rapidly reversible, at least in dogs, if correction of the stenosis removes the turbulence. The mechanism has not been determined.

REFERENCES

Aars, H. (1963). Experimental post-stenotic dilatation of the ascending aorta in rabbits. *Acta Physiol. Scand.* **59**, supp. 213, 5.

Aars, H. (1968). Aortic baroreceptor activity during permanent distension of the receptor area. *Acta Physiol. Scand.* **74**, 183–194.

Amory, H. I. and Bunch, R. F. (1948). Perivascular injection of thorotrast and its sequelae. *Radiology* **51**, 831–839.

Arvidsson, H., Karnell, J. and Möller, T. (1955). Multiple stenosis of the pulmonary arteries associated with pulmonary hypertension, diagnosed by selective angiocardiography. *Acta Radiol.* **44**, 209–216.

Banga, I. (1966). "Structure and Function of Elastin and Collagen", pp. 3–18, Akadémiai Kiadó, Budapest.

Boughner, D. R. and Roach, M. R. (1970). The effect of low frequency vibration on arterial wall elastin. AGARD Conf. Proc. No. 65 of Specialist's Meeting on "Fluid Dynamics of Blood Circulation and Respiratory Flow". Naples. May, 1970. pp. 9.1–9.8.

Boughner, D. R. "Frequency Analysis of Aortic Murmurs" (in preparation).

Brock, R. C. (1952). Congenital pulmonary stenosis. *Amer. J. Med.* **12**, 706–719.

Bruns, D. L. (1959). A general theory of the causes of murmers in the cardiovascular system. *Amer. J. Med.* **27**, 360–374.

Bruns, D. L., Connolly, J. E., Holman, E. and Stofer, R. C. (1959). Experimental observations on post-stenotic dilatation. *J. Thorac. Cardiovasc. Surg.* **38**, 662–669.

van Buchem, F. S. P. (1956). Dilatation of the pulmonary artery in pulmonary stenosis. *Circulation* **13**, 719–724.

Buck, R. C. (1961). Intimal thickening after ligature of arteries. *Circulation Res.* **9**, 418–426.

Burton, A. C. (1954). Relation of structure to function of the tissues of the wall of blood vessels. *Physiol. Rev.* **34**, 619–642.

Castellanos, A. and Hernandez, F. A. (1967). Size of ascending aorta in congenital cardiac lesions and other heart diseases. *Acta Radiol. Diag.* **6**, 49–64.

Clagett, O. T., Kirklin, J. W. and Edwards, J. E. (1954). Anatomic variations and pathologic changes in coarctation of the aorta. *Surg. Gynec. Obstet.* **98**, 103–114.

Corrsin, S. (1961). Turbulent flow. *Amer. Sci.* **49**, 300–325.

Coulter, N. A., Jr. and Pappenheimer, J. R. (1949). Development of turbulence in flowing blood. *Amer. J. Physiol.* **159**, 401–408.

D'Cruz, I. A., Arcilla, R. A. and Agustsson, M. H. (1964). Dilatation of the pulmonary trunk in stenosis of the pulmonary valve and of the pulmonary arteries in children. *Amer. Heart J.* **68**, 612–620.

DeBakey, M. E., Crawford, S., Morris, G. C., Jr. and Cooley, D. A. (1961). Surgical considerations of occlusive disease of the innominate, carotid, subclavian, and vertebral arteries. *Ann. Surg.* **154**, 698–725.

DeVries, Hk. and van den Berg, Jw. (1958). On the origin of poststenotic dilatations. *Cardiologia* **33**, 195–211.

Dryden, H. L., Murnaghan, F. D. and Bateman, H. (1956). "Hydrodynamics", pp. 451–467, Dover Publications, New York.

Dunnill, M. S. (1959). Histology of the aorta in coarctation. *J. Path. Bact.* **78**, 203–207.

Eden, K. C. (1939). The vascular complications of cervical ribs and first thoracic rib abnormalities. *Brit. J. Surg.* **27**, 111–139.

Foreman, J. E. K. and Hutchison, K. J. (1970). Arterial wall vibration distal to stenoses in isolated arteries of dog and man. *Circulation Res.* **26**, 583–590.

Frederiksen, T. and Poulsen, T. (1961). Poststenotic aneurysms complicating coarctation of the aorta. *Acta Chir. Scand.* **121**, 13–18.

Fry, D. L. (1969). Certain histological and chemical responses of the vascular interface to acutely induced mechanical stress in the aorta of the dog. *Circulation Res.* **24**, 93–108.

Gedge, S. W., Spittel, J. A., Jr. and Ivins, J. C. (1961). Aneurysm of the distal popliteal artery and its relationship to the arcuate popliteal ligament. *Circulation* **24**, 270–273.

Goldstein, S. (1938). "Modern Developments in Fluid Dynamics", Vol I, p. 311, Clarendon Press, Oxford.

Gorlin, R. and Gorlin, S. G. (1951). Hydraulic formula for calculation of the area of the stenotic mitral valve, other cardiac valves, and central circulatory shunts. I. *Amer. Heart J.* **41**, 1–29.

Gorlin, R., Haynes, F. W., Goodale, W. T., Sawyer, C. G., Dow, J. W. and Dexter, L. (1951). Studies of the circulatory dynamics in mitral stenosis. II. *Amer. Heart J.* **41**, 30–45.

Gorlin, R., McMillan, I. K. R., Medd, W. E., Matthews, M. B. and Daley, R. (1955). Dynamics of the circulation in aortic valvular disease. *Amer. J. Med.* **18**, 855–870.

Gupta, T. C. and Wiggers, C. J. (1951). Basic hemodynamic changes produced by aortic coarctation of different degrees. *Circulation* **3**, 17–31.

Halsted, W. S. (1909). Partial, progressive and complete occlusion of the aorta and other large arteries in the dog by means of the metal band. *J. Exp. Med.* **11**, 373–391.

Halsted, W. S. (1916). An experimental study of circumscribed dilation of an artery immediately distal to a partially occluding band, and its bearing on the dilation of the subclavian artery observed in certain cases of cervical rib. *J. Exp. Med.* **24**, 271–286.

Halsted, W. S. (1918). Cylindrical dilatation of the common carotid artery following partial occlusion of the innominate and ligation of the subclavian. *Surg. Gynec. Obstet.* **27**, 547–554.

Harding, J. J. (1965). The unusual links and cross-links of collagen. *Adv. Prot. Chem.* **20**, 109–190.

Harvey, E. N. (1950). Bubble formation in liquids. *In* "Medical Physics" (O. Glasser, ed.), Vol. II, pp. 137–150, Year Book Publications, Chicago.

Haust, M. D., Trillo, A. and Roach, M. R. (1972.) Histological studies on poststenotic dilatation (unpublished).

Heath, D. and Edwards, J. E. (1959). Configuration of elastic tissue of aortic media in aortic coarctation. *Amer. Heart J.* **57**, 29–35.

Holman, E. (1954a). The obscure physiology of poststenotic dilatation: its relation to the development of aneurysms. *J. Thorac. Cardiovasc. Surg.* **28**, 109–133.

Holman, E. (1954b). On the circumscribed dilatation of an artery immediately distal to a partially occluding band. Poststenotic dilatation. *Surgery* **36**, 3–24.

Holman, E. (1955). The development of arterial aneurysms. *Surg. Gynec. Obstet.* **100**, 599–611.

Holman, E. and Peniston, W. (1955). Hydrodynamic factors in the production of aneurysms. *Amer. J. Surg.* **90**, 200–209.

Imler, R. L., Jr., Hayne, R. A. and Stowell, A. (1951). Aneurysm of the subclavian artery associated with cervical rib. *Amer. Surg.* **17**, 478–485.

Jarchow, B. H. and Kincaid, O. W. (1961). Poststenotic dilatation of the ascending aorta: its occurrence and significance as a roentgenologic sign of aortic stenosis. *Proc. Mayo. Clin.* **36**, 23–33.

Jensen, O. M. and Svane, H. (1967). Aortic changes in experimental coarctation in dogs. *Acta Pathol. Microbiol. Scand.* **70**, 512–520.

Kao, K. T., Hilker, D. M. and McGavack, T. H. (1961). Comparison of synthesis and turnover of collagen and elastin in tissues of rat at several ages. *Proc. Soc. Exp. Biol. Med.* **106**, 335–338.

Keith, J. D., Rowe, R. D. and Vlad, P. (1958). "Heart Disease in Infancy and Childhood". Macmillan, New York.

Kieffer, S. A., Linde, L. M., Kegel, S. M. and Latta, N. J. (1961). Mycotic aneurysm distal to coarctation of the aorta. *J. Thorac. Cardiov. Surg.* **42**, 507–513.

Killen, D. A. and Oh, S. U. (1968). Quantitation of the severity of arterial stenosis by pressure gradient measurement. *Amer. Surg.* **34**, 341–349.

Kiloh, G. A. (1950). Pure aortic stenosis. *Brit. Heart J.* **12**, 33–44.

Kincaid, O. W. (1960). Approach to the roentgenologic diagnosis of congenital heart disease. *J. Amer. Med. Ass.* **173**, 637–647.

Kincaid, O. W. and Davis, G. D. (1961). Renal arteriography in hypertension. *Proc. Mayo Clin.* **36**, 689–701.

Kindt, G. W. and Youmans, J. R. (1969). The effect of stricture length on critical arterial stenosis. *Surg. Gynec. Obstet.* **128**, 729–734.

Kjellberg, S. R., Mannheimer, E., Rudhe, U. and Johnson, B. (1955). "Diagnosis of Congenital Heart Disease". Year Book Publications, Chicago.

Kline, J. L., Giminez, J. L. and Maloney, R. J. (1962). Post-stenotic vascular dilatation: confirmation of an old hypothesis by a new method. *J. Thorac. Cardiov. Surg.* **44**, 738–748.

MacFee, W. F. (1940). Cervical rib causing partial occlusion and aneurysm of the subclavian artery. *Ann. Surg.* **111**, 549–553.

Mann, F. C., Herrick, J. T., Essex, H. E. and Baldes, E. J. (1938). The effect on the blood flow of decreasing the lumen of a blood vessel. *Surgery* **4**, 249–252.

Martin, W. J., Kirklin, J. W. and DuShane, J. W. (1956). Aortic aneurysm and aneurysmal endarteritis after resection for coarctation. *J. Amer. Med. Ass.* **160**, 871–874.

May, A. G., van de Berg, L., de Weese, J. A. and Rob. C. G. (1963). Critical arterial stenosis. *Surgery* **54**, 250–259.

May, A. G., de Weese, J. A. and Rob, C. G. (1963). Hemodynamic effects of arterial stenosis. *Surgery* **53**, 513–524.

McDonald, D. A. (1960). "Blood Flow in Arteries". Arnold, London.

Morrow, A. G., Waldhausen, J. A., Peters, R. L., Bloodwell, R. D. and Braunwald, E. (1959). Supravalvular aortic stenosis: clinical, hemodynamic, and pathologic observations. *Circulation* **20**, 1003–1010.

Porta, L. (1845).—Cited by Halsted, W. S. (1918).

Powell, A. (1958). Theory and experiment in aerodynamic noise, with a critique of research on jet flows in their relationship to sound. *In* "Second Symposium on Naval Hydrodynamics: Hydrodynamic Noise and Cavity Flow" (R. A. Cooper, ed.), pp. 1–27, U.S. Government Printing Office, Washington.

Reid, M. R. (1916). Partial occlusion of the aorta with the metallic band. Observations on blood pressures and changes in the arterial walls. *J. Exp. Med.* **24**, 287–290.

Reid, M. R. (1924). Partial occlusion of the aorta with silk sutures, and complete occlusion with fascial plugs. The effect of ligatures on the arterial wall. *J. Exp. Med.* **40**, 293–300.

Reifenstein, G. H., Levine, S. A. and Gross, R. E. (1947). Coarctation of the aorta. *Amer. Heart J.* **33**, 146–168.

Reynolds, O. (1883). An experimental investigation of the circumstances which determine whether the motion of water shall be direct or sinuous, and of the law of resistance in parallel channels. *Phil. Trans. Roy. Soc. London* **174**, 935–982.

Roach, M. R. (1963a). An experimental study of the production and time course of poststenotic dilatation in the femoral and carotid arteries of adult dogs. *Circulation Res* **13**, 537–551.

Roach, M. R. (1963b). Changes in arterial distensibility as a cause of poststenotic dilatation. *Amer. J. Cardiol.* **12**, 802–815.

Roach, M. R. (1971). The reversibility of poststenotic dilatation in the femoral arteries of dogs. *Circulation Res.* **27**, 985–993.

Roach, M. R. and Burton, A. C. (1957). The reason for the shape of the distensibility curves of arteries. *Can. J. Biochem. Physiol.* **35**, 681–690.

Roach, M. R. and Burton, A. C. (1959). The effect of age on the elasticity of human iliac arteries. *Can. J. Biochem. Physiol.* **37**, 557–570.

Roach, M. R. and Harvey, K. (1964). Experimental investigation of poststenotic dilatation in isolated arteries. *Can. J. Physiol. Pharm.* **42**, 53–63.

Roach, M. R. and MacDonald, A. C. (1970). Poststenotic dilatation in renal arteries. *Invest. Radiol.* **5**, 311–315.

Roach, M. R. and Melech, E. (1971). Effect of sonic vibration on isolated human iliac arteries. *Can. J. Physiol. Pharm.* **49**, 288–291.

Robicsek, F. (1955). Post-stenotic dilatation of the great vessels. *Acta Med. Scand.* **151**, 481–485.

Robicsek, F., Sanger, P. W., Taylor, F. H., Magistro, R. and Foti, E. (1958). Pathogenesis and significance of post-stenotic dilatation in great vessels. *Ann. Surg.* **147**, 835–844.

Rochoff, S. D. and Austen, W. G. (1963). The hemodynamic significance of the radiologic changes in acquired aortic stenosis. *Amer. Heart J.* **65**, 458–463.

Rodbard, S., Ikeda, K. and Montes, M. (1967). An analysis of mechanisms of post-stenotic dilatation. *Angiology* **18**, 349–369.

Rudhe, U., Whitley, J. E. and Herzenberg, H. (1962). Mild pulmonary valvular stenosis studied functionally and anatomically. *Acta Radiol.* **57**, 161–171.

Skandalakis, J. E., Edwards, B. F., Gray, S. W., Davis, B. M. and Hopkins, W. A. (1960). Coarctation of the aorta with aneurysm. *Int. Abstr. Surg.* **111**, 307–326.

Slack, H. G. B. (1954). Metabolism of elastin in the adult rat. *Nature (London)* **174**, 512–513.

Spencer, M. P., Johnston, F. R. and Meredith, J. H. (1958). The origin and interpretation of murmurs in coarctation of the aorta. *Amer. Heart J.* **56**, 722–736.

Stehbens, W. E. (1959). Turbulence of blood flow. *Quart. J. Exp. Physiol.* **44**, 110–117.

Steinberg, I. (1957). Poststenotic dilatation (aneurysm) of the subclavian artery associated with cervical rib. *New Engl. J. Med.* **256**, 242–244.

Stockley, D. F. and Roach, M. R. The effect of stenosis geometry on the distal turbulent zone. (in preparation).

Vonruden, W. J., Blaisdell, F. W., Hall, A. D. and Thomas, A. N. (1964). Multiple arterial stenoses: effect on blood flow. *Arch. Surg.* **89**, 307–315.

Weintraub, A. M., Perloff, J. K., Conrad, P. W. and Hufnagel, C. A. (1964). Poststenotic dilatation of the aorta with muscular subaortic stenosis. *Amer. Heart J.* **68**, 741–747.

Wood, P. (1956). "Diseases of the Heart and Circulation", 2nd Ed., Eyre and Spottiswoode, London.

Zaroff, L. I., Kreel, I., Sobel, H. J. and Baronofsky, I. D. (1959). Multiple and infraductal coarctations of the aorta. *Circulation* **20**, 910–917.

Chapter 14

Flow Conditions at Bifurcations as Determined in Glass Models, with Reference to the Focal Distribution of Vascular Lesions†

GARY G. FERGUSON‡ and MARGOT R. ROACH§

Department of Biophysics, Faculty of Medicine,
University of Western Ontario, London, Ontario, Canada

1. INTRODUCTION

There is increasing interest in the idea that vascular bifurcations produce local disturbances of blood flow. Abnormal haemodynamic forces related to these disturbances may play an important role in the pathogenesis of focal vascular lesions such as atherosclerosis, intimal cushions, and human intracranial saccular aneurysms.

Stehbens (1959) was the first to demonstrate that bifurcations lower the critical Reynolds number for turbulence. Subsequently, he suggested that

† This work was supported by Medical Research Council of Canada Grant MA-3218.
‡ Medical Research Council of Canada Fellow.
§ Medical Research Council of Canada Scholar.

turbulence might arise normally in the cerebrovascular system, and contribute to the localization of intimal cushions and atherosclerotic plaques at intra-cranial bifurcations (Stehbens, 1961). McDonald (1960) noted that eddies could be seen with high speed movies at the aortic bifurcation of rabbits if dye was injected. In a study in rigid Y-tubes, Attinger (1964) found vortices, eddies, and turbulence in the proximal portions of branch points at low Reynolds numbers, and concluded, "that in a large portion of the arterial bed, blood flow must be disturbed over the major part of the pulsatile cycle." More recently Schroter and Sudlow (1969) have shown that complex non-parabolic flow patterns arise at junctions in perspex models of the human bronchial tree.

Gutstein and Schneck (1967) and Gutstein et al. (1968) studied boundary layer separation in branching models. They found separation at very low Reynolds numbers, and suggested that "high wall shearing stresses, trailing vortices, and scouring effects" associated with the separation could induce localized injury to the wall. Fox and Hugh (1966) developed a theory for the localization of atheroma based on the similarity between the sites of boundary layer separation in experiments using free surface flow through channels of various configurations, and the sites of atheroma in the circulation. Sub-sequently, they used this theory to explain the localization of atherosclerotic lesions at the origin of the internal carotid artery in man (Fox and Hugh, 1970).

Murphy et al. (1962) studied the focal distribution of platelet thrombi and fibrin encrustations in bifurcations placed in an extracorporeal circulation in the pig. They found that the lateral aspects of the proximal portion of the branches and the apex of the bifurcations were most frequently encrusted, and thought these were probably the result of hydraulic factors and physical stresses arising at the bifurcations.

Fry (1968) demonstrated that abnormally high shear stresses would damage vascular endothelium. On the basis of the observed topography of athero-matous lesions in the coronary arteries of hyperlipaemic dogs, he suggested that atheroma occur in areas where shearing stress is intense, such as at "the crotch of a bifurcation" (Fry, 1969a). Caro et al. (1969) have taken an opposite view, and state that the observed distribution of fatty streaking in human aortas "is coincident with regions in which the shear rate at the arterial wall is locally reduced". Better methods for measuring shear stress in vivo are needed to resolve this controversy.

In spite of the obvious haemodynamic importance of bifurcations, there has been no description of the sequence of flow patterns which arise at bifurcations with increasing flow rates, and no measurement of the effect of bifurcation angle on the critical Reynolds number. We have investigated these in glass model bifurcations.

2. FUNDAMENTAL CONSIDERATIONS

A flowing fluid experiences a combination of inertial forces and frictional (viscous) forces (Prandtl, 1952). The inertial forces per unit volume are proportional to $\bar{V}^2 \, \rho/D$ where $\bar{V}$ is the average velocity of the fluid, D is the hydraulic depth or tube diameter, and ρ is the fluid density. The frictional forces per unit volume, on the other hand, are proportional to $\bar{V} \eta/D^2$ where η is the fluid viscosity. Since the inertial forces increase as $\bar{V}^2$, whereas the frictional forces increase only as $\bar{V}$, when the fluid velocity rises a critical velocity is reached where the viscous forces are no longer able to damp out random inertial forces.

Below the critical velocity, viscous forces predominate, and flow is stream-lined, or laminar. This flow is characterized by an orderly progression of fluid particles along straight clean-cut trajectories. When the critical velocity is exceeded, inertial forces predominate, and flow becomes turbulent. Turbulent flow is characterized by chaotic, random, and disordered fluctuations in the pressure and velocity of the fluid particles within the fluid stream.

The factors determining whether flow is streamlined or turbulent are related by the Reynolds number, Re (Reynolds, 1883), which is the ratio of inertial forces to viscous forces in a fluid.

$$Re = \frac{\rho}{\eta} \times \bar{V} \times D \qquad (2.1)$$

The Reynolds number is very useful. It allows one to model hydro-dynamically and geometrically equivalent flow situations (constant Reynolds numbers) using different sizes of tubes, and different fluids. This principle of "dynamical similarity" (Prandtl, 1952) is well known to engineers who make use of it, for example, in scale models to study flow conditions in river basins. This principle is equally applicable to the study of flow conditions in the human circulation by the use of models (McKusick and Wiskind, 1959). Reynolds (1883) stressed that his measurements were made in a long straight tube, far from the inlet. Obviously a bifurcation is none of these, and flow in the branches can be considered as "inlet flow". In this region the parabolic flow profile is distorted, eddies and turbulence may arise, and there may be boundary layer separation. Further downstream, beyond the inlet, flow again becomes laminar. We have demonstrated these flow distortions with dye, and have called the flow "turbulent" if the dye was uniformly distributed across the whole diameter of the tube.

3. MATERIALS AND METHODS

The authors, Ferguson and Roach, used a modified version of Stehbens' apparatus (Fig. 1) (Stehbens, 1959) to provide constant flow through the glass models under study. Sinusoidal flow waves, produced by a Sigmamotor

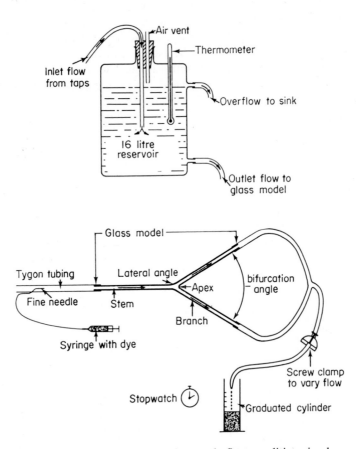

FIG. 1. Diagram of the apparatus used to study flow conditions in glass models. A 16-litre reservoir was continuously filled with water. The temperature was regulated by varying the mixture of hot and cold water. The temperature was measured both in the reservoir and in the collecting cylinder. The reservoir was vented to allow air bubbles to escape, and the overflow maintained the pressure head at 100 cm H_2O. Water flowed from the reservoir to the glass models through long straight connections of appropriately sized Tygon tubing. The flow rate was regulated by a screw clamp distal to the model, and the run off was directed by a three-way stopcock (not shown) either to the sink or to a graduated cylinder to measure flow rate, over a period of one minute, timed with a stop-watch.

The conventions used throughout the text for naming the components of a bifurcation, i.e. the stem, lateral angles, branches, apex and bifurcation angle, are shown in the lower half of the diagram.

pump, were superimposed on the steady flow. The pump rate was 70 per minute. Patterns of flow were observed by injecting, proximal to the models, a dilute solution of Evans blue dye through a fine (26 gauge, i.d. 0·010 cm) bore needle, connected to a 20 cm^3 syringe by a length of fine polyethylene tubing. Flow patterns were photographed on black and white 35 mm film. The Reynolds numbers were calculated from the dimensionless expression.

$$Re = \frac{\rho}{\eta} \times \frac{2}{\pi r} \times Q \qquad (3.1)$$

found by substituting $\bar{V} = Q/\pi r^2$ and $D = 2r$ in the original Reynolds' expression. Q is the flow rate (cm^3 s^{-1}). All Re numbers were calculated using stem radius, r(cm), rather than branch radius. The viscosity, η (poise), varies with the temperature of the perfusing water, and was obtained from the "Handbook of Chemistry and Physics". Using an Ostwald viscometer it was found that the amount of Evans blue dye used did not alter the viscosity of the mixture from that measured for water alone at the same temperature. The density, which is not very temperature sensitive, was assumed to be 1 gm cm^{-3}.

The glass models used in the experiments were five straight tubes with internal diameters (i.d.) of 7 mm and lengths of 12·5, 25, 50, 75 and 100 cm, and four symmetrical bifurcations with stems 20 cm long and 7 mm i.d., branches 15 cm long and 5 mm i.d., and bifurcation angles of 45°, 90°, 135° and 180°. All the models were made from Pyrex glass tubing by an expert glassblower.

4. Results

The apparatus provided reproducible flow, to within ±2 per cent, with repeated runs at low, moderate, and high rates, for both steady and pulsatile flow. The average critical Reynolds number (Re_c) for turbulence in the straight tubes with steady flow was 2500 ± 230 S.D.† ± 30 S.E.M.‡. The corresponding value with pulsatile flow was 2090 ± 160 S.D. ± 10 S.E.M. There was no statistically significant difference in the values for the short or long tubes. Thus it was concluded that the Tygon–glass connections were not creating a significant disturbance to flow.

A. PATTERNS OF FLOW AT THE BIFURCATIONS

Flow patterns were observed in each model, using both forward and reverse flow. With forward flow, water entered through the stem. With reverse flow, water entered the model equally through both branches and left

---

† S.D. = 1 standard deviation.
‡ S.E.M. = 1 standard error of the mean.

by the stem. As the flow rate was increased, the following sequence of patterns was seen in all the models with both steady and pulsatile flow.

(1) *Axial stream impingement*

With forward flow, at low flow rates ($Re < 200$), the axial and peri-axial streams impinged directly upon the apex of the bifurcations (Fig. 2). The incident streams were then reflected into the branches.

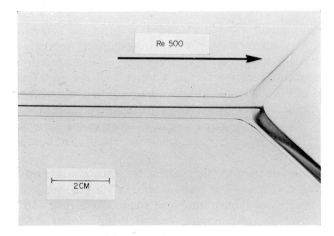

FIG. 2. Axial stream impinging upon, and rebounding from, the apex of the 90° bifurcation during steady, forward flow. The Reynolds number (Re) represents the flow rate when the photograph was taken. The direction of flow is shown by the arrow. Evans blue dye has been injected to reveal the flow pattern. All photographs have been taken using Kodak Plus X Panchromatic 35 mm film at F8 for 1/125 s.

(2) *Boundary layer separation*

At low rates of forward flow ($Re = 200–500$) the boundary layer streamline separated from the wall at the lateral angles and then reattached itself to the wall of the branch, downstream (Fig. 3). Eddy formation and turbulence occurred within the areas of separation. In general, the area of separation increased with increasing bifurcation angle, and was most prominent with pulsatile flow.

(3) *Helical flow pattern*

As the flow rate was increased, a helical pattern arose within the proximal portion of the branches. This flow pattern was particularly obvious in the wide-angled bifurcations (Fig. 4). The dye remained in orderly trajectories within the helix, which was transformed to a streamlined parabolic pattern

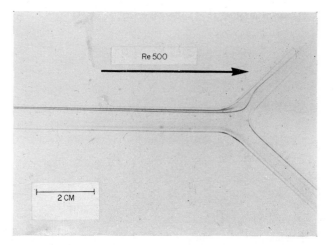

FIG. 3. Boundary layer separation at the lateral angle in the 90° bifurcation during steady flow at a low rate.

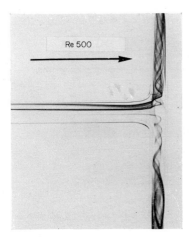

FIG. 4. Helical flow patterns in both branches of the 180° bifurcation during steady, forward flow. Scale as above in Fig. 3.

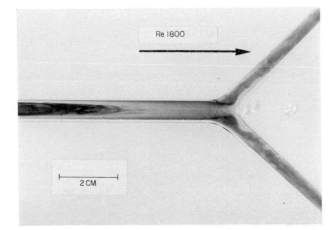

Fig. 5. Turbulence in the branches of the 90° bifurcation during pulsatile, forward flow. Turbulence can also be seen within the area of boundary layer separation at the lateral angles. Dye has cleared from the apex region because of the high flow velocity there. Flow in the stem is streamline; the next pulse of dye is seen approaching the bifurcation.

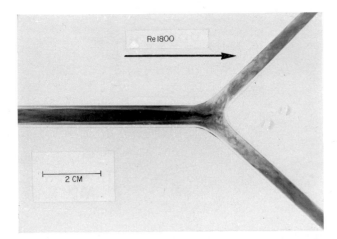

Fig. 6. Branch turbulence, as in Fig. 5, but at a later phase of the pulse cycle. The axial stream is about to impinge at the apex.

within the first few centimetres of the branch. This flow pattern was neither obviously turbulent, nor strictly laminar, but rather characterized the transition between the two.

(4) Branch turbulence

A further increase in flow resulted in turbulence, which was localized to the proximal portion of the branches, while flow distally appeared streamlined. A further increase in flow appeared to produce propagation of the turbulence to the full length of the branch, while flow in the stem and in the region of the apex remained streamlined (Figs. 5 and 6).

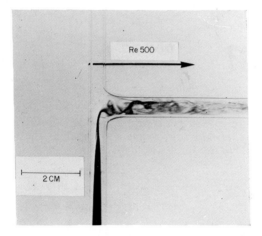

FIG. 7. Turbulence in the stem of the 180° bifurcation during steady, reverse flow. Flow is equal in both branches but dye has been injected only in one. Proximal to the junction flow is laminar, but distally it is turbulent. A remarkable feature of this turbulence, was that it arose at the junction of the two branch streams with a regular "whiplash-like" periodicity (approximately 1 s), which produced the appearance of pulsatile flow in the proximal portion of the stem.

With reverse flow, even at low flow rates, marked turbulence, with mixing of the two branch streams, occurred in the stem. This was most prominent in the wide-angled bifurcations (Fig. 7).

B. CRITICAL REYNOLDS NUMBERS AT THE BIFURCATIONS

The critical Reynolds numbers (Re_c) were measured for each bifurcation using steady and pulsatile flow, in both forward and reverse directions (Figs. 8 and 9). Each value is an average of a minimum of 20 individual measurements. This averaging was necessary because the critical flow rate corresponding to the onset of turbulence had to be judged visually with repeated injections of dye, together with a continuous adjustment of the flow rate to the critical value.

In every instance the Re_c values for the bifurcations were less than for the straight tubes. For example, the Re_c for the 90° bifurcation, with forward

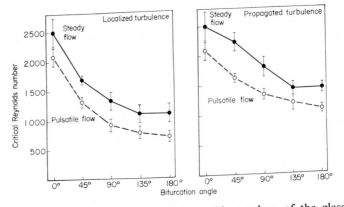

FIG. 8. Graphs comparing the critical Reynolds numbers of the glass model bifurcations during forward flow, steady and pulsatile. The bars represent ± 1 standard deviation. See text for description.

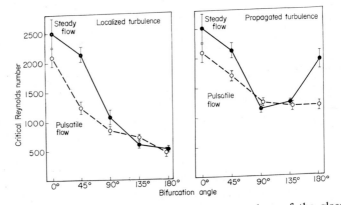

FIG. 9. Graphs comparing the critical Reynolds numbers of the glass model bifurcations during reverse flow, steady and pulsatile. See text for description.

flow and turbulence localized to the proximal portion of the branches (Fig. 8) was approximately half that for the straight tubes for both steady and pulsatile flow. The Re_c decreased with increasing bifurcation angle (Figs. 8 and 9), except in the case of the 180° bifurcation with propagated turbulence during steady, reverse flow (Fig. 9). With pulsatile flow, Re_c values were lowered by about 400. Localized turbulence arose at an Re_c approximately 25 per cent less than for propagated turbulence.

The pattern of results with reverse flow (Fig. 9) was not as simple as with forward flow. In general, the Re_c decreased with increasing angle, with the exception already noted. However, the difference between steady and pulsatile flow was much less marked than with forward flow, and was not statistically different except for the 45° bifurcation. Reverse flow usually produced turbulence at lower Re values than forward flow.

5. DISCUSSION

A. SIGNIFICANCE OF THE CRITICAL REYNOLDS NUMBER

We obtained an Re_c of 2500 for steady flow, and 2100 for pulsatile flow, in straight tubes. These are in keeping with the results of others (Prandtl, 1952). It differs from the value of 2000 originally found by Reynolds. This is to be expected, since the exact values measured vary with the magnitude of the disturbing effects produced by the apparatus. With elaborate precautions in design, Re_c values as high as 40 000 have been achieved (Prandtl, 1952).

Reynolds' result has been widely quoted for the cardiovascular system, and used in support of the argument that turbulence does not occur in the circulation under normal flow conditions (Burton, 1952). The results of this study demonstrate that bifurcations in the circulation can be expected to lower the Re_c considerably. Bifurcations represent a geometrical disturbance to flow, which increases with increasing bifurcation angle. In addition, pulsatile flow and reverse flow (analogous to flow in the venous system) lower the values even further.

Some differences in the Re_c values at bifurcations in the human circulation compared to those found for the models is to be expected, because: (1) vessels are distensible and viscoelastic rather than rigid; (2) their lining layer is not as smooth and uniform as that of the glass models; (3) the geometry of vascular bifurcations is not as simple as in the models; and (4) the contour of the pressure fluctuations produced by the Sigmamotor pump is not identical to that in the circulation. Since each of these probably represents an additional disturbing factor in the circulation, one would predict that *in vivo* Re_c values are even lower than in the models. As a first approximation, however, the trend demonstrated in the models, both in the Re_c values, and the sequence of flow patterns, will apply to the circulation.

B. REYNOLDS NUMBERS IN THE HUMAN CIRCULATION

One needs to consider whether Reynolds values comparable to those found in the model experiments occur in the human circulation. For human blood at 37°C, the Reynolds formula, based on an estimate for blood density and viscosity (Green, 1950), becomes,

$$Re = \frac{\bar{V}D}{0.027} \qquad (5.1)$$

where $\bar{V}$ is the mean flow velocity in the vessel under consideration, and D is the diameter of the vessel. If only the mean flow, Q ($cm^3 \, s^{-1}$) is known, then $\bar{V}$ can be found from $\bar{V} = Q/\pi r^2$. If calculated Re values for the circulation are greater than the Re_c values obtained in corresponding models, then turbulence is likely in the *in vivo* situation. Making use of this expression, representative Re values, from flow values published in the literature, were calculated for a variety of sites in the circulation (Table 1).

TABLE 1

Representative Reynolds numbers for major human vessels. The values of mean flow velocity have been given by the authors cited, or calculated from their mean flow data, as described in the text.

Reference	Vessel	Diameter (cm)	Mean flow ($cm^3 \, s^{-1}$)	Mean flow velocity ($cm \, s^{-1}$)	Re
Patel *et al.* (1965)	Aorta	2·5	100	22	2000
Hardesty *et al.* (1960)	Internal carotid artery	0·4	6	50	750
Patel *et al.* (1965)	Femoral artery	0·5	5	26	500
Hunt *et al.* (1964)	Renal artery	0·4	6	50	750

It is obvious that in the major distributing arteries, flow values are such that the corresponding Re values lie far below the Re_c for turbulence in a long, straight tube, but well within the range necessary for flow instability at bifurcations. As most bifurcation angles in the circulation are less than 90°, one would not expect turbulence beyond bifurcations, except possibly in the major branches of the aorta. However, it seems almost certain that axial and peri-axial stream impingement, boundary layer separation, and proximal branch helical flow will occur at most major bifurcations.

C. PATHOGENESIS OF FOCAL VASCULAR DISEASE

(1) *Topography of atherosclerotic plaques*

There is still considerable debate over the cause of the patchy distribution of atherosclerotic plaques (Rodbard, 1956; Texon, 1957; Murphy *et al.*, 1962; Mustard *et al.*, 1963; Pickering, 1968; Caro *et al.*, 1969; Fry, 1969a; Fox and Hugh, 1970). We propose that the impingement of the high velocity central streams at the apex of a bifurcation, and the occurrence of the helical flow patterns in the proximal portion of branches are important factors. Each has the effect of bringing a high velocity stream to the wall. This results in a steep velocity gradient at these sites, and consequently, a higher rate of shear than would be experienced in the main stem or distal portion of a branch (Caro et al., 1969; Fry, 1969a; Schroter and Sudlow, 1969). If high shear stress is important as Fry (1968, 1969a,b) has suggested, our model experiments show that the apex of bifurcations and the proximal portions of the branches, especially on their inner aspects, or on the lateral walls beyond the region of boundary layer separation, should be maximally involved with atherosclerotic lesions. If on the other hand, the low shear theory of Caro et al. (1969, 1970) is correct, then the lateral angle of a bifurcation, where boundary layer separation occurs and the shear rate is low, should be maximally involved.

The high shear theory is particularly attractive since Fry (1968, 1969b) has shown that an acute increase in the shear stress at the blood vascular interface in the aorta of the dog will damage the endothelial lining and expose the underlying basement membrane. If the basement membrane is exposed, platelets, fibrin, and other blood products accumulate on it (Tranzer and Baumgartner, 1967; Fry, 1968). Pathologists, and others, who favour the "encrustation" theory of atherosclerosis, originally expounded by Rokitansky (1852), believe that plaques are the end-result of such platelet-leucocyte-fibrin thrombi (Duguid, 1946; More and Haust, 1961; Murphy et al., 1962; Mustard et al., 1963; Pickering, 1968).

(2) Intimal cushions

Intimal cushions are localized areas of thickened tunica intima which occur at the lateral angles of arterial bifurcations with great frequency, particularly in the cerebral arteries (Hassler, 1961a,b; 1962a,b; Stehbens, 1960). Hassler, (1961a) considers them to be "non-atheromatous" and "physiological" in nature, the result of a "passive remodelling of the vessel wall" in response to haemodynamic forces. Others consider them to be early atherosclerotic lesions (Stehbens, 1960; Fox and Hugh, 1966; Caro et al., 1969, 1970).

Whatever their nature, there is a remarkable similarity between the location and contour of the boundary layer separation, as seen in our models, and the location and shape of intimal cushions as found in the circulation. Eddy formation and turbulence occur within an area of separation (Prandtl, 1952). This was seen in the models. Fry (1968) has shown that turbulence is as capable of damaging the endothelial lining of a vessel as shear stress. Thus, intimal cushions could well be the remnants of platelet thrombi which have occurred at the lateral angles of bifurcations secondary to damage induced by the separation.

(3) *Human intracranial saccular aneurysms*

Intracranial saccular aneurysms are abnormal pouchlike evaginations which occur in the walls of major human intracranial arteries. They invariably arise at the apex of a bifurcation (Hassler, 1961a). There is general agreement among pathologists that an acquired focal degeneration of the internal elastic membrane at the apex of the bifurcation is the necessary pathological antecedent of aneurysm formation (Forbus, 1930; Walker and Allegre, 1954; Hassler, 1961a; Stehbens, 1963; Sahs, 1966). It seems reasonable to postulate that the high local shear stresses generated by the impingement of central streams at the apex is an important factor contributing to this degeneration (Ferguson, 1970). The high shear could initiate a focal platelet thrombus, resulting ultimately in a focal plaque associated with destruction of the underlying internal elastic membrane. It is known that destruction of the elastica is an integral part of the atherosclerotic process (Friedman, 1963; Robert *et al.*, 1969).

6. SUMMARY

The patterns of flow and critical Reynolds numbers for turbulence (Re_c) in a series of glass model bifurcations with varying bifurcation angles were studied using steady and pulsatile flow. A reproducible sequence of flow patterns was found in all the models. At low flow rates ($Re < 200$) the central streams impinged at the apex of the bifurcations, and the boundary layers separated at the lateral angles. At higher flow rates ($Re = 200$–500) a helical flow pattern arose in the proximal portion of the branches which progressed to obvious turbulence at higher rates. In every case, the Re_c for the bifurcations was less than that for long, straight tubes. The exact values varied approximately inversely with the bifurcation angle, and were least with pulsatile and reverse flow. All the observed instabilities of flow, other than turbulence, arose at Re values less than 750, a range that is likely achieved at major bifurcations in the human circulation.

These findings were discussed in relation to the hypothesis that haemo-dynamic forces generated at bifurcations account, at least in part, for the focal distribution of atherosclerotic plaques, the occurrence of intimal cushions in arteries, and the pathogenesis of human intracranial saccular aneurysms.

ACKNOWLEDGEMENTS

The authors wish to express their appreciation to Miss Susan Scott who skilfully assisted in these experiments, and to Mr. Patrick Johnston, glass-blower for the Department of Chemistry, The University of Western Ontario, who made the models.

REFERENCES

Attinger, E. O. (1964). Flow patterns and vascular geometry. In "Pulsatile Blood Flow", (E. O. Attinger, ed.), McGraw-Hill, New York.

Burton, A. C. (1952). Laws of physics and flow in blood vessels. In "Visceral Circulation", (G. E. W. Wolstenholme, ed.), Churchill, London.

Caro, C. G., Fitz-Gerald, J. M. and Schroter, R. C. (1969). Arterial wall shear and distribution of early atheroma in man. Nature (London)) 223, 1159–1161.

Caro, C. G., Fitz-Gerald, J. M. and Schroter, R. C. (1970). Wall shear rate in arteries and distribution of early atheroma. AGARD Conference Proceedings No. 65 of Specialist's Meeting on "Fluid Dynamics of Blood Circulation and Respiratory Flow", Naples, May, 1970, pp. 13.1–13.8.

Duguid, J. B. (1946). Thrombosis as a factor in the pathogenesis of coronary atherosclerosis. J. Pathol. Bacteriol. 58, 207–212.

Ferguson, G. G. (1970). Physical factors in the initiation, growth and rupture of human intracranial saccular aneurysms. Ph.D. Thesis, University of Western Ontario, London, Canada.

Forbus, W. D. (1930). On the origin of miliary aneurysms of the superficial cerebral arteries. Bull. Johns Hopkins Hosp. 47, 239–284.

Fox, J. A. and Hugh, A. E. (1966). Localization of atheroma: a theory based on boundary layer separation. Brit. Heart J. 28, 388–399.

Fox, J. A. and Hugh, A. E. (1970). The precise localization of atheroma and its association with stasis at the origin of the internal carotid artery—a radiographic investigation. Brit. J. Radiol. 43, 377–383.

Friedman, M. (1963). Pathogenesis of the spontaneous atherosclerotic plaque. A study on the cholesterol-fed rabbit. Arch. Pathol. 76, 318–329.

Fry, D. L. (1968). Acute vascular endothelial changes associated with increased blood velocity gradients. Circulation Res. 22, 165–197.

Fry, D. L. (1969a). Certain chemorheological considerations regarding the blood vascular interface with particular reference to coronary artery disease. Circulation 39, Suppl. 4, 38–59.

Fry, D. L. (1969b). Certain histological and chemical responses of the vascular interface to acutely induced mechanical stress in the aorta of the dog. Circulation Res. 24, 93–108.

Green, H. D. (1950). Circulatory system: Physical principles. In "Medical Physics", (O. Glasser, ed.), Vol. 2, p. 228, Year Book Medical Publishers, Chicago.

Gutstein, W. H. and Schneck, D. J. (1967). In vitro boundary layer studies of blood in branched tubes. J. Atheroscler. Res. 7, 295–299.

Gutstein, W. H., Schneck, D. J. and Marks, J. O. (1968). In vitro studies of local blood flow disturbance in a region of separation. J. Atheroscler. Res. 8, 381–388.

Hardesty, W. H., Roberts, B., Toole, J. F. and Royster, H. P. (1960). Studies of carotid-artery flow in man. New Engl. J. Med. 263, 944–946.

Hassler, O. (1961a). Morphological studies on the large cerebral arteries with reference to the aetiology of subarachnoid haemorrhage. Acta Psychiat. Neurol. Scand. 36, suppl. 154.

Hassler, O. (1961b). Media defects and physiological intima cushions in the spinal arteries. Acta Soc. Med. Upsal. 66, 267–270.

Hassler, O. (1962a). Physiological intima cushions in the large cerebral arteries of young individuals. 1. Morphological structure and possible significance for the circulation. Acta Pathol. Microbiol. Scand. 55, 19–27.

Hassler, O. (1962b). Physiological intima cushions in the large cerebral arteries of young individuals. 2. Location. Acta Pathol. Microbiol. Scand. 55, 28–30.

Hunt, L. D., Lathem, J. E., O'Connor, F. J. and Boyce, W. H. (1964). Electromagnetic flowmeter studies of human renal arterial flow. *J. Urol.* **92**, 399–408.
McDonald, D. A. (1960). "Blood Flow in Arteries", pp. 61–65. Arnold, London.
McKusick, V. A. and Wiskind, H. K. (1959). Osborne Reynolds of Manchester. Contributions of an engineer to the understanding of cardiovascular sound. *Bull. Hist. Med.* **33**, 116–136.
More, R. H. and Haust, M. D. (1961). Atherogenesis and plasma constituents. *Amer. J. Path.* **38**, 527–537.
Murphy, E. A., Rowsell, H. C., Downie, H. G., Robinson, G. A. and Mustard, J. F. (1962). Encrustation and atherosclerosis: the analogy between early *in vivo* lesions and deposits which occur in extracorporeal circulations. *Can. Med. Ass. J.* **87**, 259–274.
Mustard, J. F., Rowsell, H. C., Murphy, E. A. and Downie, H. G. (1963). Intimal thrombosis in atherosclerosis. *In* "The Evolution of the Atherosclerotic Plaque", (R. J. Jones, ed.), University of Chicago, Chicago.
Patel, D. J., Greenfield, J. C. Jr., Austen, W. G., Morrow, A. G. and Fry, D. L. (1965). Pressure-flow relationships in the ascending aorta and femoral artery of man. *J. Appl. Physiol.* **20**, 459–463.
Pickering, G. W. (1968). "High Blood Pressure", 2nd Ed., p. 296, Grune and Stratton, New York.
Prandtl. L. (1952). "Essentials of Fluid Dynamics", pp. 98–174, Blackie and Son, London.
Reynolds, O. (1883). An experimental investigation of the circumstances which determine whether the motion of water shall be direct or sinuous and of the law of resistance in parallel channels. *Phil. Trans. Roy. Soc. London.* **174**, 935–987.
Robert, B., Legrand, Y., Dignaud, G., Caen, J. and Robert, L. (1969). Activité élastinolytique associée aux plaquettes sanguines. *Pathol. Biol. (Paris)* **17**, 615–622.
Rodbard, S. (1956). Vascular modifications induced by flow. *Amer. Heart J.* **51**, 926–942.
Rokitansky, C. (1852). "A Manual of Pathological Anatomy." Sydenham Society, London.
Sahs, A. L. (1966). Report on the cooperative study of intracranial aneurysms and subarachnoid haemorrhage. Sec. I. Observations on the pathology of saccular aneurysms. *J. Neurosurg.* **24**, 792–806.
Schroter, R. C. and Sudlow, M. F. (1969). Flow patterns in models of the human bronchial airways. *Resp. Physiol.* **7**, 341–355.
Stehbens, W. E. (1959). Turbulence of blood flow. *Quart. J. Exp. Physiol.* **44**, 110–117.
Stehbens, W. E. (1960). Focal intimal proliferation in the cerebral arteries. *Amer. J. Pathol.* **36**, 289–301.
Stehbens, W. E. (1961). Discussion on vascular flow and turbulence. *Neurology (Minneapolis)* **11**, part 2, 66–67.
Stehbens, W. E. (1963). Histopathology of cerebral aneurysms. *Arch. Neurol. (Chicago)* **8**, 272–285.
Texon, M. (1957). A haemodynamic concept of atherosclerosis, with particular reference to coronary occlusion. *Arch. Intern. Med.* **99**, 418–427.
Tranzer, J. P. and Baumgartner, H. R. (1967). Filling gaps in the vascular endothelium with blood platelets. *Nature (London)* **216**, 1126–1128.
Walker, A. E. and Allegre, G. W. (1954). The pathology and pathogenesis of cerebral aneurysms. *J. Neuropath. Exp. Neurol.* **13**, 248–259.

Chapter 15

Blood Rheology

STANLEY E. CHARM

Department of Physiology, Tufts University Medical School,
Boston, Massachusetts, U.S.A.

and

GEORGE S. KURLAND

Department of Medicine, Beth Israel Hospital
and Harvard Medical School, Boston, Massachusetts, U.S.A.

1. STRUCTURE OF BLOOD

Blood is a suspension of cells in plasma. At rest, the cells form a continuous structure, see Fig. 1 (Charm *et al.*, 1964). When the structure breaks under its own weight, sedimentation occurs. Evidence of its continuous structure can be seen when the blood structure is given sufficient support against its own

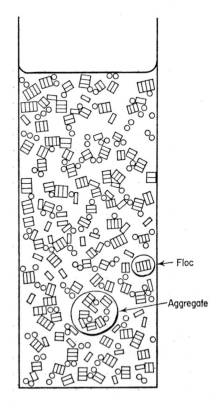

FIG. 1. A red-cell suspension at rest is a continuous structure formed from groups of cell aggregates made up of units of cells called flocs or rouleaux.

weight, e.g. by the wall of a settling tube, and settling is prevented. The viscometric behavior of blood is the result of the resistance of the blood structure to the forces attempting to deform it.

When a finite stress, (force/unit area), is applied to whole blood the continuous structure breaks. The stress required to disrupt the standing structure of blood is referred to as the yield stress. After disruption the structure appears as a cluster of cell aggregates suspended in plasma. The aggregates in turn are made up of smaller units of cells called rouleaux or flocs. As additional stress is applied, the aggregates and rouleaux become smaller. A dynamic equilibrium exists between the size of aggregates or rouleaux and the stress applied, see Fig. 2. When aggregates and rouleaux are under sufficiently high

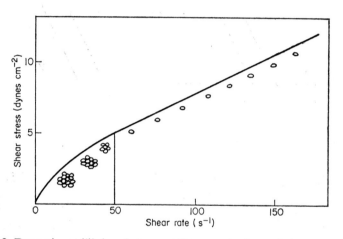

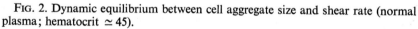

FIG. 2. Dynamic equilibrium between cell aggregate size and shear rate (normal plasma; hematocrit ≃ 45).

stress that they are reduced to individual cells, further increases in stress cannot result in changes of aggregate size. As a result the shear stress—flow rate relationship becomes a straight line at sufficiently high shear stresses, (see Fig. 2).

The nature of the attraction between cells causing them to aggregate is still not clear. Both electrostatic attraction and plasma surface tension have been suggested as mechanisms (Fahraeus and Lindquist, 1931).

In a dilute suspension containing 1 per cent cells, it requires about 30 s to achieve equilibrium when a change in stress occurs. The thixotropy or viscosity time effect is not very pronounced at this low concentration because the cells contribute so little to the suspension viscosity.

On the other hand, in more concentrated suspensions, the time required to achieve equilibrium is less. The viscosity change at low flow rates is due to changes in aggregate or rouleaux size. Since large aggregates tend to structure the suspending fluid more than smaller ones, higher apparent viscosities are associated with larger aggregates.

2. Measurement of Flow Properties of Blood

The measurement of the relationship between stress and flow is carried out on an instrument, (viscometer), designed to permit analysis of the stress acting on the fluid for a given flow condition. The principle of a viscometer

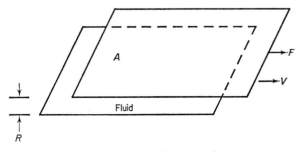

Fig. 3. Theoretical parallel plate viscometer.

may be illustrated by considering the following model: a fluid is placed between two parallel plates, (see Fig. 3). A force F is applied to the top plate, which moves with a velocity V. The distance between the plates, (R), is sufficiently small that the velocity gradient throughout $(-V/R)$ is uniform. The minus sign merely indicates that distance across the gap is measured from the moving plate. Velocity gradient is referred to as shear rate and has

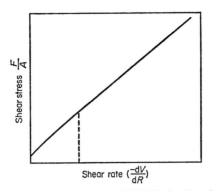

Fig. 4. Shear stress, (F/A) vs. shear rate, (dV/dR) for blood showing yield stress.

the units of 1/time. The force per unit area (F/A) is known as shear stress. Velocity and distance may be considered in terms of very small or differential elements, and designated as dV and dR respectively. The shear rate would then be $-dV/dR$. A plot may be made of F/A against $-dV/dR$ or of shear stress vs. shear rate, (see Fig. 4). Such a plot characterizes the viscometry of the fluid. The parallel plate system is not a practical viscometer for blood since the fluid could not be held in place for measurement. The shear rate ranges and volumes of blood required for commonly used blood viscometers are noted in Table 1.

TABLE 1

Commonly used viscometers for blood and plasma

Type	Shear rate range for blood (s^{-1})	Specimen volume (cm^3)
Brookfield cone and plate LVT	13–230	1
Brookfield cone and plate RVT (0·4)	5–1500	1
Weissenberg Couette viscometer with cone and plate for end effects and guarding GDM	0·01–250	14
Couette viscometer with guard	0·001–20	10
Capillary tube viscometer $(D \simeq 500 \ \mu m)$	0·01–1000	10

There are three suitable basic viscometric devices having the essential features of parallel plates which are capable of holding the fluid in place. These viscometers are (see Fig. 5): (a) cone and plate, (b) cone in cone, (c) Couette or narrow gap concentric cylinder. Shear rate ranges and volumes of blood required for commonly used blood viscometers are noted in Table 1. A guard ring is sometimes employed with a Couette viscometer to prevent the denaturation of proteins at the air-liquid interface influencing stress measurement. Capillary tube viscometers are often used in the measurement of blood viscosity. However, the tube viscometer is not truly a direct measuring viscometer in that the flow pattern associated with it is more complex than with the Couette or cone and plate viscometers. Nevertheless, it is inexpensive and capable of great accuracy under the proper conditions.

The primary condition is that the flow be uniform or homogenous through-out the tube, i.e. no differences in cell distribution with a marginal layer

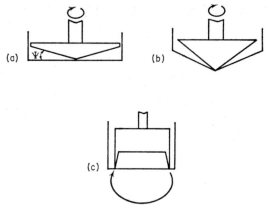

FIG. 5.   Different types of viscometer: (a) cone and plate; (b) cone in cone; (c) Couette.

develops at the tube wall. The conditions under which marginal layers develop are described later.

The flow must be also streamline, i.e. the Reynold's number for blood $D\bar{V}\rho/K^2$, must be less than 800 (Charm *et al.*, 1968), where D = tube diameter, $\bar{V}$ = mass average velocity, ρ = blood density and K^2 = "limiting apparent viscosity" for blood.

When these conditions are satisfied, a tube with $D \simeq 500\,\mu\text{m}$ is usually satisfactory as a viscometer for blood suspensions. With smaller tubes it is possible for marginal layers to occur with flowing blood. It is possible from flow rate and pressure loss information to obtain the wall shear rate, τ_w, and wall shear stress, γ_w.

The wall shear stress in a tube is

$$\tau_w = \frac{PD}{4L} \tag{2.1}$$

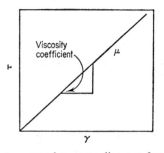

FIG. 6. Shear stress vs. shear rate diagram for blood plasma.

where P/L is pressure drop per unit length. Wall shear rate is (Rabinowitsch, 1929; Mooney, 1931)

$$\gamma_w = 2(\overline{V}/D) \left[3 + \frac{d \ln (\overline{V}/D)}{d \ln \tau_w}\right] \tag{2.2}$$

where $d \ln \overline{V}/D/(d \ln \tau_w)$ is the slope of $\ln \overline{V}/D$ vs. $\ln \tau_w$.

From a plot of τ_w vs. γ_w, the blood flow properties may be evaluated, e.g. see Fig. 4.

In general, Couette or cone and plate viscometers are preferred when they are available because of ease of measurement and the simple analysis of flow in these systems. Detailed discussion of these viscometers may be found in VanWazer et al. (1963) and Wilkinson (1960).

3. FLOW PROPERTIES OF PLASMA

A. PLASMA AS A NEWTONIAN FLUID

The shear stress ($\tau = F/A$) vs. shear rate ($\gamma = -dV/dR$) behavior of plasma is generally characterized by a straight line passing through the origin, (Charm and Kurland, 1962; Copley and Scott-Blair, 1960; Merrill et al., 1964; see Fig. 6). A fluid which exhibits such a plot is known as a Newtonian fluid. The slope of the line is the viscosity. There have however also been several reports which describe plasma as non-Newtonian (Gregersen et al., 1965; Cerny et al., 1962; Dintenfass, 1965; Shorthouse and Hutchinson, 1967). For serum and plasma viscosity, Bayliss (1952), suggests the relationship $\mu_p/\mu_w = 1/(1 - bc)$, where b = constant, c = grams of protein per 100 ml, μ_w = water viscosity and μ_p = plasma viscosity.

The viscometric plots of plasma measured in cone and plate viscometers down to shear rates of $5 s^{-1}$ often appear not to pass through the origin when extrapolated to zero shear rate. This is thought to be due to the surface denaturation at the air interface alluded to previously. This may cause a protein skin to form, but this has not been proved. Plasma does not usually exhibit this effect in Couette type viscometers which have guard rings that prevent such surface denaturation effects from influencing stress measurements.

Serum, which has a lower viscosity than plasma due to removal of fibrinogen, does not show any deviation from Newtonian behavior in cone and plate viscometers as does plasma at times. This suggests that fibrinogen plays a role in the non-Newtonian behavior of plasma.

Plasma sometimes exhibits time dependent effects which vary with respect to shear rate. If plasma is subjected to shear rates less than $5 s^{-1}$, the indicated stress will gradually fall to a minimum value. At higher shear rates, the plasma stress achieves a minimum value very rapidly. To observe these changes care must be taken not to expose the plasma to shear rates greater than $5\,s^{-1}$ when placing it in the viscometer, for these effects are not quickly reversible if at all. These observations suggest that the plasma proteins may form a network throughout the solution which is broken under stress. Attempts to make a direct measurement of strength of the plasma network have been inconclusive thus far. Plasma in both the Weissenberg Rheogoniometer with Couette attachment and the Brookfield cone and plate viscometer RVT (0·4) exhibited this time effect. The cone and plate viscometer exhibited the effect at higher shear rates than the Couette, (Charm and Kurland, unpublished data). The initial decrease in plasma viscosity has also been observed in a capillary tube viscometer (shear rate $300–500\,s^{-1}$; Scott-Blair, 1970).

The conclusion is that plasma may have transitory non-Newtonian behavior particularly at low shear rates, which is associated with fibrinogen. This change from non-Newtonian to Newtonian characteristics occurs readily *in vitro* and is not reversible. The rapid passage of plasma through a narrow hypodermic syringe is sufficient to destroy the non-Newtonian behavior of plasma. It is possible that *in vivo* the non-Newtonian character of plasma may be maintained.

It has been shown that fibrinogen in plasma which has been subjected to sufficient shear looses its ability to clot, (Charm and Wong, 1970). This indicates that plasma does undergo a shear degradation. In fact the half-life of fibrinogen in the circulation maybe explained by shear degradation.

B. EFFECT OF TEMPERATURE

The Bayliss equation for plasma viscosity noted previously provides for temperature change in the water viscosity (μ_w). Merrill *et al.* (1963a) have noted that plasma viscosity varies with temperature in the same manner as water when measured with a GDM viscometer. However, when measured in a cone and plate viscometer, it is found that this is not the case, though the reason for the discrepancy is not known.

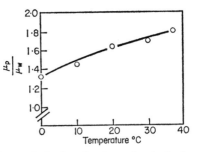

FIG. 7. Ratio of plasma (μ_p) viscosity to water (μ_w) viscosity as a function of temperature. Original data determined with cone and plate viscometer.

The ratio of plasma viscosity to water viscosity as a function of temperature is shown in Fig. 7 (Charm and Kurland, unpublished). Plasma components have a greater effect on plasma viscosity at 37° than at 0°C, i.e. plasma viscosity deviates more from water viscosity at 37° than at 0°C. Proteins and lipids in plasma may cause this difference.

C. EFFECT OF PLASMA COMPONENTS

The viscosity of plasma increases with the protein concentration as shown by the Bayliss equation. However, the various proteins have different influences on plasma viscosity depending on their shape and size. Fibrinogen is the largest of the proteins in plasma although it forms only 5.5 per cent of plasma protein. Its influence on plasma viscosity can be seen in the differences between plasma and serum viscosity, serum usually having a viscosity 20 per cent less than plasma.

The effect of globulins (usually 45 per cent of plasma protein) on viscosity is illustrated in the disease macroglobulinemia, (Somer, 1966). An increase from 1 to 4 g per 100 ml of globulin may cause a 50 per cent increase in plasma viscosity.

Albumin, the smallest plasma protein molecule is present in the largest concentration (approximately 50 per cent). Changes in albumin have the least effect of the three proteins on plasma viscosity, but it makes an important contribution to plasma viscosity through its high concentration.

A high correlation between plasma viscosity, total protein, fibrinogen and globulins has been found (Mayer, 1966; Rand et al., 1970). High albumin concentrations in plasma are accompanied at times by reduced globulin concentrations actually resulting in lowered plasma viscosities. It has also been suggested that albumin may "neutralize" the viscosity effect of other proteins in plasma, (Mayer, 1966).

Beta lipoprotein and lipalbumin have little effect on plasma viscosity. It is clear that fibrinogen and globulin concentrations have the greatest influence on blood plasma viscosity.

4. FLOW PROPERTIES OF RED CELL SUSPENSIONS

A. GENERAL EXPRESSIONS

Suspensions of cells in plasma up to a volume fraction, ϕ, of 0·05 show a constant shear stress-shear rate relationship typical of a Newtonian fluid. The viscosity of such suspensions for $\phi < 0·05$ is expressed with reasonable accuracy by Einstein's equation for spheres in suspension (Jeffery, 1922).

$$\mu_s = \mu_p \left(\frac{1}{1-\alpha\phi}\right) \tag{4.1}$$

where: μ_p = plasma viscosity
μ_s = suspension viscosity
α = shape factor, (2·5 for spheres)
ϕ = cell volume fraction.

The constant α should theoretically vary with the shape of the particles, but a value of 2·5 appears to apply to red cells when $\phi < 0.05$. The volume fraction is not only the volume fraction of the particles, but that of the particles plus any adsorbed fluid.

One of the assumptions underlying (4.1) is that the particles act as individuals and do not interact significantly. However, as ϕ increases from 0·05 the suspension viscosity departs from (4.1) because interaction between particles becomes more significant and the properties associated with the interaction, e.g. cell elasticity, aggregation, eddy flow, now influence viscosity. Eddy flow refers to the streamline flow pattern around cells or aggregates.

Many empirical equations have been suggested over the years to express blood viscosity as a function of cell concentration and plasma viscosity, (Bayliss, 1952). These generally take the form of (4.1). Thus, the Hatschek equation, determined for emulsions of tightly packed flat polyhedrical droplets,

$$\frac{\mu_s}{\mu_p} = \frac{1}{1-\phi^{\frac{1}{3}}} \tag{4.2}$$

or the expression due to Jeffery (1922).

$$\frac{\mu_s}{\mu_p} = \frac{1+\phi}{1+b\phi} \tag{4.3}$$

where b is a constant depending on shape of the particle. Cokelet (1963) has suggested that for red cell suspensions

$$\frac{\mu_s}{\mu_p} = \frac{1}{(1-\phi)^{2.5}} \tag{4.4}$$

With a cone and plate viscometer, the limiting apparent viscosity of red cell suspensions is found to be predicted up to $\phi = 0.6$ by (4.1) in which α is given by:

$$0.076 \exp\left[2.49\phi + \frac{1107}{T} \exp(-1.69\phi)\right] \tag{4.5}$$

where T = absolute temperature (°K), (Charm and Kurland, unpublished).
A plot of α against ϕ for $T = 25°$ and $37°$ is shown in Fig. 8.
Other equations similar in form to (4.1) have been proposed, e.g. Bingham and White (1911), and Hess,

$$\frac{\mu_s}{\mu_p} = \frac{1}{1-\phi} \tag{4.6}$$

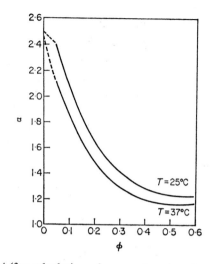

FIG. 8. α vs. ϕ (for calculation of suspension viscosity up to $\phi = 0.6$).

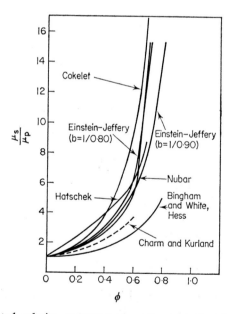

FIG. 9. Calculated relative apparent viscosity vs. cell volume fraction from various equations. (Adapted from Nubar, 1967 and calculated from (4.1) and (4.5).)

and Nubar (1967)

$$\frac{\mu_s}{\mu_p} = \frac{\lambda}{\lambda - \phi} \tag{4.7}$$

where: λ = maximum concentration of packed cells = 0·75.

A comparison of these equations is shown in Fig. 9 and it is apparent there is little agreement between them, (Nubar, 1967), and none is satisfactory for estimating limiting "apparent" blood viscosities above $\phi = 0.6$.

The fact that α varies with temperature, (4.5), suggests that either the number of cell interactions per unit time changes with temperature or the energy loss per collision changes. It is possible that the elasticity of the cells vary with temperature, thus causing changes in momentum and energy loss upon collision. A temperature related change in the internal viscosity of the cell may influence cell elasticity and hence suspension viscosity. Bayliss (1952) notes that the effect of temperature on blood viscosity may be estimated from

$$\frac{(\mu_s/\mu_w)_T}{(\mu_s/\mu_w)_{T+20}} = 1 \cdot 09. \tag{4.8}$$

However, this assumes that the relative viscosity of plasma does not vary with temperature, which has not been established, (see Fig. 7).

Merrill et al. (1963a), using a Couette viscometer (GDM) tested the viscosity of blood relative to water between 10 and 37°C, and found it to be independent of temperature at shear rates above $1 \, s^{-1}$. This is clearly in disagreement with (4.1) and (4.5), but in agreement with (4.2), (4.3), (4.4) and (4.6). Equation (4.1) with (4.7) has been tested with a cone and plate viscometer and found to be correct within 10 per cent.

A power law expression has been suggested as a means of characterizing the τ/γ relationship of blood (Charm and Kurland, 1962; Hershey and Cho, 1966):

$$\tau = b\gamma^s, \tag{4.9}$$

where b and s are constants.

It has been found that this form of equation does not hold over more than two decades of shear rates with constant values of b and s, (Charm et al., 1965), see Fig. 10. Therefore, flow constants determined from (4.9) are of limited use for application to flow analysis in capillary tubes or vessels unless it is certain that shear rates in the tube are within the experimental range measures with the viscometer.

The Herschel-Bulkley equation (4.10) has a more realistic physical basis than the Casson equation, (Scott-Blair, 1967).

$$\tau = b\gamma^s + C \tag{4.10}$$

C = the blood yield stress or shear strength.

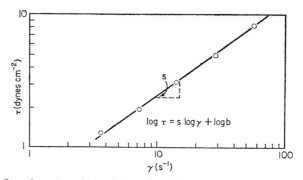

FIG. 10. Log–log plot of blood viscosity. (Adapted from Dintenfass, 1968a.)

This expression is derived by relating the stress required to break interparticle bonds and the number of bonds at any time on the assumption that doubling γ would halve the number of bonds that could reform.

However, (4.10) does not fit the flow rate-pressure relationship for blood over a wide range of shear rates (Charm et al., 1965). The methods for determining the yield stress are discussed later.

Casson (1958) derived a semi-empirical equation to describe the flow behavior of printing ink, and Reiner and Scott-Blair (1959) suggested its application to describe blood viscosity,

$$\tau^{\frac{1}{2}} = K\gamma^{\frac{1}{2}} + C^{\frac{1}{2}} \tag{4.11}$$

where: C = yield stress or shear strength of the suspension determined by extrapolation from above $1\,s^{-1}$

K = Casson "viscosity".

Casson's equation is based on the behavior of mutually attractive particles subjected to disruptive forces so that particle group size is a function of shear rate. In addition, the yield stress or shear strength of the suspension must be exceeded before the structure can be broken and flow initiated.

It has been shown that the shear stress-shear rate behavior of red cell suspensions may be expressed by this equation over a wide range of cell concentrations and shear rates (1–$100\,000\,s^{-1}$), see Fig. 10, (Charm and Kurland, 1962, 1965) and 0.1–$20\,s^{-1}$ (Merrill et al., 1964; Cokelet et al., 1963).

B. SUMMARY OF EQUATIONS DESCRIBING BLOOD SHEAR STRESS/ SHEAR RATE BEHAVIOR

Neither the power-law expression nor the Herschel-Bulkley equation may be used to express blood flow properties over more than two decades of shear rate. The Herschel-Bulkley equation had the added disadvantage of requiring three constants as compared with the power law or Casson equations which only require two.

The Casson equation appears to be the best for expressing the relationships of τ and γ for normal blood from the range of shear rates where the yield stress effects are prominent through the high shear rates where yield stress effects are negligible.

Below $1\,\mathrm{s}^{-1}$, shear-stress data may not follow Casson's equation as closely as above $1\,\mathrm{s}^{-1}$, (Merrill *et al.*, 1966), but this may be due to artifacts in low shear rate viscometry.

C. CASSON VISCOSITY, K, AND LIMITING APPARENT VISCOSITY, K^2

When the yield stress is very small compared with the shear stress, (4.11) reduces to that for a Newtonian fluid and K^2 becomes the limiting apparent viscosity or the equivalent of μ_s in (4.1). Thus,

$$K^2 = \frac{\mu_p}{1-\alpha\phi} \tag{4.12}$$

where: α is defined by (4.5). From (4.11) we have

$$K^2\gamma = C+\tau-2C^{\frac{1}{2}}\tau^{\frac{1}{2}} \tag{4.13}$$

and

$$\tau/\gamma = K^2 + \frac{2\tau^{\frac{1}{2}}C^{\frac{1}{2}} -C}{\gamma} \tag{4.14}$$

It can be seen that when the term involving C is small compared to K^2, the apparent viscosity τ/γ, is constant, and that this term becomes smaller as shear rate, γ, increases. When γ is small, this term becomes large compared to K^2 and the apparent viscosity increases. Thus, the change in apparent viscosity with shear rate is solely due to the yield stress associated with the aggregation of cells. When yield stress effects are absent, the suspension shear stress/shear rate relationship becomes that of a Newtonian fluid.

The term K^2 varies with temperature and concentration according to (4.12) where α has the relationship as shown in (4.5) or Fig. 8.

Another problem in the measurement of Casson viscosity in blood, arises from the fact that measurements with Couette viscometers and cone and plate viscometers do not agree. K^2 is 10 to 20 per cent less by cone and plate viscometry than with Couette viscometry. The reason for this is not known, (Charm and Kurland, 1968). This effect is not observed with plasma.

D. YIELD STRESS OF BLOOD

The yield stress or shear strength of blood is determined by the cell to cell contact and the cell aggregate structure (see Fig. 1).

The difficulty in measuring yield stress is due to the interaction of the

measuring instruments with the red cell structure. Little is actually understood of the detailed instrument—cell structure contact, and it is questionable
whether most direct measurements of blood yield stress are measurements
of the blood structure or the structure-instrument interface.

The methods employed for the measurement of yield stress are:

(1) *Extrapolation of $\tau^{\frac{1}{2}}$ vs. $\gamma^{\frac{1}{2}}$ plot to zero shear rate*

The intercept is the square root of the yield stress, (see (4.11) and Fig. 11).
Yield stresses obtained by extrapolation from $0 \cdot 1 \, s^{-1}$ to zero often do not
agree with extrapolation from $1 \, s^{-1}$. A 50 per cent difference in yield stress

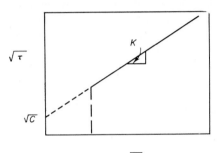

FIG. 11. Determination of blood yield stress by extrapolation.

may be expected between these two extrapolation methods (Cokelet *et al.*,
1963; Merrill *et al.*, 1966).

At finite shear rates, the shear stress is associated with suspension movement as well as the yield stress effect. In extrapolating to zero shear rate, it is
assumed that the relative effect of fluid motion on shear stress remains
constant. Hence, experiments with clay suspensions indicate that yield stress
depends on the shear pattern in the fluid, (Boardman and Whitmore, 1961).

At low shear rates the suspension may not remain uniform in the viscometer; rather it may be that two phases develop with a fluid phase at the
instrument interface. It has been observed that with very low shear rates
(e.g. $0.01 \, s^{-1}$) in blood, the $\tau^{\frac{1}{2}}$ vs. $\gamma^{\frac{1}{2}}$ curve extrapolates to the origin, and no
yield stress is evident. The effect has been observed in a Weissenberg Couette
and in the GDM viscometers, and is thought to be due to the development of a
plasma layer at the moving surface, (Chien *et al.*, 1966). A marginal plasma
layer has been observed in a GDM Couette viscometer, (Cokelet, 1963). It
has been proposed that the surfaces of the GDM viscometer be ruled with fine
grooves, to prevent the formation of two phases, but this does not appear to
help.

At low shear rates (below $0 \cdot 1 \, s^{-1}$) it has been shown that the cells in a cone and plate viscometer aggregate, "squeezing out" the plasma, (Schmid-Schönbein et al., 1968). All these effects point to the possibility of artifacts associated with low shear rate viscometry which can affect the determination of yield stress by extrapolation. To distinguish between yield stresses found from high shear rate (i.e. above $1\,s^{-1}$) and low shear rates by extrapolation, we should use C (applies to high shear rate) and τ_y (low or zero shear rate).

(2) Torque decay method

The torque decay method yields a direct measurement of blood yield stress, (Merrill et al., 1965a). The blood sample in the viscometer is stressed and allowed to come to rest, when the residual torque measures the yield stress. However, the torque reaches zero after some time and it is essential that the appropriate time for measurement be selected, i.e. when the residual torque has developed and the cell structure is still intact. Good agreement has been reported between this method and the low shear rate extrapolation method, (Merrill et al., 1965a).

(3) Pressure decay method

In principle this method is similar to the torque decay method except that a capillary tube viscometer is used together with a pressure transducer to measure the residual pressure after flow has stopped in a capillary tube. It is subject to the same problems as the torque decay method for the residual pressure may diminish rapidly to zero, because of structure breakdown or syneresis at the instrument wall. However, good agreement is reported between this method, the extrapolation method, and the torque decay method (Merrill et al., 1965a). In practice, pressure decay systems are much more difficult to operate than torque decay systems.

(4) Balance plate method

A plate immersed in a blood sample is attached to a sensitive balance. After gentle oscillation, the plate is allowed to come to rest, and the residual force acting on the plate is measured and related to the yield stress. Measurements of yield stress by this method give lower values than the torque or extrapolation methods, (Benis and Lacoste, 1968). For whole blood the yield stresses from Couette viscometry range between 0·015 and 0·05 dynes cm^{-2} while from the balance plate method the values are between 0·002 and 0·008 dynes cm^{-2}.

The repeatability of yield stress measurements by the plate method is 20 to 50 per cent. This lack of precision in yield stress measurements is thought to be due to the non-homogeneity of blood (Benis and Lacoste, 1968).

(5) Sedimentation in tapered tube

The sedimentation method for determining yield stress depends upon finding the tube diameter that just supports a column of structured cells and prevents settling, (Charm and Kurland, 1967). It assumes (as do all these methods except extrapolation), that the bonding between instrument and cells is stronger than that between cells.

In this method a microhematocrit tube is drawn to a taper and the blood sample is admitted through capillary action. The tube is taped to a microscope slide and held vertically for a few moments until the column of cells breaks. The diameter at the point of breaking, (yield diameter), is measured

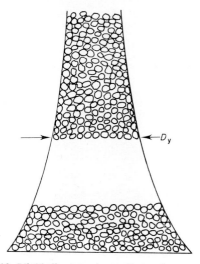

FIG. 12. Yield diameter in settling red suspension.

with a low power microscope (see Figs 12 and 13). The yield diameter is related to the yield stress in a tube with a small taper angle by,

$$\tau_y = G\phi(\rho_c - \rho_p)D_y/4 \cos \theta \qquad (4.15)$$

Where: τ_y = yield stress, (determined from shear-rates below $1 \, \text{s}^{-1}$, in this case at zero s^{-1})

G = gravitational constant, $980 \cdot 8 \, \text{cm} \, \text{s}^{-2}$

ρ_c = density of cells

ρ_p = density of plasma. (Cell and plasma density must be measured using a copper sulfate technique, Wintrobe, 1962)

D_y = diameter at point of break, cm

θ = taper angle, ($\cos \theta \cong 1$ for small angles).

In this case, it is possible to observe the cell-wall relationships at the time the cell column breaks. Before rupture of the column is complete there may be considerable disturbance in this region (Fig. 13).

This is the only method that permits direct observation of the cell structure as measurement is made. The time before the structure disintegrates com-

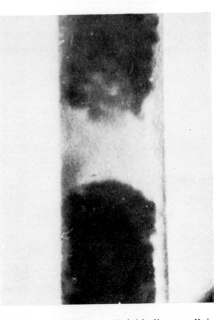

FIG. 13. Blood suspension breaking at "yield diameter" in section of vertical tapered settling tube ($\times 100$); note gap at wall in settling section.

pletely varies considerably. It is questionable whether one is measuring the strength of the cell to cell structure or of the cell to wall structure. Values of blood yield stress for this method are in the range of $0 \cdot 1$ to $0 \cdot 15$ dynes cm^{-2} and are generally in agreement with extrapolation of shear stress from above $1 \mathrm{s}^{-1}$ for data taken with a cone-plate viscometer but not with Couette viscometers, or values measured by balance plate or torque decay method; (differences between cone and plate and Couette blood viscometry were noted previously). The yield stress obtained by this method varies linearly with the hematocrit (Fig. 14), i.e. the yield diameter D_y is constant.

In summary, the yield stress of blood ranges between $0 \cdot 003$ and $0 \cdot 20$ dynes cm^{-2} depending on which method is employed for measurement. The extrapolation method using $\tau^{\frac{1}{2}}$ vs. $\gamma^{\frac{1}{2}}$ is probably the most nearly correct,

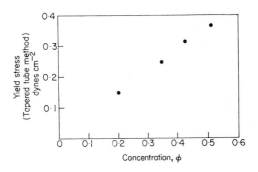

Fig. 14. Variation of yield stress by tapered tube method as function of cell volume fraction (25 °C).

although with measurements at low shear rates (below $1 s^{-1}$) artifacts may occur. Extrapolation from high shear rates has less precision because of the greater extrapolation, but avoids these low shear rate artifacts. There is no agreement as to which method is the most accurate.

5. FACTORS AFFECTING FLOW PROPERTIES OF BLOOD

A. RED CELL FLEXIBILITY

It has been suggested that cell flexibility is one of the factors influencing blood viscosity particularly at high hematocrits. Thus suspensions of cells made inelastic with acetaldehyde exhibit Newtonian properties at low shear rates, whereas normal cells do not, (Chien et al., 1967). Furthermore, at high shear rates (about $50 s^{-1}$), hardened cells show a "shear thickening" effect while normal cells exhibit "shear thinning" behavior, (Chien et al., 1969; Dintenfass, 1965; Chien et al., 1970).

Cell rigidity is related to the characteristics of the cell contents as well as the cell membrane. The cell membrane is capable of moving around the cell contents much as a tank tread would move around the wheels, (Schmid-Schönbein and Wells, 1969). The evidence for this lies in the fact that packed cells possess a viscosity much lower than would be expected, (Dintenfass, 1968a); in this case, the viscosity of the cell contents, i.e. hemoglobin, is the controlling viscosity factor.

Cells deform into prolate ellipsoids and the membrane rotates around the cell contents at shear stresses of $5 \, dynes \, cm^{-2}$ and above. Schmid-Schobein et al. (1969) showed that the deformation increases with increasing shear rate as shown by the Rumscheidt equation, (Rumscheidt and Mason, 1961).

$$D = \frac{L - B}{L + B} = \frac{\gamma_s r_c \mu_p}{\sigma} \frac{(19 \mu_p/\mu_i) + 16}{(16 \mu_p/\mu_i) + 16} \qquad (5.1)$$

where: γ_s = rate of shear

L = length and

B = breadth of ellipsoid

μ_p = viscosity of continuous medium

μ = internal viscosity

σ = interfacial tension (plasma-RBC)

r_c = cell radius.

The internal viscosity of red cells has been calculated to range between 1 and 6 cP, (Dintenfass, 1968a, b). This estimate includes cell membrane effects as well as hemoglobin viscosity.

This movement of the cell membrane around the cell contents is the mechanism by which red cells adopt themselves to flow. Hemoglobin is subjected to shear, the cell assumes the properties of a fluid drop and whole blood thus behaves as an emulsion rather than a suspension.

In pathological states, deformability may be reduced, due either to membrane defects or hemoglobin abnormality. Abnormal molecular interactions with reciprocal binding of cellular constituents represent the basic mechanism responsible for increased red cell rigidity. Intracellular reduced glutathione reduces the interactions and is the primary protective agent against loss of cell deformability. A lowered intracellular ATP level allows the formation of calcium bridges between cell constituents causing increased cell rigidity, (Teitel, 1969), and it has been shown that fresh red cells are more flexible than stored cells (Sirs, 1968). The higher viscosity associated with old stored cells might be influenced by the increased rigidity of the older cells, (Usami et al., 1969). This may be associated with change in the charge on older cells, but the effect of surface charges on cell deformability is not clear, (Danon et al., 1969).

Osmotic pressure also influences cell deformability either by changing the internal viscosity of hemoglobin or making the cell membrane more rigid. Surfactants appear to affect cell rigidity and thereby influence viscosity. Sodium oleate lowered blood viscosity in concentrations of 20–40 mg per 100 ml but raised it at 60 mg per 100 ml because of the membrane stiffening it caused, (Ehrly, 1968). Not only does cell deformability affect viscosity directly, but it may also affect plasma flow patterns between cells and their boundary layers. The flow of a rigid cell model past a stationary one has a marked effect on fluid energy loss, (Bugliarello et al., 1969).

In none of the equations presented previously for estimating blood viscosity at high shear-rates has a term for cell rigidity been included. These empirical equations were determined with normal blood where the influence of cell deformability is relatively constant. However, diseased states which affect cell flexibility would cause substantial errors in estimating blood viscosity, for example, with (4.1). Cell flexibility influences blood flow primarily through the value of α.

Cell deformability has been measured by three methods:

(a) Viscometry of a packed red cell mass.
(b) Rate of packing of a red cell column during centrifugation.
(c) Passage through polycarbonate seives.

All of these methods are indirect, difficult to analyse and influenced by factors other than those involving flexibility. For example, the plasma trapped between cells interferes with the measurement of flexibility by viscometric methods, (Jacobs, 1963; Thomas and James, 1966; Johnson, 1969).

In the centrifugal packing method, the compression of cells during centrifugation is due to the weight of the packed cells pressing down on one another. As trapped plasma is completely eliminated between the cells, the density of the column and consequently the total pressure acting on the cells is increased. However, osmotic action immediately releases water into the extracellular space. Thus, the compression force is determined by a number of factors; height of cell column, density difference between cells and plasma, centrifugal force and time applied, (Sirs, 1968). A centrifugally packed column of hardened cells appears to contain only 60 per cent of the plasma contained in normal packed cells, (Chien et al., 1968).

Measurement of cell deformability by passage through polycarbonate sieves probably lends itself to analysis more readily than other methods; however, although increases in the viscosity of cells hardened by acetaldehyde occur within 2 to 3 h, no change in flexibility is observed by the centrifugal packing method or passage through sieves for 12 h (Chien et al., 1969), which suggests the viscometric method may be the most sensitive.

B. PLASMA FACTORS

Aggregation of red cells is reflected in the yield stress. The cell aggregating capacity of plasma increases with increasing protein concentration, and it has been suggested that fibrinogen is the principal plasma protein affecting cell aggregation, (Merrill et al., 1963c). Fibrinogen shows 19 times the specific aggregating activity of normal plasma, (Hint and Arbors, 1969), and the flow properties of blood are improved by destroying fibrinogen with streptokinase, (Ehrly, 1969). Fibrinogen added to cells has less aggregating effect than does native fibrinogen, and type A cells are more affected than type 0 cells.

It has been proposed that the aggregating effect of fibrinogen is caused by the fibrinogen molecule being absorbed "end on" into crater like sites on the surface of the cell at one of its terminal ball shaped elements; the other terminal ball of the molecule is projected outward for subsequent engagement with an absorbing site on the membrane of neighboring cell (Merrill et al., 1966).

Fibrinogen added to cells in saline also produces increased aggregation. Merrill *et al.* (1965b) suggested an equation for calculating τ_y, (the yield stress determined at shear-rates below $1\,s^{-1}$).

$$\tau_y^{\frac{1}{2}} = 0.36\,B\left[\left(\frac{1}{1-\phi}\right)-1\right] \tag{5.2}$$

Where: B = function of fibrinogen concentration (see Table 2). This equation has been found to apply up to $\phi = 0.80$, (Chien *et al.*, 1966). It also agrees with yield stress values determined in a GDM Couette viscometer, but not the cone and plate viscometer.

TABLE 2

B as a function of fibrinogen concentration (Merrill *et al.*, 1965b, see (5.2))

B	Fibrinogen, g per 100 ml (plasma + ACD solution)
0·894	0·21
0·875	0·21
0·940	0·24
0·930	0·24
1·01	0·27
1·05	0·28
1·10	0·35
1·09	8·36
1·18	0·46

Red cells in serum, i.e. with no fibrinogen present, also possess a yield stress when measured in a GDM viscometer, (Chien *et al.*, 1966), although in this case it is about half that measured for cells in plasma. Minute amounts of fibrinogen—fibrin complexes lead to a dramatic increase in yield stress, (Copley *et al.*, 1967). At sufficiently high concentrations, cells in saline also show a low but definite yield stress, (Chien *et al.*, 1966).

Wells (1965) used a GDM viscometer to investigate the effect of plasma albumin, fibrinogen and globulin on blood viscosity between shear rates of 0.1 and $20\,s^{-1}$. He noted that albumin tends to decrease cell aggregation, possibly because of its strong negative charge. Fibrinogen, which has a neutral charge and is a much longer molecule than albumin, has the greatest influence in promoting cell aggregation. Globulin is also found to increase cell aggregation, but not as strongly as fibrinogen.

The importance of factors other than fibrinogen has been further investigated by Wells *et al.* (1969), who used torque decay as well as extrapolation methods to show that red cell aggregates and a finite yield stress exist in pathological sera, (all clottable proteins removed). Globulin had the most profound effect on blood viscosity, and albumin the least effect. With direct examination of flow in the bulbar conjunctiva, it is found that the relation between plasma protein levels and cell aggregation *in vivo* is considerably less predictable than that of red cell suspensions *in vitro*.

There are species differences in the hemorheological effects of serum globulins. For example, the elephant has a higher concentration of beta-2 globulin which may be similar to fibrinogen in its ability to cause rouleaux formation, (Chien *et al.*, 1969). Other plasma proteins in saline have about the same effect on cells as does saline, i.e. cell aggregation is minimal, (Merrill *et al.*, 1966).

C. EFFECTS OF OSMOTIC PRESSURE

Cell elasticity and cell shape both influence blood viscosity. The osmotic pressure difference across a red cell membrane determines to a large extent its shape, size and elasticity. It is, therefore, not surprising to find that changes in osmotic pressure will cause changes in blood viscosity.

Meiselman *et al.* (1967), measured the τ/γ relationship of red cells in hypotonic and hypertonic solutions using a GDM viscometer. In solutions with equal numbers of red cells the yield stress of the suspension increased and viscosity decreased as the solution varied from hypertonic to hypotonic. Although the number of red cells remained constant, the hematocrit varied from 34·8 at 381 mosm kg^{-1} to 72·7 at 276 mosm kg^{-1}. The increase in yield stress with increasing hematocrit could be expected, but not the decrease in viscosity with increasing hematocrit.

In a study of the mechanical properties of red cells, the erythrocyte membrane in 1·2 per cent NaCl solution (hypertonic) was found to be less resistant to deformation with only slight resistance to bending, (Rand and Burton, 1964). However, cells in isotonic or hypotonic saline (0·6 per cent NaCl) appear to have identical membrane properties, being much more rigid than those in hypertonic saline. From these observations, it seems that a hypertonic red cell suspension should have a lower apparent viscosity than either an isotonic or hypotonic suspension. This contradicts the results of Meiselman *et al.* (1967), who suggest that the differences are due to the removal of proteins and lipoproteins from saline washed membranes, which would also affect membrane characteristics.

The red cell sedimentation rate is increased in hypotonic solutions. This may be due to the increased tendency of red cells to aggregate as shown by the increased yield stress in hypotonic solutions mentioned previously. The viscosity of blood cells in hypertonic solutions, measured with an Ostwald viscometer, varies with osmolarity; for example, at 300 mosm kg^{-1} the apparent viscosity at 37°C was 1·5 cP and at 1500 mosm kg^{-1} it was 3·8 cP. It is suggested that this increase is due to an increased tendency to form a gel-like red cell aggregate, (Wells, 1968).

The increase in viscosity found by Wells is in agreement with Meiselman *et al.* (1967); however, the latter found a lower yield stress in hypertonic solutions and thus a decrease in aggregation as compared with hyptonic solutions.

The variation in cell volume with tonicity is given by Ponder (1940), as:

$$\frac{V_c}{V_{iso}} = RW[T^{-1} - 1] + 1 \qquad (5.3)$$

Where: V_c = new volume of cells

V_{iso} = volume of cells in an isotonic medium

W = the volume fraction of water in cells, generally 0·7

T = ratio of the osmolarity of the medium to that of an isotonic (0·9 per cent) NaCl solution

R = a correction factor for the non-ideal osmotic behavior of the solute—generally, R varies from 0·9 to 1·02.

From Meiselman's study, where the number of red cells was constant, the hematocrit varied with tonicity as follows: Osmolarity 276, 300, 329 and 381 mosm kg^{-2}; hematocrit 42·7, 40·1, 38·0 and 34·2, respectively. Using (5.3) with $R = 1$ and with the hematocrit at 276 mosm kg^{-1} as a standard, it is calculated that for 300 mosm kg^{-1} $H = 40·1$, and for 381 mosm kg^{-1}, $H = 34·2$. Thus Ponder's equation closely agrees with Meiselman's data and is suitable for predicting cell volume changes as a function of tonicity which in turn influences viscosity and yield stress changes as described previously.

Packed cells from hypotonic saline show a greater viscosity than normal packed cells, but crenated packed cells from hypertonic solutions show a still greater viscosity than either normal or hypertonic packed cells, (Dintenfass, 1964a).

D. EFFECTS OF ANTICOAGULANTS

The viscosity of blood with no anticoagulant remains constant at low shear-rates for two to four minutes after removal from the circulation, (Dintenfass, 1964b). Clotting starts after varying time intervals, depending not only on the intrinsic properties of the particular blood sample, but also on the shear rate used.

Blood containing citrate as an anticoagulant possesses a slightly higher apparent viscosity than blood with no anticoagulant, while the use of heparin results in a slightly lower apparent viscosity.

Rosenblum (1968), groups anticoagulants into two groups: those which shrink erythrocytes (citrate and oxalate) and those having no effect on cell size or shape (heparin, ethylene diamino tetra-acetic acid (EDTA), and acid-citrate-dextrose (ACD). Although cells shrink in citrate they do not in ACD). Accordingly the first group of anticoagulants increase viscosity, even though citrate reduces hematocrit, while those in the second group have no effect. Blood in ACD can be maintained for two days at 4°C with no change in viscosity, but the viscosity of blood in potassium oxalate changes in 2 or 3 hrs. However, blood in "balanced" oxalate, i.e. ammonium oxalate and potassium oxalate mixture, (Wintrobe, 1962), and heparinized blood is stable for one to two days at 4°C. The amounts added are critical.

Frasher et al. (1967) prepared an external arterio-venous shunt in dogs which was used as tube viscometer. The infusion of heparin caused no change in the apparent viscosity of blood. Nor do heparin or sodium EDTA alter blood viscosity as determined by a cone and plate viscometer, (Galluzzi et al., 1964), but this study did not consider storage effects. Potassium oxalate in a concentration of $2·5\,mg\,ml^{-1}$ decreased blood viscosity while heparin did not (Mayer and Kiss, 1965). It appears that conflicting results have been reported, possibly this is due to insufficient care given to the amount of anticoagulant added. In our laboratory the balanced oxalate, (Wintrobe, 1962), has been used with no changes for up to two days.

E. EFFECTS OF DEXTRAN

Although dextran is not a natural component of blood its widespread use to influence the flow properties of blood merit some discussion. Thorsen and Hint (1960) used dextrans of various molecular weights to show that cell aggregation and sedimentation is directly related to the molecular weight of plasma colloids. However, failure to appreciate the osmotic effects of the dextrans affects the original interpretations of these in vivo studies. Low molecular weight dextran (Rheomadrodex) is said to counteract disturbances in the flow properties of blood, (Gelin and Thorsen, 1961). High molecular weight dextran ($M > 80000$) increases the aggregation of red cells and low molecular dextran causes disaggregation (Bergentz et al., 1965). Both low molecular weight dextran (M 40 000, dextran 40) and high molecular weight dextran increase the electronegativity of red cells. Low molecular weight dextran causes a decrease in cell aggregation by dilution of plasma rather than by an effect on the cells (Groth, 1965; Wells, 1968). Cell aggregation is often measured by sedimentation or by a turbidometric method (e.g. Engeset et al., 1967a, b).

Both the low shear-rate Couette viscometer (GDM) and the capillary tube viscometer show that dextrans of molecular weight above 40000 increase red cell aggregation, and that all dextrans increase blood viscosity when compared with saline controls, (Meiselman and Merrill, 1968). Furthermore, no flow improvement was evident with low molecular weight dextran. It was also suggested that disaggregation might occur when suspensions previously aggregated with high molecular weight dextran ($M = 110000$) were treated with the lower molecular weight series. Infusion into humans of 10 per cent albumin or dextran 40 decreased the hematocrit, the erythrocyte aggregation, measured by sedimentation, and blood viscosity by about the same extent, (Groth, 1965).

In rabbits, dextran 40 resulted in an increased blood flow velocity, possibly due to a dilutional decrease in blood viscosity, by more than that expected from simple increase in circulatory volume. It had no effect *in vitro* on the aggregation of rabbit red cells, but counteracted intravascular aggregation by increasing the speed of circulation (Engeset *et al.*, 1967a, b).

Dextran 40 added to saline suspensions of erythrocytes increased the zeta potential (the charge difference between the diffuse, movable charge layer surrounding a particle and the bulk of the fluid), implying an increase in the electrostatic forces of repulsion acting between cells in such a suspension, (Brooks and Seaman, 1969). The mechanism of this is not clear, for the uncharged dextran molecules could not increase the negative electrokinetic charge of the cells. One possible explanation proposed by Brooks and Seaman is based on the high dielectric constant of the dextran solution. Increased electrostatic repulsion between cells, whatever the cause, reduces contacts somewhat and results in a decrease of the low shear-rate viscosity of the suspension, (Eisler and Atwater, 1963).

In summary, the effect of low molecular weight dextran appears to be due primarily to plasma dilution. In some cases dextran 40 appears to possess a specific cell dispersing property. However, it is largely through the dilution effect that the aggregation of cells and thus the blood viscosity is reduced. There is, however, no explanation as to why high molecular weight dextran increases cell aggregation. Gelin *et al.* (1968) and Engeset *et al.* (1967a) disagree with Meiselman and Merrill (1968), and find that the intravascular aggregation of human and dog red blood cells caused by high molecular weight dextran can be reversed by low molecular weight dextran.

Another starch derivative used as a plasma substitute, hydroxyethyl starch, has been compared with dextran, and it appears that low molecular weight HES is a very suitable substitute for plasma from viscosity considerations, as well as possessing suitable colloidal activity, (Cerny *et al.*, 1968).

F. EFFECTS OF OTHER CELL COMPONENTS

Platelets and white cells normally have little influence on blood viscosity. Although platelet adhesion plays an important role in clotting and seems to occupy a key position in thrombus formation, platelets are present in such a small volume fraction compared to red cells that they exert little influence on blood viscosity. However, when red and white cells are removed, the strong attraction platelets have for each other may be noted, (Swank, 1959).

In certain diseases there is a large increase in white cells. Under these circumstances the white cells appear to have the same effect on blood viscosity as red cells. In some cases, the increase in white cells is associated with a reduced number of red cells, so that the total cell volume fraction is still in the normal range and so is the apparent viscosity of blood and the yield stress. However, a suspension of white cells has a higher viscosity and yield stress than the same volume fraction of red cells, (Steinberg and Charm, 1971).

6. BLOOD FLOW AND VISCOSITY

A. POISEUILLE'S EQUATION

Poiseuille was the first to determine experimentally the correct relationship between flow rate, pressure, and tube radius, R_w. From his experiments in which blood serum and water were passed through fine bore tubes he suggested that flow rate varied as $R_w^{4\cdot2}$.

However, Hagenbach (1860) considering a homogenous, Newtonian fluid in a straight circular tube derived the expression

$$Q = \frac{\pi P R_w^{4\cdot0}}{8\mu L} \tag{6.1}$$

where P/L is the pressure gradient along the tube and Q is the volume flow rate.

This was actually the first time the viscosity coefficient, μ, was defined and recognized as a fluid property.

The simplicity of Poiseuille's equation has made it attractive, but as blood is a suspension, it does not always behave as Newtonian fluid; this can be seen from its shear stress-shear rate relationship.

Thus, red cells may aggregate together and flow as clumps which is most likely to occur at low flow rates. At high flow rates, cells may migrate away from the wall, leaving a cell poor plasma layer there which leads to further deviations from (6.1).

Nevertheless, estimates of blood flow by Poiseuille's equation are within 50 per cent of that observed experimentally. It applies exactly where yield stress effects are negligible and there is no marginal layer, and with tube diameters $> 0\cdot0500$ cm, i.e. when $PR_w/2L \gg C$.

Equations similar to Poiseuille's have been derived for blood which take into account yield stress effects for a fluid which obeys Casson's equation, (4.11).

$$\frac{32\,K^2}{D\bar{V}\rho} = \frac{PD}{\bar{V}^2\rho L} - \frac{16}{3}\frac{C}{\bar{V}^2\rho}\left[\frac{12}{7}\left(\frac{PD}{2LC}\right)^{\frac{1}{2}} - 1\right] \tag{6.2}$$

where: $\bar{V}$ = average velocity
D = diameter.

When yield stress effects are negligible, this reduces to the equivalent of Poiseuille's equation; in general when $C/\overline{V}^2\rho$ is greater than 10^{-2}, there is no development of a marginal plasma layer, and (6.2) applies.

B. NON-UNIFORM CELL DISTRIBUTION AND THE MARGINAL PLASMA LAYER

As the blood flow rate increases, it is postulated that the cells distribute themselves so that there is a higher concentration nearer the axis than at the wall. This non-uniform distribution is sometimes approximated by assuming there is a marginal layer of plasma. Although only an approximation, it does permit a convenient method for calculating pressure losses and flow rates under these conditions. The velocity profile for blood in the presence of a marginal layer is shown in Fig. 15.

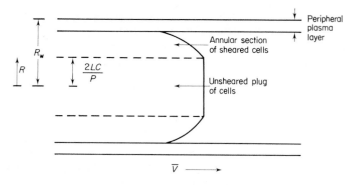

FIG. 15. Velocity profile in presence of marginal layer and yield stress effect.

The relationship between flow rate and pressure drop is given by:

$$\frac{32\,K_1^2}{D\overline{V}\rho} = \frac{PD}{\overline{V}^2\rho L}\left[\frac{1-\Delta^4}{1-\alpha\phi_1}+\Delta^4\right] + \frac{C_1\Delta^3}{\overline{V}^2\rho}\left[\frac{16}{3}-\frac{32}{7}\left(\frac{PD}{C_1L}\Delta\right)^{\frac{1}{2}}\right] \quad (6.3)$$

where $\Delta = 1-(2\delta/D)$ and where $\delta = $ width of plasma zone and K_1^2, ϕ_1, C_1 refer to the core viscosity, cell concentration and yield stress. As a first approximation these may be considered to be the same as that in the reservoir provided the marginal gap is not more than 10 per cent of the radius.

Knowing ϕ_1, it is possible to estimate K_1 and C_1. The concentration of cells in the core is found from $Q\phi = Q_1\phi_1$ where Q_1 is the flow rate of the core, and Q the flow rate in the reservoir or total flow rate. Also $Q = Q_1+Q_g$ where Q_g is the plasma flow rate in the marginal layer (Fig. 15) which may be shown to be:

$$Q_g = \frac{\pi P}{2\mu_p L}\left[\frac{R_w^2}{2} - \frac{(R_w-\delta)^2}{2}\right]^2 \tag{6.4}$$

where μ_p = plasma viscosity.

By calculating Q_g, ϕ_1 may be determined along with the other properties of the core. In order to calculate Q_g it is necessary first to measure the gap width.

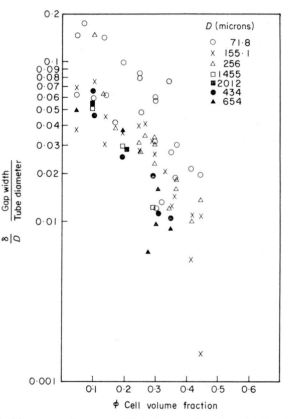

FIG. 16. Limiting or maximum gap/diameter as a function of cell volume fraction and tube diameter. (Charm *et al.*, 1968.)

Figure 16 shows δ/D for fully developed marginal layers as a function of tube diameter and cell volume fraction. The marginal layer is fully developed when $C/\bar{V}^2\rho$ is less than 5×10^{-4}, (Charm, *et al.*, 1968). When $C/\bar{V}^2\rho$ is greater than 5×10^{-4} but less than 10^{-2}, the marginal plasma layer width is a function of velocity.

C. CELL DISTRIBUTION AT BRANCHES

When a non-uniform distribution of cells exists at a branch or vessel junction, the flow entering the branch will generally be of lower hematocrit than flow in the main vessel downstream from the branch. The conditions determining the flow and hematocrit in the branch are the cell distribution, branch angle and the pressure drops along the branch and the downstream section of the main vessel.

Flow into a branch is drawn asymetrically from the parent vessel. The cell distribution in the parent vessel determines the cell concentration and thus the viscosity and flow rate in the branch. If a system consisting of a parent vessel and a branch, with both downstream ends at the same pressure is considered the flow rate must be that in which the pressure loss in the branch is equal to the pressure loss in the main vessel below the junction.

The distribution of cells in a parent vessel was studied by observing the change in hematocrit when blood was withdrawn into a branch at different flow rates from a rectangular main section $35 \mu m$ deep and $25000 \mu m$, wide (Palmer, 1965a, b). It was possible to adapt the cell distribution found in the rectangular tube to circular tubes and use this in calculations of branch flow (Charm, 1969). The flow of blood in branched circular channels (diameter 110 to $500 \mu m$) was observed to be severely disturbed at the entrance to the branch where the branch angles were $90°$ (Gelin, 1964).

A calculation using Palmer's cell distribution results with Gelin's data for a $110 \mu m$ branching system, with a reservoir hematocrit of 40, agreed with experimental data to within 10 per cent (Charm, 1969). This calculation neglected the effect of branch angle and entrance disturbances, suggesting that at such small diameters these have little effect. However, there is little experimental data available on branch flow in small tubes. The information required for the calculation, is the geometry, flow rate and hematocrit in the parent vessel, the pressure at the entrance and at the end of both vessels, plasma viscosity, and blood yield stress. It remains to be seen whether irregularities in a vessel, particularly near the mouth of the branch, cause sufficient changes in the cell distribution to alter conditions in the branch.

D. FÅHRAEUS-LINDQVIST OR SIGMA EFFECT

One of the most controversial subjects in blood flow analysis centers around the phenomenon that the apparent viscosity of blood computed from Poiseuille's equation, decreases with tube diameter when D is less than $150 \mu m$, (see Fig. 17). This behavior was reported by Fåhraeus and Lindqvist (1931) who studied blood suspensions, and by Dix and Scott-Blair (1940) who studied clay suspensions and referred to it as the Sigma effect.

The effect is controversial because certain investigators who have studied it conclude that Fåhraeus and Lindqvist merely did not recognize that the apparent viscosity of blood varies with shear-rate, and were measuring this change in viscosity rather than a change due to tube diameter *per se*, e.g. Mayer (1965). Other investigators have failed to find the effect in pressure-flow rate data for blood and have failed also to observe a marginal layer by

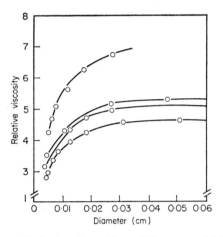

FIG. 17. Fåhraeus–Lindqvist effect. (From Fåhraeus and Lindqvist, 1931.)

direct microscopic observation (Merrill *et al.*, 1965a). However, it was pre-viously pointed out that at sufficiently low flow rates no marginal layer develops, while at higher flow rates it may, which may explain why the effect has not been observed in some cases.

The evidence in favor of a marginal layer or a cell distribution causing a dearth of cells at the wall seems overwhelming, (e.g. Fåhraeus and Lindqvist, 1931; Bugliarello *et al.*, 1965; Charm and Kurland, 1962; Thomas, 1962; Blackshear *et al.*, 1969). The observation that cells lead plasma in the circula-tion has also been explained on the basis of axial cell migration and a peri-pheral marginal layer, (Rowlands *et al.*, 1965; Thomas *et al.*, 1965).

Goldsmith and Mason (1964) and Chaffey *et al.* (1965) in model experiments observed that axial migration exists in the case of fluid drops but not with rigid particles. They also note that since erythrocytes are deformable they are analogous to fluid drops in this respect.

Cokelet (1967) analyzing the data of Fåhraeus and Lindqvist concluded that an entrance effect which reduced the main concentration of cells in the tube, could account for a change in viscosity with tube diameter. This model assumes a uniform distribution of cells in the tube and thus the absence of a marginal layer. It doesn't explain why a high cell concentration, e.g. $\phi = 0 \cdot 45$ does not result in a significant reduction of apparent viscosity in a 500 μm tube, while a low concentration, e.g. $\phi = 0.20$, does. This can be seen in Fig. 16 where the calculated gap widths are indirectly a measure of reduction in apparent viscosity. It has been observed that even at 20 μm from the entrance of a capillary tube, axial accumulations amount to about 15 per cent of the maximum (Palmer, 1969).

The reason why cells migrate away from the vessel wall under certain conditions is not yet known. However, the Fåhraeus-Lindqvist effect is due to calculating apparent viscosity from Poiseuilles equation and forcing into it pressure-flow rate information obtained in the presence of a marginal layer or its equivalent in cell distribution.

7. BLOOD FLOW PATTERNS *in vivo*

A method for measuring the velocity of fast-moving cells in blood vessels was proposed by Basler (1918). A segment of the vessel is framed by a slit oriented parallel to the direction of flow and film is run at a constant speed at right angles to the direction of flow. The moving cell photographs as a streak whose angle is related to the cell velocity. For example, a cell moving at the same apparent speed as the film produces an angle of 45°.

Monro (1964; 1965), applied this principle in an optical system which has the advantage of an immediate readout of linear velocity. His modification consisted of a rotating prism set at a right angle to the direction of flow in place of the slit. The speed of the prism is then measured with a tachometer.

In rabbit vessels, 12 to 20 μm in diameter, cells travel 0·1 to 0·5 cms^{-1} (Monro, 1965). The narrow column of cells is surrounded by a relatively wide zone of cell-free plasma. There is a rhythmical change in the blood velocity in an arteriole but this has a much longer periodicity than the pulse rate, between 10 and 30 s depending on the level of autonomic tone. Rabbit vessels of this size showed intermittent increases in cell concentration followed by cell-free plasma columns.

Intermittent corpuscular flow in rat capillaries was also noted by Palmer (1959), and a similar grouping tendency of mammalian red cells in arterioles was seen in the high speed photographs of Bloch (1962). Two hypothesis which have been offered to explain the intermittent nature of flow involve the rigidity of red cells or the presence of small aggregates. As cell aggregates pass into finer arterioles, the red cells become deformed and the diameter of the plastic masses may be reduced to less than the diameter of the red cell at rest. A flexible cell mass should move faster while a rigid mass or cell will travel more slowly and cause the more flexible ones to collect behind it (Whitmore, 1968). This may account in part for the intermittent concentration of cells observed. Palmer (1959), considered that leucocyte plugging in capillaries may also have the same effect.

By the method of Monro, the mean arterial velocity in rabbit mesentery was found to be $0.6\,\mathrm{cm\,s^{-1}}$ and in 30 to $70\,\mu\mathrm{m}$ vessels $0.36\,\mathrm{cm\,s^{-1}}$. The mean velocity in hamseter cheek pouch arterioles, averaging $34\,\mu\mathrm{m}$ in diameter, was $0.44\,\mathrm{cm\,s^{-1}}$; and in venules 24 to $74\,\mu\mathrm{m}$ in diameter the average velocity was $0.26\,\mathrm{cm\,s^{-1}}$.

Another method of measuring velocity profiles in vessels of 30 to $120\,\mu\mathrm{m}$ internal diameter is through a modification of the photometric double slit method for measuring erythrocyte velocities in capillaries (Wayland and Johnson, 1967). Two photo transistors are mounted on a screen onto which the image of the tube or vessel is projected and signals associated with the passage of red cell images are obtained. The small size allows one to make simultaneous measurements in different radial positions across the same vessel to give a velocity profile. Measurements made in vessels up to $70\,\mu\mathrm{m}$ in diameter in the cat mesentery show midline velocities of up to $3\,\mathrm{cm\,s^{-1}}$ in arterioles, and $0.6\,\mathrm{cm\,s^{-1}}$ in venules. Pulsatile flow is often observed both in arterioles and venules, (Gaehtgens et al., 1969).

Table 3 shows a typical relationship between velocity and distance from the axis in a $60\,\mu\mathrm{m}$ vessel in a hamster as measured with an instrument similar to Monro's (Berman and Fuhror, 1966).

TABLE 3

Velocity vs. distance from center, R, in 60 μm hamster vessel.
$\phi = 0.29$, $K^2 = 0.0164$ poises, $T = 37°C$, $\mu_\mathrm{p} = 0.011$ poise

R (μm)	V (cm s^{-1})
0·0	0·36
10	0·29
20	0·20
30	0·12

The viscosity term K^2 was determined experimentally in a $500\,\mu\mathrm{m}$ tube viscometer and checked by calculation using (2.1) and (4.11). It is possible from this type of velocity profile information to determine the pressure drop per unit length in the vessel and the shear rate at the vessel wall. To illustrate this, take the data in Table 3. The slope of V vs. R at some point can be determined, e.g. at $R = 20 \times 10^{-4}\,\mathrm{cm}$, $-\mathrm{d}V/\mathrm{d}R$ (the shear rate) is $90\,\mathrm{s^{-1}}$. The shear stress at that point may be estimated since $\tau/\gamma = K^2$ in the absence of a yield stress. Thus, $\tau/\gamma = 0.0164$ poises or $= 1.48\,\mathrm{dynes\,cm^{-2}}$. (This stress is about 20 times greater than the yield stress for $\phi = 0.29$, and the assumption that yield stress may be neglected is reasonable). The pressure gradient may be calculated using (2.1) and is $1.48 = (P/L)\ 20 \times 10^{-4}/2$, i.e.

$P/L = 1{\cdot}48 \times 10^2$ dynes cm^{-2}. The pressure gradient is the same at the wall and the shear stress at the vessel wall is $\tau_w = 1{\cdot}48 \times 10^3 .(30 \times 10^{-4})/2$, i.e. $2{\cdot}2$ dynes cm^{-2}.

Since there is probably a layer of plasma at the wall with a viscosity of about $0{\cdot}011$ poises, the shear rate at wall γ_w, is $\tau_w \rho_p = 2{\cdot}2/0{\cdot}011 = 200\,\text{s}^{-1}$.

If the fluid flowing in the vessel were Newtonian and followed Poiseuille's equation, the flow rate in the vessel would be $2{\cdot}87 \times 10^{-6}$ cm^3 s^{-1}, using the viscosity of whole blood with uniform cell distribution, and the average velocity would be $0{\cdot}103$ cm s^{-1}. This value is less than any of the point velocities in Table 3. Consequently, it appears that Poiseuille's equation does not apply and a uniform distribution of cells does not exist. If plasma viscosity is used instead of blood viscosity, the average velocity is about $0{\cdot}15$ cm s^{-1}, which is more reasonable.

The shear rate at the wall for a fluid in Poiseuille flow may also be found from $\gamma_w = 8\bar{V}/D$. Using a velocity of $0{\cdot}15$ cm s^{-1}, the shear rate at the wall is $(8 \times 0{\cdot}15)/60 \times 10^{-4} = 200\,\text{s}^{-1}$. This is in close agreement with the shear rate calculated from the slope of the experimental velocity profiles. The development of a marginal layer of plasma at the wall diminishes the effect of blood viscosity and would account for the increased flow rate over that predicted by Poiseuille's equation.

Estimates of wall shear rates in various vessels in man appear in Table 4. In large vessels, wall shear rates range between 100 to 200 s^{-1}, and in small vessels between 800 to 8000 s^{-1}. By freezing flowing cells in the vessels of a rabbit, it was observed that cells near the wall were preferentially oriented (Phibbs, 1967). This orientation probably influences or is due to the formation of a marginal plasma layer, and might influence cells entering branches.

TABLE 4

Estimates of wall shear rate in various vessels in man $\gamma_w = 8\bar{V}/D$

Vessel	Average velocity* (cm s^{-1})	Diameter† (cm)	γ_w (s^{-1})
Aorta	48	2·5	155
Artery	45	0·4	900
Arteriole	5	0·005	8000
Capillary	0·1	0·0008	1000
Venule	0·2	0·002	800
Vein	10	0·5	160
Vena cava	38	3·0	100

* Taken from Berne and Levy, 1967.
† Taken from Burton, 1965.

Both a marginal plasma layer and radial cell distribution were seen and the marginal layer widths observed by this method compare well with those shown in Fig. 16 (Phibbs, 1967).

There are thus several lines of evidence which lead to the conclusion that blood flow in tubes does not follow a perfect pattern of even streamlines and uniformly distributed cell concentration but rather, that at the wall of the vessel, there is a layer of decreased concentration or a plasma gap.

8. FLOW IN CAPILLARIES

Blood viscosity has no significance when considering capillary flow. Here the cell diameter is of the same order of magnitude as the vessel through which it is passing. In the analysis of capillary flow, the factors influencing flow rate and pressure loss along the capillary include, plasma viscosity, flexibility or elasticity of cells, elasticity and thickness of capillary wall, osmotic pressure in surrounding tissue and plasma, length of cell columns and pore diameter in capillary wall. These will be discussed in Chapter 16.

9. *In vitro* and *in vivo* RHEOLOGY

In vitro μm rheology has been extensively explored. However, there is a serious question about its application to *in vivo* systems. Qualitatively the indications are that it applies. However, the few quantitative attempts made to relate *in vitro* μm with *in vivo* rheology have generally failed. Take, for example, Whittaker and Winton's (1933) experiment in which the hind limb of a dog perfused with blood was used as a viscometer. The hind limb was first "calibrated" with plasma. The blood viscosity determined by this method and compared with the blood viscosity taken in a glass tube viscometer showed a lower value in the hind limb viscometer. Whittaker and Winton suggested that the difference in viscosities might be due to the Fåhraeus-Lindqvist effect.

In a modification of Whittaker and Winton's experiment, Kurland *et al.* (1968), perfused blood through a living rat tail artery. In this case, the rat artery was not only "calibrated" with plasma but was also perfused with radio-opaque solution and X-rayed to obtain the shape and diameter at various pressures.

Plasma viscosity calculated from pressure-flow rate considerations in the rat tail artery compared well with plasma viscosities calculated from tube and from cone and plate viscometers. However blood viscosities, compared in the same manner, did not agree, there were lower values in the *in vivo* system as found by Whittaker and Winton. Even after discounting the Fåhraeus-Lindqvist effect, the lack of agreement was still substantial (30 to

50 per cent difference). It was concluded that possibly some difference involving interaction of cells with the viscometer wall might explain the difference.

Bennett (1967) observed intermittent cell-wall contact in red cells flowing across a flat surface. He suggested that this behavior should be incorporated in blood flow equations.

Copley and Scott-Blair (1960) noted a lower viscosity for blood flowing in glass tubes coated with fibrin than in uncoated glass tubes. However, he also noted this same difference for plasma which is not explicable by the cell inter-action hypothesis. The influence of the vessel wall on flow does in fact seem to play a role in blood flow that is not yet defined or evaluated.

It has recently been observed in our laboratory that highly charged poly-electrolyte tubing substantially reduces the viscosity of blood as compared with uncharged polyethylene tubing. It is possible that the vessel wall has a similar effect due to electric charge. It is obvious that further work is required before *in vitro* rheology may be applied to *in vivo* systems with confidence.

10. BLOOD RHEOLOGY AND CLINICAL MEDICINE

We deal first with the effects of red blood cell concentration, then with the elasticity and other properties of the cells and finally with the influence of plasma protein and fat.

Both the red cell–red cell attraction and protein–red cell interaction are a function of red cell concentration, and both viscosity and yield stress increase as hematocrit increases. In fact, the volume fraction of red cells is the major determinant of viscosity above $1\,\mathrm{s}^{-1}$, (Fig. 9). Viscosity also varies inversely with shear-rate so that the influence of hematocrit on viscosity, which rises sharply above 58 per cent (Pirofsky, 1953; Mendlowitz, 1948) is even more significant at low shear-rate. Wells and Merrill (1961) expressed this in a family of curves showing the relation of viscosity to shear-rate becoming most sensitive at high hematocrits and low shear-rates. In parts of the venous system and in small vessels where flow velocity is low or may be phasic and even occasionally reversed, viscosity must reach very high levels with any increases in hematocrit. Recent work on the consequences of increased red cell volume fractions (Chien *et al.*, 1970; Schmid-Schoenbein *et al.*, 1969) has emphasized the importance of red cell deformation. The shear thinning behavior of blood is especially marked at high hematocrits when cell collisions are increased; the deformation of red cells becomes important and is a major factor in reducing viscosity and facilitating flow in minute vessels.

Significant elevation of hematocrit is found in primary and secondary polycythemia vera and the incidence of thrombosis is increased (Wasserman and Gilbert, 1966; Burris and Arrowsmith, 1953; Calabresi and Meyer, 1959).

The mechanisms of vascular occlusion in polycythemia include the high viscosity and high yield stress caused by the high hematocrit, the reduction in the velocity of blood flow (hence decrease in shear rate), and local vascular disease. Reduction in red cell volume in polycythemia without alteration of blood volume results in a decrease in peripheral vascular resistance and an increase in systemic blood flow and oxygen transport, probably related to the decreased blood viscosity and yield shear stress (Rosenthal et al., 1970). The converse of the rise in viscosity with polycythemia is the striking physiologic response to anemia where there is an increase in venous return and in cardiac output, which falls when hematocrit is restored (Richardson and Guyton, 1959; Guyton and Richardson, 1961). The increase in cardiac output in acute experimental anemia has been shown to be determined by the decrease in whole blood viscosity (Murray et al., 1969) and an enhancement of myocardial contractility. The frequently posed clinical problem concerns the optimal hematocrit for a patient with vascular narrowing as in coronary artery disease. Where does the harm from reduced oxygen carrying capacity exceed the benefit from improved flow resulting from decreased viscosity? (Crowell and Smith, 1967). The data of Case et al. (1955) from dogs suggest that in the presence of coronary narrowing, deterioration of ventricular function occurs at a hematocrit well avove 24 to 31 per cent, levels normally tolerable.

In addition to the influence of the volume of red cells, viscosity is influenced by the shape and elasticity of the red cell and changes in its rigidity, deformability and internal viscosity. In the smallest vessels and at high hematocrits this may be critical. For example fixed red cells are more viscous than normal cells (Chien et al., 1967, 1968; Ham et al., 1968; Schmid-Schönbein et al., 1969). Increased shear stress deforms normal erythrocytes and lowers the suspension viscosity but has no effect on the viscosity of hardened cell suspensions. A clinical counterpart of considerable significance is found in sickle cell disease. Sickle cells lie between rigid particles and normal red cells (Harris, 1950; Harris et al., 1956). Stroma-free hemoglobin solutions from homozygous sickle disease, when in the sickled form, show an extreme increase in viscosity, in resistance to packing, in mechanical fragility and in difficulty passing through microfilters (Jandl et al., 1961). The red cells in sickle-cell trait are less susceptible to the sickling process than those of homozygous disease but, even in these cells, increased viscosity resulting from hypertonicity may slow flow, permit deoxygenation and pH reduction to a level critical for sickling (Harris et al., 1956). The clinical consequences are particularly well seen in the kidney in homozygous sickle-cell disease where thrombosis often occurs.

Hemoglobin C is more viscous than normal, again leading to decreased deformability and increased blood viscosity. Significant precipitation of Heinz bodies (glutathione-hemoglobin disulfides) also makes a cell rigid, probably increases viscosity and decreases cell life span (Charache *et al.*, 1967; Murphy, 1968). Blood from patients with other types of hemolytic anemia showed no significant difference in viscosity, whether the samples were oxygenated or fully reduced (Ham and Castle, 1940). Increased hydrogen ion concentration also leads to increased internal viscosity, rigidity, aggregation of red cells and an increase in whole blood viscosity (Dintenfass and Burnard, 1966). Schmid-Schönbein and Wells (1969) have stressed the significance of the red cell membrane abnormality and changes in cell size in pathologic states, and noted a marked increase in bulk viscosity in hemolytic anemias and chronic renal and hepatic failure after allowing for the lowered hematocrit.

Alterations of other formed elements in the blood have little influence on viscosity. Red cells suspended in platelet-free plasma have the same viscosity as those suspended in normal plasma. Within the normal range the number of white blood cells has no significant influence on viscosity.

Although the major changes in blood viscosity are the result of changes in hematocrit and red cell properties, significant and critical changes may also result from alterations in the suspending plasma. To some extent these are due to changes in plasma viscosity alone but probably more significant are the effects on red cell aggregation especially at low shear. Positive correlation of plasma viscosity has been found with total protein, fibrinogen, alpha 1, alpha 2, beta and gamma globulins; an inverse relation with albumin has been noted (Mayer, 1966; Wells, 1965; Merrill *et al.*, 1963b). The extent of red cell aggregation and the anomalous flow behavior of whole blood have been ascribed to red cell-fibrinogen interaction (Replogle *et al.*, 1967; Merrill *et al.*, 1966; Chien *et al.*, 1967), the extent of the interaction being dependent on both factors. Chien *et al.* (1969) have also stressed the importance of serum globulins in shear dependent aggregation of red cells. The yield shear-stress is a function of both fibrinogen and globulin concentration (as well as hematocrit) after a minimum concentration has been reached.

Abnormal serum proteins may occasionally be of marked importance in viscosity and the physiochemical correlation of structure and viscometric effect is instructive. A hyperviscosity syndrome has been described in macroglobulinemia and in multiple myeloma (Fahey *et al.*, 1965); (Somer, 1966).

The influence of lipids on flow in the microcirculation has been repeatedly considered with conflicting results. We have studied normal students and could find no change in viscosity of plasma or whole blood $3\frac{1}{2}$ hrs after a fatty meal (Charm *et al.*, 1963). These observations confirmed those of Shearn and Gousios (1960) and Watson (1957).

In a number of important clinical states striking changes in the microcirculation have been described, but their origin is multifactorial. The increased blood viscosity of shock is a good example (Seligman *et al.*, 1946;

Berman and Fulton, 1965). Low blood pressure, slow flow (decreased rate of shear), alteration of the vascular wall, leukocytosis, platelet thromboembolism, increases in fibrinogen concentration and hematocrit, change in red cell surface, and drop in temperature may all influence microcirculatory flow, tend to increase yield stress and viscosity and to promote aggregation and sludging. Vasomotor changes (Zweifach, 1961), altered clotting and changes in vascular permeability further complicate the picture. Finally, hypoxia and metabolic alterations, particularly acidosis, would alter red cell elasticity further increase viscosity, decrease flow and impair vascular reactivity.

Alteration of microvascular flow has been noted following incompatible blood transfusion, malarial crises (Knisely, 1965) and anaphylaxis (Irwin, 1964) and many forms of tissue trauma, such as fracture, contusion, burns, cold, surgery (Gelin, 1959; 1961), myocardial infarction (Bloch, 1955) acute alcoholism (Lee *et al.*, 1968; Moskow *et al.*, 1968), bacillary pneumonia, poliomyelitis.

In view of the extensive hemodynamic and metabolic consequences which have been ascribed to intravascular erythrocyte aggregation, it is natural that efforts should have been made to improve the suspension stability of whole blood. Gelin and Thorsen (1961) noted that low molecular weight dextran (LMD) was capable of reducing the red cell loss associated with injury. The conflict is not yet resolved between those ascribing a specific disaggregating effect to LMD and those who feel that its effect is to reduce viscosity by hemodilution.

In summary, changes in viscosity and yield stress play a significant role in clinical medicine. An increased incidence of occlusive vascular disease has been demonstrated in a number of conditions characterized by increased viscosity. The rise in viscosity can result from increased hematocrit (as in polycythemia), increased rigidity of red cells (as in homozygous sickle cell disease), or altered plasma proteins (as in macroglobulinemia). In addition, increased aggregation has been associated with a variety of tissue injuries but the mechanism of this aggregation remains the subject of speculation. In some cases it is apparently related to fibrinogen, in some to other plasma proteins and in others possibly to altered properties of the red cell surface. A tendency to hyperviscosity or aggregation will be potentiated by a drop of cardiac output, velocity of blood flow, perfusion pressure or temperature or by the occurrence of acidosis. The entire picture may be further affected by vascular reactions.

REFERENCES

Basler, A. (1918). Uber die Blutbewegung in den Kapillaren. I. Mitteilung Registrierung der Stromungsgeschwindigkeit. *Pflug. Arch. ges. Physiol.* **171,** 134–135.

10*

Bayliss, L. E. (1952). Rheology of blood and lymph. In "Deformation and Flow in Biological Systems", (A. Frey-Wyssling, ed.), pp. 354–418, Interscience Publishers, New York.

Benis, A. M. and Lacoste, J. (1968). Study of erythrocyte aggregation by blood viscometry at low shear rates using a balance plate method. Circulation Res. 22, 29–41.

Bennett, L. (1967). Red cell slip at a wall in vitro. Science, N.Y. 155, 1554–1555.

Bergentz, S. E., Gelin, L. E., Lindell, S. E. and Rudenstam, C. M. (1965). The effect of trauma on equilibrium of Cr^{15} tagged red cells. 3rd European Conference on Microcirculation, Jerusalem, 1964, Vol. 7, 242–249.

Berman, H. J. and Fulton, G. P. (1965). The microcirculation as related to shock. In "Shock and Hypotensions", (L. Mills and J. H. Moyer, eds.), pp. 198–219, Grune and Stratton, New York.

Berman, H. J. and Fuhror, R. L. (1966). Personal communication.

Berne, R. M. and Levy, M. N. (1967), "Cardiovascular Physiology", p. 3, C. V. Mosby Co., St. Louis.

Bingham, E. C. and White, G. F. (1911). Viscosity and fluidity of emulsions, crystallin liquids and colloidal solutions. J. Amer. Chem. Soc. 33, 1257–1268.

Blackshear, P. L., Dorman, F. D., Madhukar, S. G. and Kihara, K. (1969). Particle motion in flowing blood. 2nd International Conference on Hemorheology, Heidelberg, p. 43, (abstract).

Bloch, E. H. (1955). In vivo microscopic observations of circulating blood in acute myocardial infarction. Amer. J. Med. Sci. 229, 280–293.

Bloch, E. H. (1962). A quantitative study of hemodynamics in the living microvascular systems. Amer. J. Anat. 110, 125–153.

Boardman, G. and Whitmore, R. L. (1961). Static measurement of yield stress. Lab. Pract. 10, 782–785.

Brooks, D. E. and Seaman, G. V. F. (1969). Role of mutual cellular repulsions in the rheology of concentrated red blood cell suspensions. Proceedings of 2nd. International Conference on Hemorheology, Heidelberg.

Bugliarello, G., Kapur, C. and Hsiao, G. C. (1965). The profile viscosity and other characteristics of blood flow in a non-uniform shear field. Symposium on Biorheology, (A. Copley, ed.), pp. 351–370. Interscience Publishers, New York.

Bugliarello, G., Hung, T. K. and James, C. E., Jr. (1969). Model studies of hydrodynamic characteristics of an erythrocyte. III. Drag in an erythrocyte–erythrocyte interaction. Proceedings of 2nd International Conference on Hemorheology, Heidelberg.

Burris, M. D. and Arrowsmith, W. R. (1953). Vascular complications of polycythemia vera. Surg. Clin. 33, 1023–1028.

Burton, A. C. (1965). "Physiology and Biophysics of the Circulation", p. 64, Year Book Medical Publishers, New York.

Calabresi, P. and Meyer, O. O. (1959). Polycythemia vera. I. Clinical and laboratory manifestations. Amer. J. Int. Med. 50, 1182–1202.

Case, R. B., Berglund, E. and Sarnoff, S. J. (1955). Ventricular function. VII. Changes in coronary resistance and ventricular function resulting from acutely induced anemia and the effect thereon of coronary stenosis. Amer. J. Med. 18, 397–405.

Casson, N. (1958). A flow equation for pigment–oil suspensions of the printing ink type. In "Rheology of Disperse Systems", (C. C. Mills, ed.), pp. 84–104, Pergamon Press, Oxford.

Cerny, L. C., Cook, F. B. and Walker, C. C. (1962). Rheology of blood. *Amer. J. Physiol.* **202**, 1188–1194.

Cerny, L. C., Grauz, J. D. and James, H. (1968). The effectiveness of plasma expanders as osmotic pressure and viscosity study. *Biorheology* **5**, 103–110.

Chaffey, C. E., Brenner, H. and Mason, S. G. (1965). Particle motions in sheared suspensions: Wall migration. *Rheologica Acta.* **4**, 64–72.

Charache, S., Conley, C. L., Waugh, D. F., Ugoretz, R. J. and Spurrell, J. R. (1967). Pathogenesis of hemolytic anemia in homozygous hemoglobin C Disease. *J. Clin. Invest.* **46**, 1795.

Charm, S. E. (1969). Calculation of branch flow. *2nd International Conference on Hemorheology*, Heidelberg, (abstract).

Charm, S. E. and Kurland, G. S. (1962). The flow behavior and shear–stress shear–rate characteristics of canine blood. *Amer. J. Physiol.* **203**, 417–421.

Charm, S. E. and Kurland, G. S. (1965). Viscometry of human blood for shear-rates of 0–100 000 s⁻¹. *Nature, Lond.* **206**, 617–618.

Charm, S. E. and Kurland, G. S. (1967). Static method for determining blood yield stress. *Nature, Lond.* **216**, 1121–1123.

Charm, S. E. and Kurland, G. S. (1968). The discrepancy in measuring blood in Couette, cone and plate and capillary tube viscometers. *J. Appl. Physiol.* **25**, 786–789.

Charm, S. E. and Wong, B. L. (1970). Shear degradation of fibrinogen in the circulation. *Science, N.Y.* **170**, 466–468.

Charm, S. E., Kurland, G. S. and Brown, S. L. (1968). The influence of radial distribution and marginal plasma layer on the flow of red cell suspensions. *Biorheology* **5**, 15–43.

Charm, S. E., McComis, W., Tejada, C. and Kurland, G. S. (1963). Effect of a fatty meal on whole blood and plasma viscosity. *J. Appl. Physiol.* **18**, 1217–1219.

Charm, S. E., Kurland, G. S., McComis, W. and Song, C. (1965). Energy losses in steady and pulsatile blood flow. *Bibl. Anat.* **17**, 340–345.

Charm, S. E., McComis, W. and Kurland, G. S. (1964). Rheology and structure of blood suspensions. *J. Appl. Physiol.* **19**, 127–133.

Chien, S., Dellenbeck, R. J., Usami, S., Seaman, G. V. F. and Gregersen, M. I. (1968). Centrifugal packing of suspensions of erythrocytes hardened with acetaldehyde. *Proc. Soc. Exp. Biol.* **127**, 982–985.

Chien, S., Usami, S. and Dellenbeck, R. J. (1967). Blood viscosity: Influence of erythrocyte deformation. *Science, N.Y.* **157**, 827–831.

Chien, S., Usami, S., Dellenbeck, R. J., Bryant, C. A. and Gregersen, M. (1969). Change of erythrocyte deformability during fixation in acetaldehyde. *Proceedings of 2nd International Conference on Hemorheology*, Heidelberg.

Chien, S., Usami, S., Dellenbeck, R. J. and Gregersen, M. (1970). Shear dependent deformation of erythrocytes in rheology of human blood. *Amer. J. Physiol.* **219**, 136–142.

Chien, S., Usami, S., Taylor, H., Liniberg, J. S. and Gregersen, M. (1966). The effects of hematocrit and plasma protein on human blood rheology at low shear rates. *J. Appl. Physiol.* **21**, 81–87.

Cokelet, G. R. (1967). Comments on the Fåhraeus–Lindqvist effect. *Biorheology* **4**, 123–126.

Cokelet, G. R. (1963). The rheology of human blood. Doctoral Dissertation. M.I.T., Cambridge, Mass.

Cokelet, G. R., Merrill, E. W., Gilliland, E. R., Shin, H., Britten, A. and Wells, R. E. (1963). Rheology of human blood: Measurement near and at zero shear rate. *Trans. Soc. Rheol.* **7**, 303–317.

Copley, A. L. and Scott-Blair, G. W. (1960). Apparent viscosity and wall adherence of blood vessels. In "Flow Properties of Blood and Other Biological Systems", (A. Copley and G. Stainsby, eds.), pp. 97–117. Pergamon Press, Oxford.

Copley, A. L., Luchini, B. W. and Whelan, E. W. (1967). On the role of fibrinogen–fibrin complexes in flow properties and suspension-stability of blood systems. *Biorheology* **4**, 87, (abstract).

Crowell, J. W. and Smith, E. E. (1967). Determinant of the optimal hematocrit. *J. Appl. Physiol.* **22**, 501–504.

Danon, D., Marikovsky, Y. and Skutelsky, E. (1969). The sequestration of old erythrocytes and expulsed nuclei from the circulation of mammalians. *Proceedings of 2nd International Conference on Hemorheology*, Heidelberg.

Dintenfass, L. (1964a). Rheology of packed red blood cell containing hemoglobins A–A–S–A and S–S. *J. Lab. Clin. Med.* **64**, 594–600.

Dintenfass, L. (1964b). Viscosity and clotting of blood in venous thrombosis and coronary occlusion. *Circulation Res.* **14**, 1–16.

Dintenfass, L. (1965). Some observations on the viscosity of pathological human blood plasma. *Thrombosis et Diathesis Haemorrhagica* **13**, 492–499.

Dintenfass, L. and Burnard, E. D. (1966). Effect of hydrogen in the *in vitro* viscosity of packed red cells and blood at high hematocrits. *Med. J. Aust.* **1**, 1072.

Dintenfass, L. (1968a). Internal viscosity of the red cell and a blood viscosity equation. *Nature, Lond.* **219**, 956–958.

Dintenfass, L. (1968b), Blood viscosity internal fluidity of the red cell, dynamic coagulation and the critical capillary radius as factors in physiology and pathology or circulation and microcirculation. *Med. J. Aust.* **1**, 688–696.

Dix, F. S. and Scott-Blair, G. W. (1940). On the flow of suspensions through narrow tubes. *J. Appl. Physics.* **2**, 575–581.

Ehrly, A. M. (1968). Reduction in blood viscosity at low rates of shear by surface active substances: A new hemogheologic phenomenon. *Biorheology* **5**, 299–314.

Ehrly, A. M. (1969). Desaggregation of erythrocyte aggregates and decrease of the structural viscosity of human blood by 2-phenyl-benzyl-aminomethyl imidazolidine (antozolin). *Proceedings of 2nd International Conference on Hemorheology*, Heidelberg.

Eisler, A. J. and Atwater, J. (1963). Effect of mean corpuscular hemoglobin concentration of viscosity. *J. Lab. Clin. Med.* **62**, 401–406.

Engeset, J., Stalker, A. L. and Matheson, N. A. (1967a). Effects of dextran 40 on red cell aggregation in rabbits. *Cardiovasc. Res.* **1**, 379–384.

Engeset, J., Stalker, A. L. and Matheson, N. A. (1967b). Objective measurements of the dispersing effect of dextran 40 on red cells from man, dog and rabbit. *Cardiovasc. Res.* **1**, 385–388.

Fahey, J. L., Barth, W. F. and Solomon, A. (1965). Serum hyperviscosity syndrome. *J. Amer. Med. Assoc.* **192**, 464–467.

Fåhraeus, R. and Lindqvist, R. (1931). Viscosity of blood in narrow capillary tubes. *Amer. J. Physiol.* **96**, 562–568.

Frasher, W. G., Wayland, H. and Meiselman, H. J. (1967). Outflow viscometry in native blood. *Bibl. Anat.* **9**, 266–271.

Gaehtgens, P., Meiselman, H. J. and Wayland, H. (1969). Evaluation of the photometric double slit velocity measuring method in tubes 25 to 130 μ bore. *Bibl. Anat.* **10**, 571–578.

Galluzzi, N. J., Delashmutt, R. E. and Connolly, V. J. (1964). Failure of anticoagulants to influence the viscosity of whole blood. *J. Lab. Clin. Med.* **64**, 773–777.

Gelin, L. E. (1959). The significance of intravascular aggregation of blood cells following injury. *Bull. Soc. Int. Chirg.* **18**, 4–19.

Gelin, L. E. (1961). Disturbances of the flow properties of blood and its counteraction in surgery. *Acta. Clin. Scand.* **122**, 287–293.

Gelin, L. E. and Thorsen, O. K. A. (1961). Influence of low viscous dextran on peripheral circulation in man. *Acta. Clin. Scand.* **122**, 303–308.

Gelin, L. E. (1964). A method for studying the aggregation of bloodcells erythrostatis and plasma skimming in branching capillary tubes. *Bibl. Anat.* **4**, 362–375.

Gelin, L. E., Bergentz, S. E., Helander, G. C., Linder, E., Nilsson, N. J. and Rudenstam, C. M. (1968). Hemodynamic consequences from increased viscosity of blood. *In* "Hemorheology", (A. Copley, ed.), pp. 721–728, Pergamon Press, Oxford.

Goldsmith, H. L. and Mason, S. G. (1964). Some model experiments in haemodynamics. *Bibl. Anat.* **4**, 462–478.

Gregersen, M. I., Branko, P., Chien, S., Duncan, S., Chang, C. and Taylor, H. (1965). Viscosity of blood at low shear rates: Observations on its relation to volume concentration and size of red cells. *In* "Symposium on Biorheology", (A. Copley, ed.), pp. 613–628. Interscience Publishers, New York.

Groth, G. G. (1965). Disturbances in the flow properties of blood. Ph.D. Thesis, Karolinska Institute Serafirmerlasarettet, Stockholm.

Guyton, A. C. and Richardson, T. Q. (1961). Effect of hematocrit on venous return. *Circulation Res.* **9**, 157–164.

Hagenbach, E. (1860). Über die Bestimmung der Zahigkeit einer Flussigkeit durch den Ausfluss aus Rohren. *Pogg. Ann.* **109**, 385–427.

Ham, T. H. and Castle, W. B. (1940). Relation of increased hypotonic fragility and erythrostasis to the mechanisms of hemolysis in certain anemias. *Trans. A. Am. Physicians* **50**, 127–132.

Harris, J. W. (1950). Studies in the destruction of red blood cells: VIII.Molecular orientation in sickle-cell hemoglobin solutions. *Proc. Soc. Exp. Biol.* **75**, 197–201.

Harris, J. W., Brewster, H. H., Ham, T. H. and Castle, W. B. (1956). Studies in the destruction of red blood cells—The biophysics and biology of sickle-cell disease. *Arch. Int. Med.* **97**, 145–168.

Hershey, D. and Cho, S. J. (1966). Laminar flow of suspensions (blood): Thickness and effective slip velocity of the film adjacent to the wall. *In* "Chemical Engineering in Medicine", Chem. Eng. Progress Symposium Series 62, (E. F. Leonard, ed.), pp. 139–145. Amer. Inst. of Chem. Engineers, Philadelphia.

Hint, H. and Arbors, K. E. (1969). Specific red cell aggregating activity in normal blood donors and in patients with high sedimentation rate. *Proceedings of 2nd International Conference of Hemorheology*, Heidelberg.

Irwin, J. W. (1964). The living microvascular system during anaphylaxis. *Ann. Allergy* **22**, 329–333.

Jacobs, H. R. (1963). The deformability of red cell packs. *Biorheology* **1**, 233–238.

Jandl, J. H., Simmons, R. L. and Castle, W. B. (1961). Red cell filtration and the pathogenesis of certain hemolytic anemias. *Blood* **18**, 133–148.

Jeffery, G. B. (1922). The motion of ellipsoidal particles immersed in a viscous fluid. *Proc. Roy. Soc. A.* **102**, 161–179.

Johnson, P. C. (1969). Hemodynamics. *Ann. Rev. Physiol.* **31**, 331–352.

Knisely, M. H. (1965). Intravascular erythrocyte aggregation (blood sludge). *In* "Handbook of Physiology", (P. Dow and W. F. Hamilton, eds.), pp. 2249–2292. Section 2, Vol. 3. Amer. Physiol. Soc., Washington.

Kurland, G. S., Charm, S. E., Brown, S. L. and Tousignant, P. (1968). A comparison of blood flow in a living vessel and in glass tubes. *In* "Hemorheology", (A. Copley, ed.), pp. 609–614. Pergamon Press, Oxford.

Lee, W. H., Najib, A., Weidner, M., Clowes, G. H. A., Murner, E. S. and Vujovic, V. (1968). The significance of apparent blood viscosity in circulatory hemodynamic behavior. *In* "Hemorheology", (A. Copley, ed.), pp. 587–607, Pergamon Press, Oxford.

Mayer, G. A. (1965). Anomalous viscosity of human blood. *Amer. J. Physiol.* **208**, 1267–1269.

Mayer, G. A. (1966). Relation of the viscosity of plasma and whole blood. *Amer. J. Clin. Path.* **45**, 273–276.

Mayer, G. A. and Kiss, O. (1965). Blood viscosity and *in vitro* anticoagulants. *Amer. J. Physiol.* **208**, 795–797.

Meiselman, H. J., Merrill, E. W., Gilliland, E. R., Pelletier, G. A. and Salzman, E. W. (1967). Influence of plasma osmolarity on the rheology of human blood. *J. Appl. Physiol.* **22**, 772–781.

Meiselman, H. J. and Merrill, E. W. (1968). Observations on the rheology of human blood: Effect of low molecular weight dextran. *In* "Hemorheology", (A. Copley, ed.), pp. 421–432, Pergamon Press, Oxford.

Mendlowitz, M. (1948). The effect of anemia and polycythemia on digital intravascular blood viscosity. *J. Clin. Invest.* **27**, 565–571.

Merrill, E. W., Cokelet, G. R., Britten, A. and Wells, R. E. (1964). Rheology of human blood and the red cell plasma membrane. *Bibl. Anat.* **4**, 51–57.

Merrill, E. W., Gilliland, E. R., Cokelet, G. R., Shin, H., Britten, A. and Wells, R. E. (1963a). Rheology of human blood: Effect of temperature and hematocrit. *J. Biophysics* **3**, 199–213.

Merrill, E. W., Gilliland, E. R., Cokelet, G. R., Shin, H., Britten, A. and Wells, R. E. (1963b). Rheology of blood and flow in the microcirculation. *J. Appl. Physiol.* **18**, 255–260.

Merrill, E. W., Cokelet, G. R., Britten, A. and Wells, R. E. (1963c). Non-Newtonian rheology of human blood: Effect of fibrinogen deduced by subtraction. *Circulation Res.* **13**, 48–55.

Merrill, E. W., Benis, A. M., Gilliland, E. R., Sherwood, R. K. and Salzman, E. W. (1965a). Pressure-flow relations of human blood in hollow fibers at low flow rates. *J. Appl. Physiol.* **20**, 954–960.

Merrill, E. W., Margetts, W. G., Cokelet, G. R. and Gilliland, E. W. (1965b). The Casson equation and rheology of blood near zero shear. *In* "Symposium on Biorheology", (A. Copley, ed.), pp. 135–143, Interscience Publishers, New York.

Merrill, E. W., Gilliland, E. R., Lee, T. S. and Salzman, E. W. (1966). Blood rheology: Effect of fibrinogen deduced by addition. *Circulation Res.* **18**, 437.

Monro, P. A. G. (1964). Visual particle velocity measurement: For fast particles and blood cells *in vivo* and *in vitro*. *Proceedings of 2nd European Conference on Microcirculation*, (Harders, ed.), p. 34, Karger, Basel.

Monro, P. A. G. (1965). Visual particle velocity measurements in fluid streams. *In* "Symposium on Biorheology", (A. Copley, ed.), pp. 439–449, Interscience Publishers, New York.

Mooney, M. (1931). Explicit formulas for slip and fluidity. *J. Rheology* **2**, 210.

Moskow, H. A., Pennington, R. C. and Knisely, M. H. (1968). Alcohol, sludge and hypoxic areas of nervous system, liver and heart. *Microvasc. Res.* **1**, 174–185.

Murphy, J. R. (1968). Hemoglobin CC disease: Rheologic properties of erythrocytes and abnormalities in cell water. *J. Clin. Invest.* **47**, 1483.

Murray, J. F., Esobar, E. and Rapaport, E. (1969). Effects of blood viscosity on hemodynamic responses in acute Normovolemic anemia. *Amer. J. Physiol.* **216**, 638–642.

Nubar, Y. (1967). Effect of slip on the rheology of a composite fluid: Application to blood. *Biorheology* **4**, 113–150.

Palmer, A. A. (1959). A study of blood flow in minute vessels of the pancreatic region of the rate with reference to intermittent corpuscular flow in individual capillaries. *Quart. J. Exp. Physiol.* **44**, 149–159.

Palmer, A. A. (1965a). Axial drift of cells and partial plasma skimming in blood flowing through glass slits. *Amer. J. Physiol.* **209**, 1115–1122.

Palmer, A. A. (1965b). Plasma skimming in human blood flowing through branching glass capillary channels. *In* "Symposium on Biorheology", (A. Copley, ed.), pp. 245–253, Interscience Publishers, New York.

Palmer, A. A. (1969). The influence of length of a capillary channel on the axial accumulation of red cells. *Proceedings of 2nd International Conference on Hemorheology*, Heidelberg, (abstract).

Phibbs, R. A. (1967). Personal communication.

Pirofsky, B. (1953). The determination of blood viscosity in man by a method based on Poiseuille's law. *J. Clin. Invest.* **32**, 292–298.

Ponder, E. (1940). Red cell as osmometer. *Cold Spr. Harb. Symp. Quant. Biol.* **8**, 133–143.

Rabinowitsch, B. (1929). Uber die viskositat and elastizitat von solen. *Z. Phys. Chem.* **2**, 1–26.

Rand, R. P. and Burton, A. C. (1964). *Mechanical properties of the red cell* membrane. *Biophys. J.* **4**, 115–136.

Rand, P. W., Barker, N. and Lacombe, E. (1970). Effects of plasma viscosity and aggregation on whole blood viscosity. *Amer. J. Physiol.* **218**, 681–688.

Reiner, M. and Scott-Blair, G. W. (1959). The flow of blood through narrow tubes. *Nature, Lond.* **184**, 354–355.

Replogle, R. L., Meiselman, H. J. and Merrill, E. W. (1967). Clinical implications of blood rheology studies. *Circulation* **36**, 148.

Richardson, T. Q. and Guyton, A. C. (1959). Effects of polycythemia and anemia on cardiac output and other circulatory factors. *Amer. J. Physiol.* **197**, 1167–1170.

Rosenblum, W. I. (1968). *In vitro* measurements of the effects of anticoagulants on the flow properties of blood: The relationship of these effects to red cell shrinkage. *Blood* **31**, 234–241.

Rosenthal, A., Nathan, D. G., Marty, A. F., Button, L. N., Mietinnen, O. S. and Nadas, A. S. (1970). Acute hemodynamic effects of red cell volume reduction in polycythemia of cyanotic congenital heart disease. *Circulation* **42**, 297–307.

Rowlands, S., Groom, A. C. and Thomas, H. W. (1965). The difference in circulation times between erythrocyte and plasma *in vivo*. *In* "Symposium on Biorheology", (A. Copley, ed.), pp. 371–379, Interscience Publishers, New York.

Rumscheidt, F. D. and Mason, S. G. (1961). Particle motions in sheared suspensions. XII. Deformation and burst of fluid drops in shear and hyperbolic flow. *J. Colloid Sci.* **16**, 238–261.

202 S. E. CHARM AND G. S. KURLAND

Schmid-Schönbein, H., Gaehtgens, P. and Hirsch, H. (1968). On the shear-rate dependence of red cell aggregation in vitro. J. Clin. Invest. 47, 1447–1454.

Schmid-Schönbein, H. and Wells, R. E. (1969). Red cell deformation and red cell aggregation: Their influence in blood rheology in health 'and disease. Proceedings of 2nd International Conference on Hemorheology, Heidelberg.

Schmid-Schönbein, H., Wells, R. E. and Goldstone, J. (1969). Influence of deformability of human red cells upon blood viscosity. Circulation Res. 25, 131–143.

Scott-Blair, G. W. (1967). A model to describe the flow curves of concentrated suspensions of spherical particles. Rheologica Acta 6, 201–202.

Scott-Blair, G. W. (1970). Personal communication.

Seligman, A. M., Frank, H. A. and Fine, J. (1946). Traumatic shock. XII. Hemodynamic effects of alterations of blood viscosity in normal dogs and in dogs in shock. J. Clin. Invest. 25, 1–21.

Shearn, M. and Gousios, A. (1960). Effect of intravenous fat emulsions on human blood viscosity. Arch. Int. Med. 106, 619–621.

Shorthouse, B. O. and Hutchinson, M. T. (1967). Investigation into the viscoelasticity of cell free plasma using the Bio-rheogoniometer. Bibl. Anat. 9, 232–239.

Sirs, J. A. (1968). The measurement of the hematocrit and flexibility of erythrocytes with a centrifuge. Biorheology 5, 1–14.

Somer, T. (1966). The viscosity of blood, plasma and serum in Dys and Paraproteinemias. Acta. Med. Scand. (Suppl. 456) 180, 1–97.

Steinberg, M. H. and Charm, S. E. (1971). Effect of high concentrations of leukocytes on whole Blood Viscosity. Blood 38, 299–301.

Swank, R. L. (1959). Changes in blood of dogs and rabbit by high fat intake Amer. J. Physiol. 196, 473–477.

Teitel, P. (1969). A haemorheological view on the molecular interactions between red cell constituents in the pathogenesis of constitutional haemolytic anaemias. Proceedings of 2nd International Conference on Hemorheology, Heidelberg.

Thomas, H. W. (1962). The wall effect in capillary instruments. Biorheology 1, 44–56.

Thomas, H. W., French, R. J., Groom, A. C. and Rowlands, S. (1965). The flow of red cell suspensions through narrow tubes: The extracorporeal determination of the difference in mean velocities of red cells and their suspending phase. In "Symposium on Biorheology", (A. Copley, ed.), pp. 381–391, Interscience Publishers, New York.

Thomas, H. W. and James, D. E. (1966). The trapped supernatant in the packed red cell column on centrifugation of bovine red cell suspensions and its relation to the deformability of the red cell. In "Hemorheology", (A. Copley, ed.), pp. 569–583, Pergamon Press, Oxford.

Thorsen, G. and Hint, H. (1960). Aggregation, sedimentation and intravascular sludging of erythrocytes. Acta. Chir. Scand. Suppl. 154, 6–51.

Usami, S., Chien, S. and Gregersen, M. I. (1969). Viscometric behavior of young and aged erythrocytes. Proceedings of 2nd International Conference on Hemorheology, Heidelberg.

VanWazer, J. R., Lyons, J. W., Kim, K. Y. and Colwell, R. T. (1963). "Viscosity and flow measurements", p. 201, Interscience Publishers, New York.

Wasserman, L. R. and Gilbert, H. S. (1966). Complications of polycythemia vera. Seminars in Hematology 3, 199–208.

Watson, W. C. (1957). Lipemia, heparin and blood viscosity. Lancet 273, 366–367.

Wayland, H. and Johnson, P. C. (1967). Erythrocyte velocity measurement in microvessels by a correlation method. *Bibl. Anat.* **9,** 160–163.

Wells, R. E. (1965). The effects of plasma proteins upon the rheology of blood in microcirculation. *In* "Symposium on Biorheology", (A. Copley, ed.), pp. 431–435, Interscience Publishers, New York.

Wells, R. E. (1968). Hemorheologic effects of the dextrans on erythrocyte aggregation: Hemodilution versus disaggregation. *In* "Hemorheology", (A. Copley, ed.), pp. 415–419, Pergamon Press, Oxford.

Wells, R. E. and Merrill, E. W. (1961). The variability of blood viscosity. *Amer. J. Med.* **31,** 505–509.

Wells, R. E., Schmid-Schoenbein, H. and Goldstone, J. (1969). Flow behavior of red cells in pathologic sera: Existence of a yield stress in absence of fibrinogen. *Proceedings of 2nd International Conference on Hemorheology*, Heidelberg.

Whittaker, S. R. F. and Winton, F. R. (1933). The apparent viscosity of blood flowing in the isolated hind limb of the dog, and its variation with corpuscular concentration. *J. Physiol.* **78,** 339–369.

Whitmore, R. L. (1968). "Rheology of the Circulation", p. 128, Pergamon Press, Oxford.

Wilkinson, W. L. (1960). "Non-Newtonian Flow", p. 39, Pergamon Press, Oxford.

Wintrobe, N. M. (1962). "Clinical Hematology", p. 323, Lea and Febiger, Philadelphia.

Zweifach, B. W. (1961). "Functional Behavior of the Microcirculation", Charles C. Thomas, Springfield, Illinois.

Chapter 16

The Mechanics of Capillary Blood Flow

J. M. FITZ-GERALD

Department of Mathematics, University of Queensland,
St. Lucia, Brisbane, Australia

1. INTRODUCTION

A. MORPHOMETRY

The mechanics of flow of a complex, particulate suspension depends largely on the morphometry of the channelling system through which it passes. In particular, the relation of particulate diameter to vessel lumen, the arrangement of vessel elements, the characteristics of the suspending fluid, the Reynolds number of the flow, and the physical properties of the particulates all need to be considered when the flow dynamics are discussed. Capillary motion therefore presents problems quite different from those associated with larger vessels. Red cells have diameters very similar to those of the capillary lumens; they are highly deformable and they move at velocities characteristic of very small Reynolds' numbers. It is expected that the flow will be essentially that of tightly-fitting elastic particles through tubes filled with fluid in slow viscous motion.

Most workers now accept that true capillaries may be defined as vessels whose walls are devoid of smooth muscle. They range in diameter from a lower limit of about 3·0 µm up to perhaps 15 µm; that is, approximately 0·5 to 2·0 unstressed RBC diameters. Lengths may range from 100 µm to 1 mm or more (Fung, 1968), and branched networks are usually formed, with anastomoses every 100 µm or so. Cross-sections are roughly circular, although the walls are by no means smooth and regular, and in some cases considerable deviations from circularity are observed. Between muscle fibres, for example, the cross-section tends to be flattened to an elliptic shape (Wiedeman, 1963).

Since the discovery of capillaries by Malpighi, considerable efforts have been made to elucidate the structure and function of capilliary networks in various organs. Excellent reviews of such work are available (Wiedeman, 1963). In this chapter, however, the main objective is to discuss the features of flow through a typical capillary element, that is, to gain understanding of the fluid mechanics underlying capillary flow in general. Regional, large-scale differences due to vascular organization may then be assessed in the light of this knowledge.

There will, inevitably, be some exceptions. The capillaries in the septa of the alveoli of the lung form a complex "marsh", which Weibel and Gomez (1962) have idealized to a hexagonal network of very short elements. Recently Sobin et al. (1970) have introduced the "sheet flow" concept for the pulmonary alveolar microcirculation. The blood is considered to be flowing in the space between two surfaces separated by irregular posts; the flow should be characterized, not by the relation between red cell diameter and capillary lumen, but by the surface separation and the ratio of post volume to total volume available, both considered in relation to RBC size.

The splenic microvasculature follows yet another pattern. It is still an open question as to whether there is a continuous, closed-channel pathway from artery to vein through the red pulp, or a diffusion-like system with RBC's and plasma migrating to the venous side through openings in capillary walls. Sinuses occur in the capillaries, and diameter may become as small as 3·0 µm. It has been speculated (Burton, 1968) that these extremely narrow vessels play some role in removing aged RBC's from the circulation.

Other examples of specialized morphometry may be cited; virtually all, however, are variations on a theme in that they involve the passage of suspensions of relatively large particles at high concentrations through narrow vessels. The description of such a flow must be the cornerstone of any discussion of capillary fluid mechanics and function.

B. PRINCIPAL PHENOMENA

Many features of capillary flow may be observed or noted even before detailed knowledge of the physics of the flow is available. These phenomena must guide the construction of any theoretical model, and a description of the flow which does not adequately include and explain them should be regarded very critically.

The prime function of any capillary network is the exchange of nutrients and metabolites between blood and tissue (see Chapter 17). Design of the capillaries should induce flows which optimize these exchange processes; further, the pathways may be different for gases, water and solutes such as ions, proteins and fats. Moreover, sensitive control of perfusion is needed over a large range, in order that considerably varying requirements may be met. Perhaps for this reason, most of the pressure drop in the cardiovascular system occurs in the microcirculation, some 60 per cent in the arterioles and 20–30 per cent in the capillaries; these figures depend to a large extent on arteriolar muscular tone. Pressure losses in the large arteries and the veins, which are merely high-volume supply and collection lines, are much smaller. A useful analogy here is the distribution of domestic electricity supplies; this also suggests that the ability of capillaries to sustain a high pressure gradient (defined as pressure change per unit length, not merely pressure drop), i.e. the high resistance of capillaries, is an important feature. The wide range of control required also indicates that non-linear responses to perfusion control mechanisms may occur.

Red cells have a shorter residence time in capillaries than does the surrounding plasma. Capillary haematocrits are correspondingly lower than those in larger vessels. A proportion of the plasma "leaks out" of the vessels near the arterial end and returns in the distal zones; some of the flow is therefore extracapillary, and Howe and Sheaffer (1967) have suggested that this helps to explain the RBC's shorter residence time. Filtration rates for plasma components, in particular water, vary considerably from organ to organ; for water, from $2 \cdot 5 \times 10^{-4} \, \mu m^3 \, s^{-1}$ $\mu m^{-2} \, (cmH_2O)^{-1}$ in muscle to $3 \times 10^{-2} \, \mu m^3 \, s^{-1} \, \mu m^{-2} \, (cmH_2O)^{-1}$ in renal glomeruli. This range of filtration rates does not appear to affect markedly the flow characteristics of capillaries, although abnormally high rates occurring at damage sites may cause bunching of the RBC's and cessation of flow.

C. EARLY STUDIES

Most of the early work on capillary flow, as mentioned above, was concerned with morphology and morphometry. Krogh (1922) was also interested in the supply and removal role of blood in capillaries, and pioneering studies by Fåhraeus and Lindqvist (1931) showed the anomalous

"viscosity" of blood flowing in small tubes, of diameter down to about
40 μm or so. Virtually all of the work on flow mechanics in vascular beds
was of an indirect nature, due in no small measure to the extreme difficulty
of measuring pressure differences accurately in very small vessels without
disturbing the flow.† Measurements of resistance and capacitance effects in
relatively large vascular beds characterized the performance of an entire
network, and often included the effects of vasomotion and autoregulation
in the muscular-walled vessels. Such studies gave little or no information
about the mechanics of flow in individual capillaries, nor did they relate
the fluid dynamics to observed phenomena.

2. THE NATURE OF THE FLOW

As blood passes into vessels of ever-decreasing diameters, its particulate
nature becomes more important. In large vessels under relatively high shear
conditions, whole blood viscosity may be taken to be sensibly constant, and
a Newtonian-fluid approximation is very reasonable. RBC concentrations
are virtually uniform except for a layer a few microns thick at the wall. The
effect of this cell-poor layer becomes more important in very small arteries
and veins, and contributes to the Fåhraeus–Lindqvist effect. Whitmore
(1967) refers to this as a "sheared-core" flow; there is a high velocity gradient
in the plasma zone near the wall, but additional velocity gradients (shears)
are present in the cell-rich core. Relative motions of red cells are
facilitated by the lubricating action of plasma in the core. Depending on
vessel diameter, a core cross-section may contain several red cells (see
Charm and Kurland, Chapter 15).

As capillary diameters decrease further, the sheared-core flow changes to
an "axial train" configuration, with the red cells moving in single file
surrounded by a plasma zone. Whitmore envisaged this as occurring
gradually as the lumen diameter fell below about 15 μm. Filmed studies by
Monro (1964), however, indicate that a sheared-core type of flow, albeit
involving only two or three cells in the core cross-section, occurred for
capillary diameters as low as 12 μm. This is permitted by the extreme
deformability of red cells, to be discussed later. True axial-train motion occurs
in capillaries of diameter smaller than about 10 μm or so. (See Fig. 1.)

The high rates of shear on those parts of cells (in axial trains) near the
vessel wall will cause considerable deformation and reduction in effective
cell diameter, the amount depending on the flow velocity. Thus even in a
capillary of diameter 8 μm, approximately equal to the diameter of an un-

---

† Wiederhielm and Rushmer (1962) have developed a micropipette pressure transducer,
which allows pressure measurements in small vessels, but to the author's knowledge, no
data are yet available on pressure gradients vs. blood velocity in individual capillaries.

stressed red cell, we would expect to find a plasma layer, perhaps 1 μm thick, between vessel wall and cell. Further decreases in diameter will cause more and more deformation of the cells, and reduction in thickness of the surrounding plasma layer. Monro (1964) and Palmer (1959) have shown

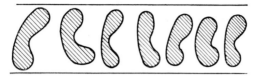

FIG. 1. Axial train motion of red cells in 8–10 μm diameter capillaries.

that this is usually accompanied by a gradual evening out of the spacing between neighbouring cells. As the diameter becomes very small indeed, a stage is reached where no more deformation of the cells is possible without cell rupture.

In these axial train configurations, the motion of the plasma is quite unusual. Prothero and Burton (1961) pointed out that, relative to the train of red cells, the plasma in the inter-cell spaces must perform a "circus-like" motion, with the fluid at the tube walls moving backwards (relative to the cells) and the fluid on the axis moving forward to compensate. This has been termed "bolus flow" by Prothero and Burton (Fig. 2). Lighthill (1968)

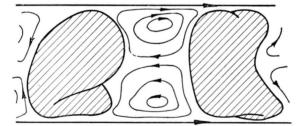

FIG. 2. Bolus flow streamlines between two deformed red cells in a narrow capillary.

has shown that there must also be a "leakback" of plasma past each cell; this will contribute to the higher mean velocity of cells than of plasma in such vessels. This leakage effect also applies in non-tightly-fitting cases, although there the two types of plasma motion are closely connected, with a relatively small bolus flow near the axis (Wang and Skalak, 1969).

To sum up then, it appears as if most capillary flow can be described in terms of an axial train motion of cells in the plasma, with the ease or tightness of fit of the cells determined by lumen diameter and amount of cell deformation due to viscous drag. The shearing-core behaviour, typical of the largest capillaries, may be thought of as an easily-fitting modification of the axial train idea; the general sheared-core case is treated elsewhere, and the present paper will be devoted to a discussion of the axial train configuration.

The fluid dynamics of these flows are largely determined by the Reynolds number, which measures the relative importance of viscous and inertial effects in controlling the motion. It is defined by

$$Re = \frac{LU}{\nu}, \tag{2.1}$$

where L is a typical length scale (here taken as capillary radius), U is a typical velocity (mean flow velocity), and ν is the kinematic viscosity of the plasma, taken as 1·85 cP (Gabe and Zatz, 1968). RBC velocity is a convenient measure of mean flow, and ranges from 0 to 1000 μm s^{-1} in most capillaries; unfortunately, little information is available about the variation of RBC velocities with capillary diameter, and of course these depend on pressure gradient. Fulton and Lutz (1957) give a value of 10–20 RBC diameters per second for capillaries in the 7 μm diameter range, say 100–200 μm s^{-1}.[†] Reynolds numbers therefore range from 0 to approximately 10^{-2}. This places the motion firmly in the slow, viscous regime; inertial effects are negligible, and pressure gradients are balanced by viscous forces only.

This has several important implications. Results such as Bernoulli's equation do not apply here; "dynamic pressure" is the same as "static pressure". Centrifugal forces are completely negligible, and flow proceeds with equal ease around a sharp bend as along a straight tube (for the same cross-sections). Turbulence is never generated, separation does not occur, wakes and jets can never exist. In general the flow is relatively insensitive to details of geometry, although broad geometric features can create important effects, such as the lubrication pressure developed in a convergent channel; this will be considered in some detail later.

Pressure-flow relationships in narrow capillaries will be affected by the haematocrit, since the type of flow at any point, and hence the local resistance, depends very much on whether or not a red cell is present there. As mentioned earlier, capillary haematocrits are expected to be smaller than arterial values because of the greater mean velocity of red cells than of plasma. Obviously the haematocrit will depend on capillary diameter, blood velocity and local functional peculiarities; Gibson et al. (1946), for example, report that mean small-vessel haematocrits are approximately 0·7 times arterial. Haematocrit

---

[†] Johnson and Wayland (1967) quote mean velocities from 150 μm s^{-1} to 1·8 mm s^{-1}, although no indication is given of capillary diameter.

reduction might be expected to be greatest in vessels where the leakback is greatest; Whitmore (1967) suggests that this occurs at about 15 μm diameter, or slightly less if erythrocyte deformation is allowed for. The figure reported by Gibson *et al.*, therefore, is probably too low as far as small capillaries are concerned, and a reasonable value is likely to be in the vicinity of 0·8–0·9 times arterial haematocrit. Indeed, pulmonary capillary haematocrit has been found (Fishman, 1963) to be some 13–17 per cent lower than large-vessel values.

Direct measurement of pressure gradients in capillaries during flow has not yet been achieved, and only indirect values are available. Between 20 and 30 per cent of the pressure drop in the systemic circulation occurs in the capillaries (Fung, 1968; Landis and Pappenheimer, 1963; Prothero and Burton, 1962a), i.e. about 20–30 mmHg. This occurs over distances of the order of 0·1 to 1 mm, so that pressure gradients might be estimated to lie in the range 20–80 mmHg mm^{-1}, with the upper limit reduced to allow for pressure losses in metarterioles, precapillaries, etc. The pressure gradient required to produce a mean velocity of, say, 500 μm s^{-1} in a 7μm capillary, supposing blood were a Newtonian fluid with a viscosity of 5·5 cP (the high-shear bulk viscosity of blood), is only about 7 mmHg mm^{-1}. Thus any theory of capillary flow will need to explain a considerable enhancement of "apparent blood viscosity" in very small vessels.

An interesting feature of capillary flow is that velocities are very intermittent, and may vary considerably in a random manner. Studies by Palmer (1959) indicate that the variation is usually greatest in the narrowest capillaries, suggesting that flow in these is most sensitive to changes in the applied local pressure gradient. Palmer's results also show that the intermittancy is frequently of the "stick-slip" type, with a sudden transition from motion to no-motion situation; very low velocities are seldom observed. In larger capillaries, "drifting" can occur as the local pressure gradient becomes very small; this suggests that the resistance offered by a capillary which does not markedly compress the red cells is smaller and less sensitive than that of a very small capillary.

Palmer proposes that these intermittent velocities are caused by leucocyte plugging, by plasma skimming, and by variations in flow pattern elsewhere producing changes in local pressure gradient. Plasma skimming, which usually occurs when a small capillary opens directly off a considerably larger vessel, creates a local sharp decrease in haematocrit, and a corresponding increase elsewhere. Thus although mean microcirculatory haematocrits are smaller than large-vessel ones, it would seem to be advantageous to study separately the fluid mechanics of a single red cell passing through a capillary, and the dynamics of plasma boli between adjacent red cells with various cell spacings, in order that suitable combinations of these may be used to discuss flow properties over a wide range of local haematocrits.

3. THEORETICAL CONSIDERATIONS

All the models for the fluid dynamics of capillary flow proposed since the pioneering work of Prothero and Burton have sought to explain the interaction between red cell, surrounding plasma, and the capillary wall; that this is the core of the problem has been strongly suggested by the discussion of the previous sections. Since the motion is intimately concerned with the extremely flexible erythrocyte, the first aspect to be considered will be the mechanics of its deformations during capillary flow.

A. ERYTHROCYTE MECHANICS

A currently-accepted, simple model of the erythrocyte is that of a thin, very flexible, slightly elastic membrane in the form of a biconcave disc, about 8 μm in diameter and 2 μm thick at the rim (Ponder, 1948; Rand and Burton, 1964), membrane thickness of the order of 10 nm (Canham, 1970; Fung and Tong, 1968), containing an incompressible medium, principally liquid (Fung, 1969). The forces which maintain the shape are at present imperfectly understood, but several suggestions merit comment.

Fung and Tong (1968) give an exhaustive analysis of a pressurized non-uniform shell, with maximum elastic stiffness in the equatorial zone. Much of the justification is based on the problem of sphering; and it is suggested that a known (Murphy, 1965) preferential distribution of cholesterol in the red cell, around the equator, might assist in producing the additional stiffness required there. Lopez et al. (1968) propose an equilibrium between electrostatic potential of the charged membrane, a uniform, inwardly-directed pressure difference, and a uniform elastic tension. This is perhaps preferable on at least one count; it has been observed that after sphering or crenation, a red cell does not necessarily return to exactly its original form, i.e. the equator and the dimples may occur at different positions on the cell surface. There may, of course, be rapid rearrangement of the stiffness distribution in Fung and Tong's model.

Canham (1970) has examined a model based on a minimum principle for bending energy of the membrane, assumed uniform. The principle is actually stated as one of a minimum total curvature, and interpreted to mean least bending energy for a linear, isotropic thin shell; the possibility that the stress-strain relation is non-linear is not included. Predicted shapes for normal cells and for a swelling sequence in hypotonic media, however, agree well with observation (Rand, 1964). A further recent proposal (Shrivastav and Burton, 1969), a development of earlier work (Rand, 1964; Rand and Burton, 1964), indicates that the cell contents may form bonds which hold the two dimpled surfaces together.

Clearly, more information is needed before the problem can be resolved;

what emerges, however, is that some combination of elastic tension, bending stiffness, pressure difference, and possibly electrostatic charge and interior bonding, produces the observed shape for given surface area and volume. The exact mechanism will determine the deforming effect of stresses applied to the cell; very little work has been done on this problem. Fung (1966) has pointed out that if bending stiffness plays any role, that is if the cell membrane can be considered to be a thin shell, then application of a large external hydrostatic pressure will probably lead to modes of buckling; since the interior of the cell is incompressible, Fung considers that such deformations will be isochoric and applicable, i.e. preserving

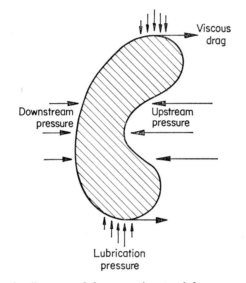

FIG. 3. Schematic diagram of forces acting to deform a red cell in narrow-capillary flow.

volume and surface area. If, on the other hand, the cell membrane possesses no bending moment, then increases in uniform external pressure are immediately transmitted to the interior, the pressure difference across the membrane remains the same, and no buckling will occur.

Deformation is more likely to result from the application of non-uniform stresses. In capillary flow, these will be of two types (Fitz-Gerald, 1969a; Lighthill, 1969) (see Fig 3): large-scale bending or "bowing" due to the combined effect of a pressure difference across the cell and drag around the rim from the sheared, viscous plasma; and additional local "squashing" because of the close proximity of part of the membrane to the endothelium. What Lighthill (1969) calls the "bowing stress" will reduce the effective diameter of the RBC in a sheared flow (e.g. capillary flow), and enable the cell to fit more easily into a vessel of given diameter. The deformation mode which actually occurs may well be very complex.

Fitz-Gerald (1969a, 1970) assumed a simple "parachute" shape as a first approximation, in order to obtain some quantitative values for effective RBC diameters under various conditions. With this assumption, it is possible to relate the pressure drop across the cell,

$$\Delta p = p \text{ (upstream)} - p \text{ (downstream)},$$

to the effective radius. Consider a very simple red cell model (Fig. 4), where the pressure difference Δp causes curvature of the cell membrane, and viscous stresses adjust to produce equilibrium of forces. Using the well-known result

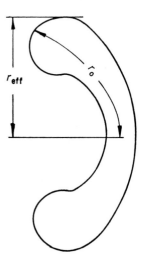

FIG. 4. Reduction of effective red cell radius in a simple "parachute" configuration.

that the pressure difference across a curved membrane under tension is proportional to the total curvature, Fitz-Gerald (1969a) finds that the effective cell radius is given by, essentially,

$$r_{\text{eff}} \approx \frac{8S}{\Delta p} \sin \frac{r_0 \Delta p}{8S}, \qquad (3.1)$$

where r_0 is the unstressed cell radius, and S is the "resistance to bending" measured by Rand and Burton (1964); this includes both effects of elastic surface tension and bending moment. The constants are obtained by taking a probable value for the ratio of inner and outer radii of curvature for the two sides of the cell, and assuming that the unstressed shape is maintained by bonds exerting forces on the inner face of each membrane. The formula is very approximate, giving order-of-magnitude information only. In particular, the deformation of the rim section is ignored, and the configuration is supposed to be almost symmetrical.

Studies of large-scale models (Fitz-Gerald, 1969b; Hochmuth and Sutera, 1968, 1970; Lee and Fung, 1969), however, do not support this axisymmetric mode of deformation for very tightly-fitting capillaries. While Fitz-Gerald's formula gives the correct qualitative behaviour, namely that r_{eff} decreases with increasing Δp, the analysis is inapplicable to very narrow capillaries. Instead of the parachute shape, a more commonly-observed configuration involves curling-up of opposite sides of the RBC into a modified "crepe-suzette" (Prothero and Burton, 1961) form, which progresses with its long axis tilted at an angle to the vessel axis. In addition, creases and kinks are frequently observed in the constricted regions, (Fig. 4). A narrow plasma-filled gap occurs between endothelium and cell around most of the cell's circumference, although the creases allow part of the rim to have comparatively high clearance (easy fit) for quite a small applied pressure difference; other such gaps may also occur due to uneven rolling-up.

Equation (3.1) should therefore be modified, for such cases, in two ways; firstly, the parameter $8S$, which depends on equal curvature contributions from two directions, is probably more like $4S$, since the longitudinal curvature in the crepe suzette shape is much less than the transverse curvature. Further, since r_{eff} must be regarded as a mean value for the red cell, the relatively free sections referred to above will reduce the effective radius by an amount b, say, practically independent of Δp since it is largely geometrically determined. Thus a more realistic expression for the effective radius might be

$$r_{eff} = \frac{4S}{\Delta p} \sin \frac{r_0 \Delta p}{4S} - b. \tag{3.2}$$

This type of formula is later shown to be in reasonable agreement with model experiments.

Additional "squashing" deformation due to local pressure changes in the constricted zones around the rim may also be treated semi-quantitatively, although again order-of-magnitude information only can be expected. While the elastic behaviour of the cell membrane during variations in RBC size is probably quite non-linear (Fung and Tong, 1968), the cell is so flexible that little change in membrane area or tension might be expected during deformation in narrow capillaries. Under these circumstances, Fitz-Gerald (1969a) has shown that a reasonable approximation to the membrane distortion is to assume a linear dependence of local cell diameter (or plasma gap width) on local pressure. The elastic compliance β, defined as the radius decrease per unit pressure increase, is shown to be approximately

$$\beta \approx r_{\text{eff}}^2/15S. \tag{3.3}$$

This formula is derived from the law of pressure difference across a membrane under tension, used above. Several errors inherent in its use have been discussed (Fitz-Gerald, 1969b); experimental data on the elastic behaviour of the red cell are so meagre, however, that it does not seem at present worthwhile to use a more complicated analysis. It should be pointed out that the pressure variations producing the radius changes required for the (stressed) cell to fit inside the capillary may be provided either by lubrication-type pressure forces in a plasmatic gap, or by direct contact between RBC membrane and endothelium. This question is discussed below.

B. RESISTANCE-FREE RBC MOTION CONCEPT

Once some knowledge of the mechanics of deformation of the red cell is available, the more difficult problem of the cell-plasma-endothelium interaction may be studied. Published work falls into two main categories; those which consider the red cell to have no appreciable interaction with the endothelium, and those where a large part of the resistance to flow occurs in a narrow plasma gap between red cell and vessel wall. The first type of theory postulates that almost all of the resistance is due to the plasma flow between adjacent red cells. The earliest serious exponents were Prothero and Burton (1961, 1962a,b); their pioneering work was of considerable importance, and is worth discussing in some detail.

The first step was to show that the resistance of a fluid bolus is greater than that due to a similar length of Poiseuille flow. This was done using a large-scale model, with an alcohol bolus between two long air bubbles. Results showed that the resistance depended inversely on the ratio of bolus length to tube radius; for conditions approximating those of capillary flow, a resistance increase of 30 per cent or less was obtained for the plasma sections of the flow, due to the bolus motion. Supposing that whole blood had a bulk, high-shear viscosity about twice that of plasma, and that the plasma boli occupied about half the length of the tube, then the mean apparent viscosity of a length of capillary flow would be only about 65 per cent of the bulk viscosity of whole blood, provided the red cells did not contribute appreciably to the resistance.

Resistance measurements were then carried out on whole blood flowing through micropipettes, whose tip diameters were of order 5 μm. Results from these experiments agreed well with the model results; Prothero and Burton deduced that the red cells offered no appreciable frictional resistance during capillary flow, and that the necessary deforming forces on the cell could be provided by direct contact with the vessel wall as the fatty-acid coated cell membrane slid easily over the endothelial surface. This hypothesis was apparently confirmed by the ease with which red cells passed through millipore filters, of mean pore diameter as low as 3 μm, under small driving pressures, of the order of 1 cmH$_2$O. The final conclusion was that the viscosity of blood in narrow capillaries may be taken to be about 2·0 cP, slightly higher than that of plasma alone, and considerably less than the bulk high-shear whole blood value. This low apparent viscosity might be considered as a limiting case of the Fahreus–Lindquist effect for somewhat larger vessels.

Several points need further discussion. Firstly, the Reynolds number used in the model and whole blood pressure-flow measurements was considerably higher (some 500–1000 times) than values characteristic of capillary flow. Erythrocytes in the micropipette experiments would therefore have been subjected to far greater deforming shear forces than they experience *in vivo*. As mentioned in the previous section, this would considerably reduce their effective diameter, and made it improbable that any but the briefest contact between red cell and tube wall occurred. The experiment thus eliminated from consideration any possible red cell resistance effects. It is interesting that these experimental results agree well with the theoretical predictions of Whitmore (1967) for unstressed red cells in considerably larger vessels; the results may perhaps be interpreted as a measurement of the Fåhraeus–Lindqvist effect for vessels of the order of 15 μm diameter.

In a previous section, it was pointed out that for the pressure to drop the required amount in the capillaries, enhanced apparent viscosities should occur. A calculation based on the value 2 cP, using the formula derived for Poiseiulle flow

$$\frac{\mathrm{d}p}{\mathrm{d}n} = \frac{8\mu U}{a^2},\qquad(3.4)$$

where dp/dn is the pressure gradient, U is the mean velocity (red cell velocity) and a is capillary radius, shows that, for a capillary of 7 μm diameter, a velocity as high as 1 mm s^{-1} requires a pressure gradient of only 7 mmHg mm^{-1}, well outside the range suggested earlier.

The apparent anomaly of the ease of passage of RBC's through millipore filters is resolved by recalling that it is the pressure gradient, not absolute pressure, that determines the deformation and relative clearance of an RBC in a vessel of given diameter. Prothero and Burton (1961, 1962a,b) do not quote a thickness for their filters, making pressure gradients difficult to estimate. The experiments have been repeated, however, by Gregersen and Bryant (1966), who give sufficient data for detailed analysis. Using a 12 μm thick nuclepore filter, they find that pressures of the order of 1–2 cmH$_2$O are sufficient to force even packed red cells through pores of 4 and 5 μm diameter. A simple calculation shows, however, that this represents a pressure gradient of some 50–100 mmHg mm^{-1}, well in the upper range of physiological values, and far in excess of that required should the red cells offer no resistance to motion.

Although the flow of plasma in the inter-RBC spaces will be discussed in detail later, it is pertinent at this point to consider some recent work on the pressure drop expected in bolus flow (Lew and Fung, 1969a, 1970). Lew and Fung (1969a) present an analytic solution of the problem for the comparatively tightly-fitting case, and find that the mean pressure gradient in a bolus dp/dx, for a given tube diameter and velocity, is related to the bolus length l by a curve which may be represented, to a good approximation by

$$\frac{dp}{dx} = a + \frac{b}{l}, \tag{3.5}$$

where a and b are constants. It is a matter of simple algebra to convince oneself of an important fact. For a given haematocrit, i.e. a given total length of fluid-filled space in fixed length of capillary, the total pressure drop in the plasma is *independent* of the red cell arrangement; a long bolus followed by a series of short ones represents the same total pressure drop as a group of uniform boli, provided that the number of boli is the same in each case. Suppose in a section of capillary flow the total plasma bolus length is L, and that there are n individual boli with lengths $l_1, \ldots, l_n$. Then the pressure drop Δp_n in each bolus is

$$l_n \frac{dp}{du_n} = l_n(a + b/l_n) = al_n + b,$$

and the total pressure drop is

$$\Delta p = \sum \Delta p_n$$
$$= \sum (al_n + b)$$
$$= a \sum l_n + nb$$
$$= aL + nb,$$

independently of the individual lengths l_n. Rouleau formation (seldom observed in narrow capillaries) would tend to reduce the total plasma pressure drop by reducing the number of individual boli.

The effect of decreasing bolus length by increasing the haematocrit is more complex, and is discussed later; it is sufficient here to point out that Lew and Fung's results show that, in general, an increase in haematocrit above normal values implies a decrease in total pressure drop, in a given length of capillary, due to the plasma-filled regions. The maximum possible pressure drop in the plasma boli, in fact, is very little more than the value expected for an equivalent length of cell-free plasma, under any circumstance of haematocrit and RBC distribution. Numerical calculations by Bugliarello et al. (1966) confirm these results.

C. RED CELL RESISTANCE

In view of the need to explain enhanced apparent viscosity effects, it seems desirable to reconsider the problem of RBC contributions to flow resistance. It might be suggested that frictional forces would not present a serious obstacle to the motion of erythrocytes, since the membranes are coated with layers of "slippery" phospholipids. However, the coatings may well depend for their "slipperiness" on the presence of water; Lighthill (1969) has cited the analogy of the large frictional forces associated with a dry cake of soap. In any case, completely dry membranes probably do not occur in vivo. The presence of a thin layer of fluid (presumably plasma) in the narrow gap between cell and endothelium, while reducing the frictional resistance by a lubrication-like mechanism, implies much larger viscous forces than those present in the plasma-filled spaces; this is due to the much greater velocity gradients required in the constriction zone.

Bloor (1968) modelled the flow by a series of rigid cylinders, with simple Couette flow in the annular spaces. His calculations showed that, while some enhancement of resistance occurred due to the formation of bolus flow, most of the resistance contributions came from the Couette flow regimes. Lew and Fung (1970) included the possibility of red cell resistance in their formula for apparent viscosity, but made no attempt to compute its value. This rigid-cell model has at least one serious flaw. In narrow capillaries, although some deformation of the RBC is caused by the large-scale bowing stresses described earlier, additional local "squashing" around the rim is almost certainly necessary to ensure sufficient ease of fit. The uniformly-decreasing pressure in the Couette flow is unable to provide these deforming forces.

Barnard et al. (1968) discussed a model of narrow capillary flow where the red cell was considered to be a thin sheet supporting no bending moment, but opposing the viscous shear stresses with elastic tension. The final shape of the RBC sheet was calculated, and the apparent viscosity of the suspension was found to be 1·05, relative to plasma. While this figure is in agreement with Prothero and Burton (1962a), it is almost certainly too low; neglect of the thickness of the red cell does not seem justifiable, since it is of the order of size of the other dimensions being considered. The elastic sheet RBC model is considerably more deformable than a thick cell, since it ignores the stresses associated with the distorted upstream section of the membrane, and the difficulty of fitting a finite-volume cell into a narrow space.

Similar apparent viscosities were obtained by Wang and Skalak (1969) for non-tightly-fitting cases; in that calculation, the red cell suspension was modelled by a line of rigid spheres. Viscosities of 1·5 relative to plasma were obtained for spheres 20 per cent smaller than the tube diameter, and even less for smaller spheres. All this work seems to confirm the predictions of Whitmore (1967), that the Fåhraeus–Lindqvist viscosity reduction effect continues to vessels of perhaps 10 μm diameter, with a minimum viscosity, achieved at perhaps 12 μm diameter, very little more than that of plasma alone. As the axial train flow gives way to constricted, tightly-fitting narrow capillary flow, with enhanced apparent viscosity, none of the approaches so far considered seem likely to remain valid.

D. ELASTOHYDRODYNAMIC LUBRICATION

Lighthill (1968) recognized the need to consider a flow regime capable of supporting normal loads, i.e. of providing the necessary forces to compress the rim of the RBC sufficiently to allow the film of plasma to flow through the constriction zone. A local maximum of pressure is needed near the point of tightest fit, maintained by the relative motion of cell and wall and by the geometry of the deformable narrow gap. Such flows are very well-known in lubrication theory, and Lighthill proposed the important concept, that the RBC is lubricated by the plasma during passage through narrow capillaries. The type of lubrication involved here is a very unusual one; there are three essential features which must be retained in any analysis of the flow.

Firstly, a pressure distribution with a local peak in the lubrication gap must be elastically demanded to allow free passage of the cell. Secondly, there must be a strong coupling between the geometry of the gap and the pressure distribution, each markedly affecting the other, in such a way that the viscous forces on the fluid within the gap balance the gradient of the pressure distribution. Thirdly, the driving pressure forces and the viscous forces must be in equilibrium. The first two conditions imply that a form of elastohydrodynamic lubrication is present; its analysis requires that one equation connecting pressure and gap width be obtained from the Navier–Stokes equations of fluid motion, another from the elastic properties of the cell membrane (and possibly of the vessel wall, if significant deformations occur there). The third condition above supplies a boundary condition, enabling one to select, from all the possible solutions of the two equations, that one which gives equilibrium of forces on the RBC.

While Lighthill's calculations qualitatively revealed many of the interesting features of this lubricated motion, some of his concepts were refined and extended in the more sophisticated analysis of Fitz-Gerald (1969a), who obtained better quantitative agreement with experimental results. The latter work forms the basis of the discussion which follows.

Under the usual assumptions of thin-film lubrication theory, the equations of fluid motion may be integrated to obtain a Reynolds equation, relating pressure gradient to gap thickness. For this configuration, the equation is very non-linear; it is easier to interpret in Lighthill's approximate form

$$\frac{dp}{dx} = -\frac{6\mu U}{h^2} + \frac{12\mu Q}{h^3}, \tag{3.6}$$

where p is the pressure, x the axial coordinate, μ the coefficient of viscosity, U the velocity, h the gap thickness (a function of x and p), and Q is the "leakback". This quantity Q is the flux of fluid back past the red cell per unit length of circumference of vessel. Non-zero values of Q are essential for lubrication, implying that the red cell has a higher mean velocity than the plasma. This is in accord with experiment (Groom, 1967; Groom $et\ al.$, 1957).

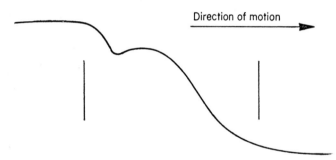

Direction of motion

FIG. 5. Typical low-clearance pressure profile in the lubrication gap; the vertical lines show the approximate limits of the constricted zone.

The first term here is a negative gradient due to relative motion of red cell and vessel; the second term is an additional positive gradient required to force fluid back through the gap. Together they produce a maximum of pressure near the point of greatest "unsquashed" red cell diameter, and a corresponding minimum near the upstream end of the gap. A typical pressure profile is shown in Fig. 5. The maximum occurs where $h = 2Q/U$; this is used as a measure of typical gap thickness, and is expressed as a ratio of the unstressed vessel radius to:

$$C = \frac{2Q}{Ur_0}, \tag{3.7}$$

where C is the "gap thickness parameter". It also measures the fractional difference between RBC velocity and mean plasma velocity. Thus if, for a solution of the equations, $C = 0.05$, the gap thickness is typically 5 per cent of the vessel radius, and the red cells are travelling 5 per cent faster than the plasma.

As discussed earlier, the gap thickness h at any point is assumed to depend linearly on the local pressure:

$$h = f(x) + \alpha(p - p_0). \tag{3.8}$$

Here $f(x)$ is some reference gap thickness function; it is that profile which would exist if the pressure were everywhere equal to the reference level p_0. This reference pressure is defined as that pressure which, when applied to the constriction zone, compresses the red cell just sufficiently for the maximum red cell diameter to equal the vessel diameter. It depends on both vessel diameter and the pressure difference applied across the red cell, since the unsquashed cell diameter is still reduced by the bowing stresses described earlier. Thus in a narrow capillary, a red cell with a given applied pressure difference across it (and hence a given unsquashed diameter) will require more pressure to deform it sufficiently to just fit inside than it would in a

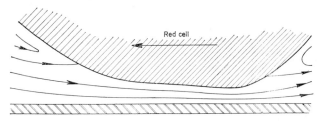

FIG. 6. Streamlines in a lubrication gap, showing the "necking".

larger vessel. Similarly, if the applied pressure difference is reduced, and the unsquashed diameter increased in consequence, more pressure is again required to ensure a fit.

Where the reference pressure p_0 is greater than the mean pressure on the cell in the absence of additional lubrication pressures, the cell is said to be in a negative clearance situation, and correspondingly for positive clearance. Since greater lubrication pressures are required to allow free movement for negative clearances, it might be expected that the additional stresses generated will lead to an increased resistance in these circumstances. A typical lubrication gap, and corresponding streamlines, is shown in Fig. 6. Notice that some of the flow which intrudes from the plasma-filled region between successive RBC's is turned back, rather than contributing to the leakback.

The value of the leakback Q, a priori unknown, may be determined by requiring that the driving force, provided by the pressure difference acting over the area of the tube, be just equal to the viscous resistance built up in the lubrication zone. Iterative, numerical techniques were used by Fitz-Gerald (1969a) to obtain a large number of solutions.

Results are obtained in terms of relationships between clearance, velocity, pressure gradient, gap thickness and resistance. If it is also known how the clearance depends on tube diameter and pressure gradient, pressure-flow curves for red cells in capillaries of various diameters may be plotted. Several interesting features of the results are summarized by Fitz-Gerald (1970), who introduces some convenient notation for this purpose. The resistance to flow of the RBC suspension is expressed as a ratio D of the resistance expected for a corresponding homogeneous Newtonian fluid (CHNF), where "corresponding" is used to imply a fluid having viscosity typical of whole blood in the bulk under high shear, and moving with the same mean velocity. An alternative interpretation of D is that it represents an apparent viscosity for the flow. A velocity reduction factor R_V is the ratio of red cell velocity to the mean velocity expected for CHNF under the same pressure gradient. It is found that:

(1) Velocities are considerably smaller than those expected if the pellet-fluid character of the flow were ignored.

(2) R_V depends sensitively on the pressure gradient, implying a non-linear dependence of velocity on pressure gradient. Over a large range of capillary diameter it is found that, approximately

$$R_V \propto \text{(pressure gradient)}^{\frac{1}{4}}.$$

(3) For positive clearances film thickness and leakback are relatively insensitive to changes in the velocity.

(4) For negative clearance, (narrow capillaries and small velocities), film thickness decreases markedly with velocity (or pressure gradient): in fact

$$C \propto \text{(velocity)}^{\frac{1}{4}}.$$

As velocity, and film thickness, decrease, it is suggested (Fitz-Gerald, 1969a; Lighthill, 1968) that failure of lubrication may occur, leading to greatly increased resistance at some finite pressure gradient. Lighthill (1968) refers to this as "seize-up". Such an effect would tend to explain Palmer's results (1959) for narrow-capillary flow described earlier. Experiments by Dintenfass (1966) also suggest that such a seize-up mechanism operates; his results may, however, have been affected by his use of glass channels for measurement of apparent viscosities.

(5) At a given clearance, D increases as velocity decreases; D also increases as clearance decreases. Fitz-Gerald finds values of D ranging from 2 to 20 for conditions typical of capillary flow. Approximately, for a given clearance,

$$D \propto \text{(velocity)}^{-\frac{1}{3}}.$$

Fitz-Gerald's calculations were made for an axisymmetric model with no fluid leakage through the walls of the capillary. However, he shows that the effects of asymmetry and filtration on the pressure-flow relations and other results are negligible to the approximation being used.

E. IMPLICATIONS OF THE LUBRICATION THEORY

Fitz-Gerald's numerical results (1970) applying the lubrication theory to capillary flow phenomenon were obtained using a very crude "parachute" or "thimble" RBC deformation model. Subsequent large-scale model studies (Fitz-Gerald, 1969b; Lee and Fung, 1969), however, have shown that this mode seldom occurs in narrow-capillary flow. For other modes (e.g. buckled or "crepe-suzette"), a smaller pressure gradient is required to produce deformation to a given effective diameter. Better clearance, with correspondingly less resistance, would be expected for these modes, under a given applied pressure gradient, than for the parachute mode. Thus while the model experiments confirm the basic lubrication theory, some of the numerical predictions quoted (Fitz-Gerald, 1970) for actual red cell movement are probably in error, particularly those concerning the spectacularly high apparent viscosities expected for low-velocity flow in very narrow capillaries. Qualitatively, however, the applications are valid, and the predictions agree reasonably well with most of the available experimental data.

The principal application is to the pressure-flow relations, and the related phenomena of enhanced apparent viscosity and perfusion control. Fitz-Gerald produces curves of predicted red cell velocities against applied pressure gradients, and although these gradients are probably somewhat higher than actually needed, they fall well within the range suggested earlier. Emphasis is placed on the point that not only does the resistance increase as velocity decreases for a given clearance, but the drop in pressure gradient also reduces the large-scale deforming stresses on the RBC; the cell consequently has a larger effective diameter and a smaller clearance, with additional resistance increase. It is expected, therefore, that these combined effects produce a sensitive, non-linear dependence of RBC velocity on applied pressure gradient, with the sensitivity increasing as vessel diameter decreases. It is suggested that control of perfusion by variations in muscular tone in the arterioles and pre-capillary sphincters is thereby facilitated by a kind of amplification process.

Such non-linear effects may be interpreted as a velocity-dependent apparent viscosity. Whitmore's (1967) theory shows how the apparent viscosity begins to rise as vessel lumen approaches effective cell diameter; Fitz-Gerald's (1970) viscosity curves fit well to Whitmore's in the intermediate region, with viscosities that continue to rise to values as high as 10–20 times bulk blood viscosity for very small capillaries and low pressure gradients. A series of viscosity curves is required, since there is dependence on both vessel diameter and pressure gradient.

F. PULMONARY MICROCIRCULATION

Pulmonary capillary flow presents problems of a unique character. Zone I, (see Milnor, Chapter 18) where both arterial and venous pressure are less than alveolar, has no flow. Zone II, with alveolar pressure between arterial and venous, exhibits patchy, unsteady flow in the complex maze of capillaries surrounding the alveolus. In such a network, some pathways will offer less resistance than others because of greater diameter or shorter path length, or both. Flow in these principal channels might be expected to be fairly stable. The possibility of seize-up when the pressure gradient falls below some threshold value, and the sensitive, non-linear dependence of velocity on pressure gradient, may well account for the patchy, unstable flow observed in the smaller, more resistive capillary sections, particularly when blockage at some point by leucocytes is considered.

In zone III, however, where both arterial and venous pressures are higher than alveolar, the networks are fully extended, and the flow should rather be thought of in terms of the "sheet flow" concept of Fung and Sobin (1969). Although typical dimensions of the flow spaces are still very similar to red cell diameter, the geometry is so irregular that Fitz-Gerald's lubrication theory results cannot be applied except in a very qualitative way. In that sense, the non-linear resistance enhancement effects will still occur, but account must now be taken of the complicated, non-constant clearance under these conditions. Pressure drops due to the motion of the plasma must also be considered. Fung and Sobin (1969) have considered the slow viscous flow of a Newtonian fluid through a very simplified model of the septum. They obtain results which are a good agreement with data from experimental studies on an appropriate model. They ignore in their analysis the presence of the posts and the resistance due to the red cells, and the results should be viewed as being suggestive rather than quantitative. Subsequently Lee and Fung (1969) analysed viscous flow between two sheets, past a post, and this work was extended by Lee (1969) to include an array of posts.

It was shown that local resistance to flow is considerably enhanced by posts whose diameter is large compared with sheet thickness, but that this effect fell off rapidly as post diameter decreased. Reasonably simple equations were presented, governing the distribution of pressure, velocity and sheet thickness, in a simple alveolar model when boundary conditions are known. Little attempt was made to apply these results to physiological situations nor was any account taken of the presence of red cells.

A further problem which should receive attention is that of the transmission of pressure waves through the pulmonary microcirculation. Although in the systemic microcirculation pulsatile pressures die away rapidly through viscous damping, Maloney *et al.* (1968) have demonstrated that pressure pulses may be transmitted, albeit considerably reduced in amplitude, to the venous side of the lung. The transmission coefficient falls with increasing frequency, as expected; however, in view of the very low Reynolds numbers characterizing alveolar blood flow, it might be assumed that no transmission at all should occur. These experimental findings have been confirmed, e.g. Kaplan and Kimbel (1970), but no theoretical work on the problem has appeared.

4. MODEL STUDIES

Experimental verification *in vivo* of a theory of capillary flow is extremely difficult. Simultaneous measurements of pressure gradient and velocity must be obtained in individual vessels without disturbance to flow, and such techniques are not yet available. Landis (1933) measured the velocity of red cells by microcinematography, in vessels of various diameters (down to 7 μm), and estimated the pressure gradients needed to cause such flows if the apparent viscosity were the same as the bulk, high-shear value. His computed results of a few $cmH_2O\ mm^{-1}$ for narrow capillaries were much less than those he expected from other considerations, and he concluded that the viscosity of blood in very small vessels is considerably higher than that in large vessels. Although this is in accord with a lubrication theory of red cell movement, it can hardly be accepted as confirmation.

In vitro experiments using actual red cells present difficulties which, although not as daunting, are still formidable. The work of Prothero and Burton (1962b), for example, was hindered by problems of manufacture of suitable artificial capillaries, and measurement at physiological values of velocity. Most of the available experimental information on capillary fluid mechanics has therefore had to be obtained with large scale models. The basic technique is well known; a flow system is constructed using similarity principles, duplicating as many as possible of the non-dimensional parameters of the original system.

Two obvious parameters here are the Reynolds number, and the ratio of cell diameter to vessel lumen. A sophisticated model duplicating these parameters, but ignoring the elastic properties of the red cell, was constructed by Hochmuth and Sutera (1968, 1970). They used neutrally-buoyant, rigid caps (truncated spheres) and investigated their behaviour in low Reynolds number tube flow. Diameter ratios (cap diam. to tube diam.) ranged from 0·723 to 0·998, with caps of thickness 0·16 to 0·5 diameters, i.e. from a thin' 'new moon" profile to hemispheres. The experiments were designed to test orientation stability, and measure pressure-drop and velocity characteristics. The results are quite significant.

It was found that non-hemispherical caps quickly took up stable orientations with their axes parallel to the tube axis (i.e. normal to the flow). Hemispheres with diameter ratio close to unity moved with their axes of revolution at an angle of about 20° to the tube axis. Smaller hemispheres rotated very slowly as they moved along the tube. These observations are probably not very relevant to capillary flow, since the elastic, flexible nature of red cells will modify their stability properties considerably.

The pressure drop due to the presence of a single cap was obtained from appropriate formulae, using measurements made with a number of caps in the tube. It was found that, provided the spacing between caps exceeded about 0·3 tube diameters, the results were independent of spacing. This feature of bolus-flow pressure gradients has already been mentioned in a theoretical context, and will be discussed further in a later section.

For diameter ratios markedly less than unity (below about 0·8), pressure drop data agree well with theoretical prediction (Wang and Skalak, 1969; Whitmore, 1967). Effective viscosities, interpreted in terms of actual blood flow, are well below that of bulk whole blood, in agreement with the Fåhraeus–Lindqvist effect. For larger diameter ratios, significant increases in resistance occur. For these cases, the additional pressure drop associated with a single cap, over that expected for Poiseuille flow of the surrounding fluid in the absence of the cap, may be considered to have two components: that associated with the maintenance of a bolus flow, and that due to the high-shear zone in the region of relative constriction. As the cap thickness increases, and the constricted, lubrication zone becomes longer, an increasing contribution to the resistance will occur from the second effect mentioned above. Hochmuth and Sutera found that, for a diameter ratio about 0·875, with a thickness of 0·35 diameters (a reasonable figure for a red cell under similar circumstances), the effective viscosity for a 50 per cent "haematocrit" was approximately double the fluid viscosity. This agrees very well with Whitmore's theoretical prediction from his axial train model, and with the calculations of Wang and Skalak for a row of rigid spheres. Applied to capillary flow, this indicates that for a capillary of some 10 μm diameter, the effective viscosity is approximately equal to the bulk whole blood viscosity; the reversal of the Fåhraeus–Lindqvist effect has already commenced. Such an application is probably useful, since the elastic effects due to the flexible red cell do not become important until narrower capillaries are reached.

For increasing diameter ratios, effective viscosity increases, reaching a value of about six times fluid viscosity for hemispheres of diameter about 0·996 tube diameters, again at a haematocrit of 50 per cent. This corresponds to an analogous blood viscosity of three times the bulk value. Hochmuth and Sutera (1970) note that even this figure is insufficient to account for the viscosity enhancement required by Landis (1933); the explanation lies in the neglect of the elastic nature of the red cell. A lubrication analysis based on the rigid cell model (Hochmuth and Sutera, 1968) is in agreement with the experimental data; however, the increased pressure in the constricted zone does not now have to provide any normal support to deform the erythrocyte. In fact, the situation corresponds very closely to a positive clearance situation, in Fitz-Gerald's terminology, one where the lubrication "squashing" effect is not strictly necessary to allow the erythrocyte to fit the vessel. True negative clearances are not reproduced in this rigid cap model; and it was seen in the previous discussions that the high resistance effects are most evident under negative clearance conditions. Furthermore, such extremely small gap thicknesses as 0·004 diameters do not occur for positive clearance at physiological cell velocities. The enhanced viscosities observed by Hochmuth and Sutera for diameter ratios very close to one therefore correspond to actual red cell flow in very narrow capillaries at un-physiologically high applied pressure gradients, where sufficient "bending" has occurred to produce positive clearance.

The above rather detailed discussion serves to emphasize yet again the necessity to include the elastic properties of the red cell in any work on narrow-capillary flow. Lee and Fung (1969) made a number of thin-walled biconcave rubber red cell models, filled with liquid, and tested them in a series of tubes filled with a high-viscosity (295 poise) silicone fluid. Reynolds numbers in the range 4×10^{-4} to 4×10^{-2} were obtained; diameter ratios (cell to tube) ranged from 1·7 to 0·85, modelling all but the very smallest observed capillaries. The thickness of the rubber wall was chosen to give the model similar non-dimensional elastic properties as a red cell; it was noted, however, that lack of detailed information about the red cell membrane made the last similarity agreement of doubtful validity.

Modes of deformation depended to a large extent on the diameter ratio. When the cell was considerably larger than the tube, ratios 1·7 and 1·36, the cell entered the tube sideways, buckling in at the equator and out at the poles (dimples). Although the cells almost completely filled the tube, photographs showed that a thin lubricating layer of fluid was present at all times during motion. The clearance (in Fitz-Gerald's sense) is very difficult to estimate under these circumstances, since no simple membrane theory suffices to determine the effective cell diameter in the absence of the lubrication "squashing" forces. It will be negative, and presumably slightly greater than the theoretical value for a crepe-suzette configuration. The availability of these higher-clearance buckling modes may well allow the red cell to maintain clearance, and hence resistance to flow, at acceptable levels even in the very narrowest capillaries. It should be pointed out, however, that although the deformations observed by Lee and Fung (1969) on their models agreed with many published red cell modes (e.g. Branemark and Johnson, 1963), not all of those reported could be duplicated.

At a diameter ratio of 1·1, some buckling occurred, but the crepe suzette (folded) mode became evident. For a ratio of unity, the parachute shape was noted; at very low velocities, an edge-on, slightly buckled configuration also occurred. In all cases, the models showed little tendency to align themselves perpendicular to the direction of motion.

It was found that in most cases, the cell velocity was greater than the mean flow velocity, as predicted by both the lubrication theory and the axial train theory for higher clearances. Values obtained for the ratio of velocities are in semi-quantitative agreement with both theories.

Pressure-flow characteristics provide good qualitative support for some of the predictions of the lubrication theory. Non-linear curves of pressure gradient versus cell velocity were obtained, the effect being much more pronounced at lower clearances (diameter ratio 1·36). A record of the pressure variations at a point as a cell passes shows clearly the maximum required to cause squashing, followed by a minimum at the end of the lubrication zone, where the "necking" occurs. A calculation of pressure drop for the cell train as a ratio of the Poiseuille value for the fluid showed enhanced resistance due to the cells, but comparison with either *in vivo* measurements or theory could be made at a qualitative level only, because of the difficulty of evaluation of the elastic behaviour of an erythrocyte.

Fitz-Gerald (1969b) produced a model system very similar to that of Lee and Fung. Fluid-filled, latex-walled cell models were forced along a tube filled with a high-viscosity silicone fluid. Similar deformations were observed (at the same diameter ratio), although there was less tendency to buckle and more to fold or roll; this was almost certainly due to differences in elastic behaviour between the two systems. The elastic parameter used by Fitz-Gerald was the "natural" one from the lubrication theory; it compares the viscous resistance of the lubricating fluid over the length of the lubrication zone with the elastic resistance of the cell membrane. Again difficulties occurred in attempts to compare the elastic behaviour of model and actual cell, and the results obtained, although providing, again, confirmation of the lubrication theory, probably represented only quali-tative information on capillary mechanics *in vivo*.

Resistance was found to increase with decreasing velocity at the rate predicted by theory; and for very small velocities, corresponding to only a few tens of $\mu m\,s^{-1}$ in very narrow capillaries, very high effective viscosities were observed. The variation of clearance with pressure gradient was also in agreement with theory, provided the calculation was performed for a crepe-suzette type of deformation. The clearance rose, and hence resistance fell, as the applied pressure gradient was increased. Attempts to introduce the cells in the parachute mode failed, showing that this is a very low clearance, high-resistance configuration, probably absent in the narrower capillaries.

Indirect evidence was also found for the "necking" phenomenon, and increase of resistance was observed when a cell was accidentally forced through a very narrow end section (diameter ratio 2·2). Very small bubbles in the fluid were used as tracers to observe the fluid streamlines; Lee and Fung (1969) used suspended particles, and in both experiments the streamlines agreed well with theory.

It seems, then, as if the lubrication concept of red cell motion is valid. Most of its predictions have been verified at least qualitatively by flexible-cell model experiments; non-linear dependence of velocity on pressure gradient and vessel diameter, viscosity enhancement, the form of the pressure variation in the lubrication zone, and the predicted relationships between resistance, clearance and velocity have all been demonstrated. The value of further model studies must depend on a more accurate comparison between the elastic properties of cell and model, and their relation to the other flow parameters.

5. Plasma Motions

Although an understanding of the pressure-flow relationships, and their implications, is essential to any theory of capillary flow, a discussion of the supply and removal role of capillary networks requires a knowledge of the detailed flow patterns of plasma between the red cells and endothelium. Nutrients and metabolites carried in the blood have a wide range of diffusion coefficients, and mass transport of slowly-diffusing species may well be considerably influenced by convection. While it is not proposed to include exchange mechanisms in this chapter, the discussion which follows will be partly directed towards the diffusion-convection problem. Moreover, the pressure drops occurring in the plasmatic gaps may be significant particularly in the larger capillaries, and may be computed from the streamline data.

As mentioned earlier, the first qualitative discussion, by Prothero and Burton (1961), showed that in narrow capillaries plasma must perform a circulating motion relative to the red cells, called "bolus flow"; this is because the fluid near the wall slows down due to viscous drag, and must then move towards the axis, as the next cell approaches, and rapidly catch up the preceding cell to maintain mean plasma velocity equal to red cell velocity. Even when leakback is present, a modified form of this pattern exists; a thin layer of fluid from the lubrication zone, remains near the wall, lubricating successive cells as they pass, and the bolus flow occurs inside this. Constant diffusional exchange occurs between the two regions.

Several attempts have been made to model the bolus flow mathematically; both numerical and analytical techniques have been used (Aroesty and Gross, 1970; Bloor, 1968; Bugliarello *et al.*, 1966; Bugliarello and Hsaio, 1970; Fitz-Gerald, 1969b; Lew and Fung, 1969a; Wang and Skalak, 1969; Zien, 1969). All agree on the basic form of the flow, as indeed they must, but show some lack of agreement on the details, both of streamline pattern and the associated pressure drop.

Since the Reynolds number is small, the flow may be described in terms of a stream function ψ, which may easily be shown to satisfy the equation

$$\left(\frac{\partial^2}{\partial r^2} - \frac{1}{r}\frac{\partial}{\partial r} + \frac{\partial^2}{\partial z^2}\right)^2 \psi = 0. \tag{5.1}$$

In axisymmetric cylindrical coordinates r, z (used in all analyses), ψ is related to the velocity components u (axial) and v (radial)

$$u = \frac{1}{r}\frac{\partial \psi}{\partial r}, \qquad v = -\frac{1}{r}\frac{\partial \psi}{\partial z}. \tag{5.2}$$

It can be shown that ψ, at any point (r, z), represents the volume flux of fluid through the circle centred on the z-axis, perpendicular to it, passing through the point in question, apart from a constant multiplying factor of 2π.

Pressure gradients may be computed from the low-Reynolds number Navier–Stokes equation

$$\nabla p = \nu \nabla^2 \mathbf{u}, \tag{5.3}$$

where ν is the kinematic viscosity, and $\mathbf{u}$ is the vector expression for the velocity:

$$\mathbf{u} = u\hat{\mathbf{z}} + v\hat{\mathbf{r}}; \tag{5.4}$$

$\hat{\mathbf{z}}$ and $\hat{\mathbf{r}}$ represent unit vectors in the axial and radial directions respectively. In component form, the equation becomes

$$\frac{\partial p}{\partial z} = \nu \left(\frac{\partial^2 u}{\partial r^2} + \frac{1}{r}\frac{\partial u}{\partial r} + \frac{\partial^2 u}{\partial z^2}\right)$$
$$\frac{\partial p}{\partial r} = \nu \left(\frac{\partial^2 v}{\partial r^2} + \frac{1}{r}\frac{\partial v}{\partial r} + \frac{\partial^2 v}{\partial z^2} - \frac{v}{r^2}\right). \tag{5.5}$$

It should be noted that the important quantity here is the pressure gradient ∇p, i.e. pressure change per unit length in an appropriate direction; this should not be confused with pressure difference (often denoted by Δp) between two points in the flow, which is meaningless unless the distance between the points is also specified. Unfortunately, there is a widespread tendency to use the term "pressure gradient" loosely, in a context where "pressure drop" is meant. The effectiveness of a pressure difference as a driving force on a fluid flow depends solely on the pressure gradient it sets up. Clearly, a pressure difference of only 1 cmH_2O has little effect applied to the ends of a 1 mm length of capillary (pressure gradient less than 1 mmHg mm^{-1}); when, however, the same pressure difference is applied across a nuclepore filter 20 μm thick, the resulting pressure gradient is about 20 mmHg mm^{-1}, comparatively high on the physiological scale.

The plasma gap is usually considered to consist of a short, hollow cylinder, partially or completely blocked at either end by rigid walls, representing the red cells. These end walls are usually considered to be plane, to facilitate solution of the equations; although this is a very simplified model, it will still provide useful information. Minor variations in geometry should not influence the flow greatly, except possibly near singularities. Complete blocking means that leakback is ignored and assumes that the red cell extends over the entire capillary lumen. In this case the boundary conditions are that the velocity is zero on the capillary walls (the no slip and no penetration conditions) and equal to the red cell velocity at the ends. A convenient coordinate system is one moving with the red cell, so that the end velocity is zero, and the walls move backwards at cell speed. This is the reference frame in which the circulating bolus flow occurs.

When partial blocking is assumed, the end boundary condition is more complex. Zero velocity still occurs on the cell face, while in the leakage gap a velocity profile is imposed, consistent with the flow assumed in the thin layer between red cell and capillary wall; essentially the two flows are "patched together" where the leakback flow enters the plasma-filled, cell-free region. If a rigid, pill-box model is used for the red cell, a Couette profile results (Bloor, 1968); this has the disadvantage of ignoring elastic control of leakback. An improvement is to use the lubrication theory velocity profile, for a range of values of the film thickness parameters (Fitz-Gerald, 1969b). A typical geometry, together with the associated streamlines, is shown in Fig. 7.

This matching technique is used because of the difficulty of solving the flow globally in the tightly-fitting case. For larger capillaries, however, where a considerable gap may occur between cell and endothelium, it is possible to obtain the whole flow in one calculation. Wang and Skalak (1969) show that the bolus flow still occurs, on a reduced scale, surrounded by a wide "leakback zone" outside the core region occupied by the cells. Apparent viscosities lie between plasma and whole-blood values; the Fåhraeus–Lindqvist effect is operating, and the flow is essentially that considered by Whitmore (1967), in his axial train analysis. Leakback is considerably greater than in the narrow vessels where cell lubrication is required, and it is probable that most of the differential in residence times between cells and plasma occurs in these larger capillaries.

Numerical solutions (Aroesty and Gross, 1970; Bloor, 1968; Bugliarello and Hsaio, 1970) of (5.1) for the completely blocked case give streamline patterns very similar to that proposed by Prothero and Burton (1961). Bloor proposed that for small values of bolus length/diameter ratio λ, two or more concentric circulation cells were formed; however, these have not

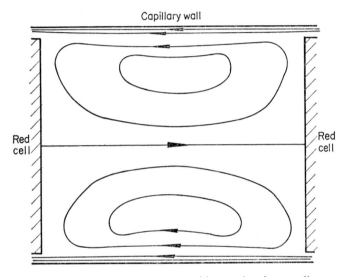

FIG. 7. Model of a plasma space, with associated streamlines.

been confirmed in other work. Analytical solutions (Fitz-Gerald, 1969b; Lew and Fung, 1969a, 1970) show the single-bolus flow pattern; in the partially-blocked case, a leakback zone occurs along the capillary wall, outside the circulation cell. Fitz-Gerald (1969b) also found, from an analytical solution, small additional cells very close to the cell face, near the axis. In any case, the velocities associated with these multiple-cell patterns are very small, except in the main circulation; such low velocity, secondary cells might well be missed by a numerical solution procedure. It should be pointed out, that relative to the vessel wall, no circulation occurs; streamlines then begin and end on the cell faces.

An analytical solution of the problem involves expansion, in terms of eigenfunctions, of the disturbance to the Poiseuille flow caused by the blocking effect of the cells. All of these perturbation functions decay away from the cell face; it may be shown (Fitz-Gerald, 1969b) that the most persistent one decays approximately as $\exp(4 \cdot 4z/a)$, where z is the distance from the cell face and a the vessel radius. For $z = a$, therefore, the disturbance should decay to about 1 per cent of its value at the cell face; this implies that in boli where $\lambda \geqslant 1$, say, the disturbance to the Poiseuille profile at either end will be virtually independent of the other, as will its effect on the pressure drop. Alternative eigenfunction expansions, in sinusoidal functions rather than exponential (Lew and Fung, 1969a, 1970) confirm these decay rates. Aroesty and Gross (1970) find, numerically, near-parabolic velocity profiles at the midpoint for large λ, but find that for very small λ (e.g. 0·2), the velocity is almost constant over most of the cross-section, and equal to the red cell velocity. The disturbance is thus confined to a boundary layer near the wall, with a very slow circulation inside. A similar dependence of flow pattern on cell spacing is found by most other authors.

This suggests that the pressure drop due to the plasma surrounding a train of tightly-fitting row of n cells is that due to a similar length of plasma alone (i.e. a length equal to the sum of lengths of the boli) in Poiseuille flow, together with n times the additional pressure drop due to the disturbance caused by an isolated cell. It is not necessary to have uniform spacing, provided no space is sufficiently small to allow interaction; hence it is to be expected that the resistance due to plasma in a given length of capillary containing a given number of cells is not particularly sensitive to variations in relative cell positions. When any space becomes very small, interaction between the two disturbances should reduce the pressure drop due to each, since the velocity profile would not then need to decay completely to the Poiseuille value, thus decreasing the magnitude of each disturbance.

For a given haematocrit, then, a maximum pressure drop is expected for equal spacing; spacing variations should produce little change, until some spacings become very small. Minimum pressure losses should occur when the cells clump together in long trains. Lew and Fung (1969a) confirm these predictions; for a partially blocked case with a cell diameter nine-tenths vessel diameter, they find a pressure drop of 1·5 to 2·0 times the Poiseuille value for typical capillary haematocrits (30–45 per cent). Variation of individual bolus lengths from $\lambda = 0·5$ to 4·0, for any mean value of λ, produces negligible change of pressure drop. If the cells clump together, so that the mean λ increases, the pressure drop decreases progressively as cell trains become longer, tending to the Poiseuille value as $\lambda \to \infty$. Pressure drops of this magnitude are negligible compared with resistance offered by tightly fitting red cells in narrow capillaries, but may well be significant in larger capillaries, where positive clearance conditions obtain, and red cell resistance is correspondingly less.

Moreover, it might be expected that a large part of the disturbance pressure loss for the completely occluded case is due to the presence of the flow singularity at the cell-wall junction. If this singularity is removed by replacing the model by a partially occluded one, the pressure loss decreases markedly (Lew and Fung, 1970). Bugliarello and Hsaio (1970) also find that varying the character of the singularity, for example by curving the cell faces, alters the pressure drop. In some sense, the effect of this singularity may be compared with the viscous resistance from the narrow lubrication film around the cell. The development from completely occluding cells, to rigid cells with leakback, to flexible, lubricated cells represents progressively closer approach to reality.

Convective enhancement of mass transfer in capillaries depends on the transported material. Movement of gases between tissue and red cell probably occurs principally across the narrow lubrication zone; diffusion paths are much longer in the bolus, and Aroesty and Gross (1970) have shown that the circulating flow there has little convective influence on the transfer rate. However, high shear regions around the entrance to the lubrication zone (Bugliarello and Hsaio, 1970; Fitz-Gerald, 1969b) may increase the cell area available for rapid transport. For slower-diffusing, high molecular weight species, the bolus flow may well serve to move fluid with a good concentration of the material near the high-shear region along the capillary wall.

Apart from the basic bolus flow, other plasma motions have been considered. Howe and Sheaffer (1967) discussed pericapillary flow, in which some plasma was assumed to diffuse out through the wall, move slowly through the surrounding tissue, and return at the distal end. This explained the variation in residence times between cells and plasma, although such an explanation is unnecessary in view of the conclusions of the axial train and lubrication theories. Several analyses of the sheet-flow pulmonary capillary flow have been made (Fung and Sobin, 1969; Lee, 1969; Lee and Fung, 1969), in which the effects of red cells have been ignored. Lew and Fung (1969b) have considered flow in occluded vessels with permeable walls, again in the absence of red cells.

6. Future Developments

Although semi-qualitative agreement with experiment has been obtained in a variety of circumstances, much remains to be done. Erythrocyte lubrication is still imperfectly understood, principally because of a lack of knowledge of cell membrane mechanics, and modes of deformation of the cell in narrow vessels. A particular problem is to calculate the clearance of an erythrocyte in a vessel of given size and at a given velocity; the resistance, and hence the apparent viscosity, depends quite sensitively on clearance, particularly in narrower vessels. Model studies can provide little more than qualitative confirmation of theory until more accurate modelling of the elastic behaviour is achieved. These model studies must also be supplemented by direct measurement of pressure-flow relationships, preferably *in vivo*. Flow mechanics in specialized, complex geometries are virtually unknown. Sheet flow in alveolar septa, in the presence of relatively large, flexible red cells, must be analysed; presumably some modification of both lubrication and bolus flow is involved, superimposed on the general flow already obtained. Little attention has been paid to the distribution of velocities in networks, or to flows in the presence of large osmotic pressures and high filtration, in the concentrating regions of the kidney. Effects of pathological conditions such as tissue damage, sickle cell anaemia, and pulmonary oedema have been discussed only qualitatively. Finally, the complex mass transfer processes, perhaps involving chemical reactions, diffusion and convection, have yet to be analysed in the light of capillary mechanics and plasma flow patterns.

REFERENCES

Aroesty, J. and Gross, J. F. (1970). Convection and diffusion in the microcirculation. *Microvascular Res.* 1, 247–268.

Barnard, A. C. L., Lopez, L. and Hellums, J. D. (1968). Basic theory of blood flow in capillaries. *Microvascular Res.* 1, 23–24.

Bloor, M. I. G. (1968). The flow of blood in the capillaries. *Phys. Med. Biol.* 13, 443–450.

Branemark, P. I. and Johnson, I. (1963). The shape of circulating blood corpuscles. *Biorheology* 1, 139–142.

Bugliarello, G., Day, H. J., Brandt, A., Eggenburger, A. J. and Hsaio, G. C. C. (1966). Model studies of the hydrodynamic characteristics of an erythrocyte. *In* "Hemorheology" (A. L. Copley, ed.), pp. 305–319. Pergamon Press, Oxford (1968).

Bugliarello, G. and Hsaio, G. C. C. (1970). A mathematical model of the flow in the axial plasmatic gaps of the smaller vessels. *Biorheology* 7, 5–36.

Burton, A. C. (1968). Role of geometry, of size and shape, in the microcirculation. *Fed. Proc.* 25, 1753–1760.

Canham, P. B. (1970). The minimum energy of bending as a possible explanation of the biconcave shape of the human red blood cell. *J. Theoret. Biol.* 26, 61–81.

Dintenfass, L. (1966). Viscosity of blood at high haematocrits measured in microcapillary (parallel-plate) viscometers of $r = 3$–30 μm. *In* "Hemorheology" (A. L. Copley, ed.), pp. 297–309. Pergamon Press, Oxford (1968).

Fåhraeus, R. and Lindqvist, T. (1931). The viscosity of the blood in narrow capillary tubes. *Amer. J. Physiol.* 96, 562–568.

Fishman, A. P. (1963). Dynamics of the pulmonary circulation. *In* "Handbook of Physiology", Vol. 2, Section 2, pp. 1667–1743. American Physiology Society, Washington, D.C.

Fitz-Gerald, J. M. (1969a). Mechanics of red-cell motion through very narrow capillaries. *Proc. Roy. Soc. B.* 174, 193–227.

Fitz-Gerald, J. M. (1969b). Blood flow in narrow capillaries. Doctoral Dissertation, University of London.

Fitz-Gerald, J. M. (1970). Implications of a theory of erythrocyte motion in narrow capillaries. *J. Appl. Physiol.* **27,** 912–918.

Fulton, G. P. and Lutz, B. R. (1957). The use of the hamster cheek pouch and cinephotomicrography for research on the microcirculation and tumour growth, and for teaching purposes. *Boston Medical Quart.* **8,** 1–7.

Fung, Y.-C. (1968). Biomechanics: its scope, history and some problems of continum mechanics in physiology. *Appl. Mechs. Revs.* **21,** 1–20.

Fung, Y.-C. (1966). Theoretical considerations of the elasticity of red cells and small blood vessels. *Fed. Proc.* **25,** 1761–1772.

Fung, Y.-C. (1969). Blood flow in the capillary bed. *J. Biomechanics* **2,** 353–372.

Fung, Y.-C. and Sobin, S. S. (1969). Theory of sheet flow in lung alveoli. *J. Appl. Physiol.* **26,** 472–488.

Fung, Y.-C. and Tong, P. (1968). Theory of the sphering of red blood cells. *Biophys. J.* **8,** 175–198.

Gabe, I. T. and Zatz, L. (1968). Studies of plasma viscosity under conditions of oscillatory flow. *Biorheology* **5,** 86–87.

Gibson, J. G. II, Seligman, A. M., Peacock, W. C., Aug, J. C., Fine, J. and Evans, R. D. (1946). The distribution of red cells and plasma in large and minute vessels of the normal dog, determined by radioactive isotopes of iron and iodine. *J. Clin. Invest.* **25,** 848–857.

Gregersen, M. I. and Bryant, C. A. (1966). Evaluation of deformability of red cells by sieving tests. *In* "Hemorheology" (A. L. Copley, ed.), pp. 539–549, Pergamon Press, Oxford (1968).

Groom, A. C. (1967). Transit times of cells and albumin through the vascular bed of skeletal muscle. *Biorheology* **4,** 98.

Groom, A. C., Morris, N. B. and Rowlands, S. (1957). The difference in circulation times of plasma and corpuscles in the cat. *J. Physiol.* **136,** 218–225.

Hochmuth, R. M. and Sutera, S. P. (1968). Large scale model studies of apparent viscosity and erythrocyte velocity in capillaries. *In* "Proceedings 5th European Conference Microcirculation, Gothenburg" (H. Harders, ed.), pp. 113–123. Karger, Basel and New York (1969).

Hochmuth, R. M. and Sutera, S. P. (1970). Spherical caps in low Reynolds-number tube flow. *Chem. Eng. Science* **25,** 593–604.

Howe, J. T. and Sheaffer, Y. S. (1967). Analysis of a recent hypothesis of plasma flow in pericapillary spaces. *Circulation Res.* **21,** 925–934.

Johnson, P. C. and Wayland, H. (1967). Regulation of blood flow in single capillaries. *Amer. J. Physiol.* **212,** 1405–1415.

Kaplan, A. S. and Kimbel, P. (1970). Pulmonary capillary blood flow waves in subjects with abnormal pulmonary haemodynamics. *J. Appl. Physiol.* **28,** 793–801.

Krogh, A. (1922). "The Anatomy and Physiology of Capillaries", Yale University Press, New Haven.

Landis, E. M. (1933). Poiseuille's law and the capillary circulation. *Amer. J. Physiol.* **103,** 432–443.

Landis, E. M. and Pappenheimer, J. R. (1963). Exchange of substances through the capillary walls. *In* "Handbook of Physiology". Vol. 2, Section 2, pp. 961–1034. American Physiology Society, Washington, D.C.

Lee, J. S. (1969). Slow viscous flow in a lung alveoli model. *J. Biomechanics* **2,** 187–198.

Lee, J. S. and Fung, Y.-C. (1969). Stokes flow round a circular cylindrical post confined between two parallel plates. *J. Fluid Mech.* **37,** 513–528.

Lee, J. S. and Fung, Y.-C. (1969). Modelling experiments of a single red blood cell moving in a capillary vessel. *Microvascular Res.* **1,** 221–243.

Lew, H. S. and Fung, Y.-C. (1969a). The motion of the plasma between the red cells in the bolus flow. *Biorheology* **6,** 109–119.

Lew, H. S. and Fung, Y.-C. (1969b). Flow in an occluded circular cylindrical tube with permeable wall. *Z. Angew. Math. Phys.* **20,** 750–766.

Lew, H. S. and Fung, Y.-C. (1970). Plug effect of erythrocytes in capillary blood vessels. *Biophys. J.* **10,** 80–99.

Lighthill, M. J. (1968). Pressure-forcing of tightly-fitting elastic pellets along fluid-filled elastic tubes. *J. Fluid Mech.* **34,** 113–143.

Lighthill, M. J. (1969). Motion in narrow capillaries from the standpoint of lubrication theory. *In* "Circulatory and Respiratory Mass Transport" (G. E. N. Wolstenholme and J. Knight, eds.), pp. 85–96, Churchill, London.

Lopez, L., Duck, I. M. and Hunt, W. A. (1968). On the shape of the erythrocyte. *Biophys. J.* **8,** 1228–1235.

Maloney, J. E., Bergel, D. H., Glazier, J. B., Hughes, J. M. B. and West, J. B. (1968). Transmission of pulsatile blood pressure and flow through the isolated lung. *Circulation Res.* **23,** 11–23.

Monro, P. A. G. (1964). The deformation of red cells and groups of cells in blood flowing in small vessels. *Bibl. Anat.* **7,** 376–382.

Murphy, J. R. (1965). Erythrocyte metabolism VI: cell shape and the location of cholesterol in the erythrocyte membrane. *J. Lab. Clin. Med.* **65,** 756–774.

Palmer, A. A. (1959). A study of blood flow in minute vessels of the pancreatic region of the rat with reference to intermittent corpuscular flow in individual capillaries. *Quart. J. Exp. Physiol.* **44,** 149–159.

Ponder, E. (1948). "Hemolysis and Related Phenomena", Grune and Stratton, New York.

Prothero, J. W. and Burton, A. C. (1961). The physics of blood flow in capillaries: I. The nature of the motion. *Biophys. J.* **1,** 565–579.

Prothero, J. W. and Burton, A. C. (1962a). The physics of blood flow in capillaries: II. The capillary resistance to flow. *Biophys. J.* **2,** 199–212.

Prothero, J. W. and Burton, A. C. (1962b). The physics of blood flow in capillaries: III. The pressure required to deform erythrocytes in acid–citrose–dextrose. *Biophys. J.* **2,** 213–222.

Rand, R. P. (1964). Mechanical properties of the red cell membrane. II. Visco-elastic breakdown of the membrane. *Biophys. J.* **4,** 303–316.

Rand, R. P. (1967). Some biophysical considerations of the red cell membrane. *Fed. Proc.* **26,** 1780–1784.

Rand, R. P. and Burton, A. C. (1964). Mechanical properties of the red cell membrane. I. Membrane stiffness and intracellular pressure. *Biophys. J.* **4,** 115–135.

Shrivastav, B. B. and Burton, A. C. (1969). Evidence from studies of birefringence of structure across the dimple region of red cells. *J. Cell. Physiol.* **74,** 101–114.

Sobin, S. S., Tremer, H. M. and Fung, Y.-C. (1970). Morphometric basis of the sheet-flow concept of the pulmonary alveolar microcirculation in the cat. *Circulation Res.* **26,** 397–414.

Wang, H. and Skalak, R. (1969). Viscous flow in a cylindrical tube containing a row of spherical particles. *J. Fluid Mech.* **38,** 75–96.

Weibel, E. R. and Gomez, D. M. (1962). Architecture of the human lung. *Science, N.Y.* **137**, 577–585.

Whitmore, R. L. (1967). A theory of blood flow in small vessels. *J. Appl. Physiol.* **22**, 767–771.

Wiedeman, M. P. (1963). Patterns of the arteriovenous pathways. *In* "Handbook of Physiology", Vol. 2, Section 2, pp. 891–933. American Physiology Society, Washington, D.C.

Wiederhielm, C. A. and Rushmer, R. F. (1962). Pre- and post-arteriolar resistance changes in the blood vessels of the frog mesentery. *Bibl. Anat.* **4**, 234–243.

Zien, T.-F. (1969). Hydrodynamics of bolus flow—an analytical approach to blood flow in capillaries. *Bull. Math. Biophys.* **31**, 681–694.

Chapter 17

Flows across the Capillary Wall

C. C. MICHEL

Fellow of The Queen's College, Oxford:
University Laboratory of Physiology, Oxford, England

LIST OF SYMBOLS

A	= area across which diffusion or flow is occurring
A_m, A_p, A_s, A_w	= total membrane area, total pore area, total area available to solute, total area available to solvent
a	= effective molecular radius, usually taken as Stokes–Einstein radius
C	= concentration
$C_s, C_p, C_a, C_v,$ $C_t, C_l, C_e,$	= concentrations in solute, plasma, arterial blood, venous blood, tissue, lymph and interstitial fluid, respectively
dC/dx	= concentration gradient within a solution in the direction x
ΔC	= concentration difference across a membrane
D_s	= diffusion coefficient of solute, s
η	= coefficient of viscosity
f_{sm}, f_{sw}, f_{wm}	= frictional coefficients for solute and membrane, solute and solvent and solvent and membrane
J_s	= net mass flow of solute
$J_v, J_{v_L}, J_{v_F},$	= net volume flow, lymph flow, net capillary filtration
J_D	= net diffusion flow (i.e. volume flow of solute relative to solvent)
K_s	= diffusional conductivity of solution to solute
L_D	= phenomenological coefficient of solute diffusional flow in membrane
L_P	= phenomenological coefficient of volume flow in membrane
L_{PD}, L_{DP}	= Onsager cross coefficients of solute flow and solvent flow
M_s	= membrane permeability expressed as $J_s/\Delta C$
μ_s, μ_w	= chemical potential of solute, water
$\partial \mu_s/dx$	= gradient of chemical potential in the direction x
n	= number of pores
P	= hydrostatic pressure
π	= osmotic pressure

$\Delta P, \Delta \pi$	= hydrostatic pressure gradient and osmotic pressure gradient across a membrane
$\dot{Q}$	= blood flow, volumetric
R	= universal gas constant
r	= membrane pore radius
ρ_r	= post capillary resistance
σ_s	= osmotic reflection coefficient of membrane to solute, s
T	= absolute temperature
t	= time
v_s, v_w	= mean net velocity of solute or solvent
w	= membrane slit width
ω	= membrane permeability defined as $J_s/\Delta \pi$ when $J_v = 0$.

1. INTRODUCTION

The ultimate flows of the circulation occur across the walls of the exchange vessels of the capillary beds. That these flows are occurring can be deduced from the concentration changes which occur when blood flows through a capillary bed and may be visualized by the way in which some dye substances are able to leave the circulation and stain the extravascular tissues. Experiments with dyes have suggested that not only the anatomical "true" capillaries are involved in blood-tissue exchange, but the walls of venular capillaries and small venules are at least as permeable if not more permeable than the smallest vessels. In this review the term capillary is used in a functional sense to include all these types of vessels.

The most important structure of the capillary is a single layer of flattened endothelial cells, in fact one or two endothelial cells are the only structures undeniably visible when true capillaries are viewed with the light microscope. For substances which can enter and leave cells easily (e.g. lipid soluble molecules including the respiratory gases) the layer of endothelial cells offers no barrier to flow between the blood and the tissues. Where the capillary wall differs from the cell membrane is in its high permeability to low molecular weight lipid insoluble molecules and ions, combined with a finite but very low permeability to protein molecules of size equal to or greater than serum albumin. It is with the flow of water and water soluble molecules across the capillary wall that this review is largely concerned partly because the available quantitative data on capillary permeability has concerned them and partly because the pathway taken by these substances implies a specialized structural pathway which has given rise to much controversy.

The most simple structures to account for capillary permeability would be water-filled pores which penetrated the endothelium or lay between adjacent endothelial cells. This hypothesis, which is almost as old as the postulate of the capillaries themselves, has sustained many attacks made upon it and in recent years direct evidence has accumulated in its favour. Before we consider this evidence let us briefly summarize the present views on capillary structure.

2. THE STRUCTURE OF THE CAPILLARY WALL AND DIRECT EVIDENCE FOR ITS POROUS NATURE

A. THE STRUCTURE OF THE CAPILLARY WALL

The light microscopists of the last century showed that the thin walls of capillaries were made up of a single layer of flattened endothelial cells which was continuous with the layer lining the larger blood vessels. The nuclei of these cells could be stained and the intercellular junctions could be demonstrated by a silver method devised by von Recklinghausen. This argentophilic nature of the cell junctions led to a belief that the endothelial cells were held together by a cement-like substance. It also seemed likely that the cell junction might be a pathway for the movement of water and solutes between the blood and the tissues fluids. Some workers were prepared to go even further in their views. The changes in capillary permeability which were known to occur in injured tissue were believed by some to result from a loosening of the intercellular regions and Julius Arnold (1875) described the emigration of white cells from inflamed capillaries as occurring between the endothelial cells.

The importance of the intercellular cement in regulating the permeability of capillaries has been revised and restated in this century by Chambers and Zweifach (1940, 1947). Their views were based on a large number of observations made on living tissues which indicated the $[Ca^{++}]$ and pH dependence of capillary permeability. The uptake of carbon particles was increased when the $[Ca^{++}]$ was low or zero and the pH of the perfusate and superfusate was also low. It is worth pointing out that Chambers and Zweifach (1940) suggested the cement substance covered the entire surface of the endothelial cell as well as being present in the junctional region.

The introduction of the electron microscope has greatly increased our knowledge of the capillary wall during the past twenty years. In addition to the endothelial cells, basement membrane of thin electron dense material has been shown to be a consistent feature of capillaries. Such a structure had been described by some of the early light microscopists but many eminent histologists regarded it as an artefact. The electron microscope left no doubt about its existence but its dimensions suggest that it is unlikely to have been seen with the light microscope.

Three types of capillary have been described. In muscle, skin, the central nervous system, lung and mesentery, the endothelial cells form a continuous layer and are surrounded by a continuous basement membrane. These vessels, which are the group we shall be most concerned with in this review, are said to be "continuous" capillaries (Fig. 1). In the sinusoids of the liver, spleen and bone marrow, large gaps can be seen between the endothelial

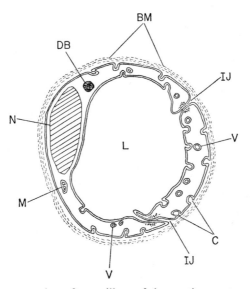

FIG. 1. Transverse section of a capillary of the continuous type (e.g. a capillary of mammalian skeletal muscle) showing the appearance seen in electron micrographs. The nucleus (N) of one endothelial cell, and several vesicles (V) and caveoli (C) in both cells are shown. At the intercellular junction (IJ), the outer membranes of the adjacent endothelial cells appear to come into contact with one another. The basement membrane (BM) forms a continuous electron-dense layer around both endothelial cells. L, lumen; M, mitochondria; DB, dark body.

cells and the basement membrane in these vessels are said to be "discontinuous" (Fig. 2). In the capillaries of the intestine, renal glomerulus and tubules, endocrine glands, choroid plexus and ciliary body and the *retia mirabilia*, the endothelium is thinned in certain special regions to form a single electron-dense layer. These regions have been called fenestrae and the capillaries are said to be of a "fenestrated" type (see Fig. 3).

Endothelia have been found to contain the various inclusions common to most cells, e.g. mitochondria, Golgi apparatus, centrosomes etc. but their most conspicuous cytoplasmic structures are large numbers of vesicles which are clustered particularly around the borders of the cell. The vesicles appeared to rise from or fuse with the cell membranes forming flask-shaped bodies called *caveoli intracellulares*. The openings of the caveoli on the

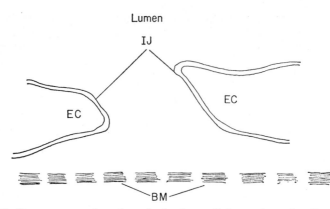

FIG. 2. Transverse section through the intercellular region of a discontinuous capillary (e.g. from liver). Note the large gap between the two cells (IJ) and the discontinuous basement membrane, BM; EC, endothelial cell.

endothelial surface are 15–40 nm in diameter. The neck is up to 20 nm in length, and opens into the cavity of the vesicle, 60–70 nm diameter, which approximates to the average size of the vesicles enclosed in the cytoplasm (Bruns and Palade, 1968a).

Several specialized forms of vesicle have been described. The moderately rare acanthosome is a vesicle, the cytoplasmic borders of which are covered by an electron-dense material which gives it a bristled appearance. A commonly occurring structure is the multivesicular body which consists of a large vesicle bounded by a unit membrane and enclosing numerous small vesicles also with unit membranes. Other inclusions which are found in endothelial cells are the dark bodies which have a uniformly dense structure and the Weibel Palade bodies which appear as elongated structures composed of parallel tubules.

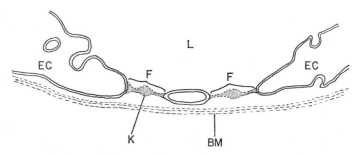

FIG. 3. Transverse section through the fenestrated region of a fenestrated capillary (e.g. from intestinal mucosa). F, fenestrae; K, central knob; BM, basement membrane; L, lumen; EC, endothelial cell.

The cell junctions of continuous and fenestrated capillaries did not appear to be particularly patent pathways. Although the intercellular space consists of a narrow cleft (about 20 nm wide for most of its length) filled with electron-dense material, it usually showed a region of narrowing in the luminal third for a length of 20–40 nm.

Palade and his co-workers have argued this "tight" region of the junction represents a region of fusion of the outer leaflets of the cell membranes somewhat like a gasket sealing the vascular lumen from the extracapillary space. Such seals between adjacent cells or *zonulae occludentes* have been described in epithelia by Farquhar and Palade (1963) and have shown to present a formidable barrier to the diffusion of particles as small as the extracellular ions (Loewenstein, 1966).

This view held precedence until 1967 when M. J. Karnovsky published a most important paper on capillary structure and function. Karnovsky made a very careful examination of the intercellular region in mouse heart capillaries. Using the high powers of the electronmicroscope he concluded that in most cases a gap of approximately 4 nm in width could be observed between the adjacent cells. In some rarer instances the intercellular space appeared to be obliterated by touching or fusing of the external leaflets of cell membrane but Karnovsky preferred to interpret this as evidence for a series of *maculae occludentes* which might hold the cells together but not provide a continuous seal. Between the points of fusion Karnovsky proposes the existence of oval slits, and, although hesitant to be quantitative about their geometry, he suggests their maximum width may be 4 nm.

In a detailed study of fenestrated capillaries of the rat intestine Clementi and Palade (1969) have shown that the fenestrae are circular, being about 40 nm in diameter, and the membrane or "diaphragm" covering them has a central blob 15 nm in diameter. Clementi and Palade have suggested that the fenestrae are formed by the progressive thinning of opposing regions of inner (luminal) and outer cell membranes of endothelium and they have described cylindrical structures in intestinal endothelium which they believe represent embryonic fenestrae.

The only muscle capillaries which have been shown to possess fenestrae are those of the external eye muscles (Collin, 1969).

B. DIFFUSION PATHWAYS ACROSS THE CAPILLARY

As mentioned earlier, substances such as oxygen and carbon dioxide which can readily enter cells should be able to cross the entire wall of the capillary. This is presumably also true of many low molecular weight lipid-soluble substances and may also be true to a limited extent to water. The movement of water down a given gradient of hydrostatic or osmotic pressure is twice as great across the capillary wall than it is across the most permeable cell membrane (the red cell) and furthermore water soluble substances of low molecular weight such as ions, sugars, amino acids etc. pass more easily across capillary walls than cell membranes by several orders of magnitude.

Several attempts to identify the diffusion pathway for these substances have been made by light microscopists. Florey (1926) used a technique whereby mutually precipitating ions were placed on either side of capillary endothelium. He found precipitation occurring in the endothelial cytoplasm and in the intercellular junctions. Several workers have extended and repeated this work, notably Mende and Chambers (1958) who observed (in vivo) lines of precipitation along the cell junctions. This work has been criticized on the grounds that the endothelial cells took up Trypan blue and the capillary wall was probably damaged.

The combination of electron-opaque tracers and electron-microscopy deflected interest away from the intercellular junction to the vesicle system. Palade (1960) was able to show particles of gold and ferritin particles (diameter 11 nm) inside the cytoplasmic vesicles and outside the capillaries after they had been added to the blood. There was no evidence for the passage through the intercellular junction.

Florey (1964) and Jennings and Florey (1967) investigated the capillaries of the rat coronary circulation using saccharated iron oxide and ferritin as electron opaque tracers. These capillaries appeared to be more permeable to the saccharated iron oxide than to the ferritin and more permeable to both substances when the vessels were perfused with a balanced salt solution than when the tracers were injected intravenously into the intact animal. Whereas both types of tracer particle were found in the cytoplasmic vesicles only iron particles were seen in the junctional regions.

In a later study, Bruns and Palade (1968b) found that ferritin crossed the capillary walls of the rat diaphragm within two minutes of the suspension being injected into the circulation, Ferritin was regularly seen in the vesicles but never in the intercellular junctions.

In the unfenestrated "continuous" capillaries it would appear that a molecule the size of ferritin is transported across the endothelial cell via the cytoplasmic vesicles and excluded from the cell junctions. In terms of molecular dimensions, however, ferritin is a large particle, much larger than many of the plasma proteins which leave the circulation only very slowly, and it is not necessarily a good indicator of pathways available to much smaller molecules.

The fenestrated capillaries of the intestinal mucosa are more permeable to plasma proteins than muscle capillaries. Clementi and Palade (1969a) have used ferritin and a smaller tracer, the enzyme horse-radish peroxidase (see below), to investigate diffusion pathways across these capillary walls in the mouse. Ferritin appeared in the spaces surrounding the capillaries three minutes after injection. It could be seen in the cytoplasmic vesicles and also appeared to cross the capillary wall through a small number of the fenestrae which appeared to be highly permeable to the tracer. Although the structural details of the permeable fenestrae were not clear, the authors suggested that their fenestral diaphragms were partially or entirely missing. The smaller tracer, horse-radish peroxidase, crossed through all the fenestrae and entered the vesicles in the earliest pictures. There was some evidence that the peroxidase entered the luminal part of the intercellular junction only as far as the "tight" region.

A major re-interpretation of the ultrastructural basis of capillary permeability was made in 1965 by J. H. Luft. He believed that the tight regions between the endothelial cells might represent the fusion of adjacent cell membranes but might still be permeable to water and low molecular weight water-soluble molecules. Luft also drew attention to the electron-dense material which fills the intercellular space of the junction. This, he suggests, is a mucopolysaccharide on the evidence that it can react with ruthenium red to form an electron-dense residue.

Luft's views which emphasized the importance of the intercellular junction as the pathway for transcapillary exchange were voiced to a wider public by Majno (1965) in his monumental review of vascular ultrastructure. To a large extent this prepared the way for Karnovsky who, in 1967, presented powerful evidence in favour of the diffusion pathway being located in the junction.

Karnovsky developed a method for detecting an intermediate molecular weight tracer (mol. wt. 40 000), horse-radish peroxidase, using the electron microscope. Studying the permeability of the capillaries of mouse heart, Karnovsky was able to show reaction product of horse-radish peroxidase in the intercellular regions and in the endothelial vesicles in preparations fixed a few minutes after the injection of the tracer into the circulation. Although there was no evidence of hindrance to the passage of the tracer through the junctional region, Karnovsky drew attention to the possible criticism that in most of his pictures, the appearance of tracer in the junction did not necessarily mean that it had traversed the capillary wall by this route. Since the vesicles were also loaded with reaction product it seemed conceivable that the intercellular cleft could have filled secondarily to the passage through the vesicle system.

Furthermore it was argued that no gradient of tracer could be seen extending away from the junctions on the outside of the capillaries and such gradients might be expected if the junctions were the principal transport pathway.

After raising these questions Karnovsky was able to partially answer them.

A few of his pictures showed junctions containing reaction product throughout their length, whereas only the vesicles on the luminal side of the capillary appeared to contain tracer.

More recently Karnovsky (1970) has been able to use a tracer of lower molecular weight (12 000), cytochrome peroxidase. This molecule appears more rapidly outside the capillaries than horse-radish peroxidase and the preferential filling of the intercellular junctions together with a density gradient receding from them in the extracapillary space seems now to have answered the major criticisms of the earlier work. It is worth noting that the later studies were carried out on skeletal muscle capillaries as well as cardiac capillaries.

It is perhaps worth noting that the morphological evidence for there being a formidable barrier at the tight junction arose largely from the studies of Muir and Peters (1962) on cerebral capillaries. That such a barrier does exist between cerebral endothelial cells has now been supported by histochemical studies. Reese and Karnovsky (1967) were unable to detect the penetration of horse-radish peroxidase across this barrier and more recently Brightman et al. (1970) have found that these tight junctions are a barrier to the very much smaller tracer, microperoxidase (mol. wt. < 2000), in mammals if not in all vertebrates. It would seem that Muir and Peters' interpretation of their own evidence was substantially correct. It was the extrapolation to other types of capillary—without reference to function—which led to confusion.

Recent observations on the permeability of living capillaries to dye substances also suggest that the diffusion pathway for low molecular weight water soluble molecules is located in the intercellular junctions. Michel (1969, 1970) has followed the passage of Patent Blue V out of the microcirculation in frog mesentery. The coloured anion of this dye has an equivalent weight of 559 and it binds only slightly with plasma and tissue proteins. In order to obtain a step change in dye concentration within a vessel, Michel used a micropipette to perfuse individual capillaries. During the first few seconds of the perfusion the dye appeared to leave the capillary to a varying extent along the length of the vessel. An objective record of the uneven permeability was obtained by measuring the optical density of photographs taken during the early stages of perfusion. Michel has argued that uneven permeability of the capillary at a microscopic level would be a consequence of a pore system located only in the intercellular region. Using the silver method to stain the cell junctions, the number of cell junctions per unit area of capillary wall has been found to vary with a similar spatial frequency to the variation in permeability to dye.

On its own this would be very strong circumstantial evidence for the dye passing across the capillary wall through pores or slits located between the endothelial cells. Taken along with the evidence from electronmicroscopy it would appear that the intercellular regions are indeed the principal diffusion pathway for those water soluble molecules so far investigated and that the endothelial cells are relatively impermeable to these substances.

If pores are defined as regions of high permeability separated by regions of low permeability it can be said that direct evidence for pores in the capillary wall does exist.

3. PRINCIPLES GOVERNING FLOW ACROSS MEMBRANES AND THE THEORY OF RESTRICTED DIFFUSION THROUGH MEMBRANE PORES

With the possible exception of transport via cytoplasmic vesicles, the flows across the capillary wall are passive. By this it is meant that no energy for transport is supplied within the capillary wall, net flow being the result of differences in chemical potential at its inner and outer surfaces. A quantitative description of these flows of solute and water should relate to the forces (i.e. the gradients of chemical potential) which are responsible for them, through a series of coefficients. If such a description is complete, the coefficient should account for the interactions between solute and solvent and the membrane structure. If we possessed an accurate picture of the diffusion pathway, and if we were certain of the laws governing molecular movements through this pathway, the nature of the membrane coefficients could be determined.

Although there is evidence in favour of a system of pores or slits between the endothelial cells, our information about this pathway is qualitative and we cannot be certain that the junctional regions are the only route for many of the small water soluble molecules. The evidence in favour of pores or slits, however, does provide a basis for a quantitative model of the capillary wall which assumes that the passive flows of water and solute occur through pores. Such a model was devised by Pappenheimer *et al.* (1951) long before the recent evidence for the intercellular diffusion pathway became available.

But before the pore theory is discussed, we should consider some general principles which apply to the passive movements of water and solutes across membranes. These principles were first clearly formulated by Kedem and Katchalsky in 1958 and have considerably influenced the design and interpretation of experiments on membrane permeability. The account of these principles given below is a simplified version of that outlined by Kedem and Katchalsky (1958, 1961) and Katchalsky and Curran (1965). We shall begin by considering the process of the simple diffusion of an uncharged solute in aqueous solution.

A. BULK FLOW AND DIFFUSION IN SIMPLE DILUTE SOLUTION

The bulk flow of a solution, as its name suggests, involves the total transport of solute and solvent together. If a solution of initially uniform concentration flows down a tube, solute and solvent travel with equal velocities and no change in concentration occurs. The mass transport of the solute is equal to the product of its concentration and the volume flow.

Transport by net diffusion is a rather different process involving the dissipation of gradients of chemical potential within the solution. If net diffusion is regarded as a flow, then the force responsible for it is the gradient of chemical potential. The mean net velocity of the diffusing solute is directly proportional to this driving force and the constant of proportionality, K_s, is the conductance of the solution to the solute molecules.

$$\text{i.e. mean net velocity} = \bar{v}_s = -K_s(\partial\mu_s/\partial x) \tag{3.1}$$

It is perhaps easier to think of resistances rather than conductances and K_s may be thought of as the reciprocal of the coefficient of friction between solute and solvent molecules in the solution (f_{sw}):

i.e.
$$K_s = 1/f_{sw}. \tag{3.2}$$

If the solution is maintained at a constant temperature, the chemical potential of the solute is related to the mole fraction of solute, or the molar concentration of solute when the solution is dilute, C_s. The chemical potential of a solute in any particular solution, μ_s, is defined with reference to the chemical potential of a molar solution μ_s°

i.e.
$$\mu_s - \mu_s^\circ = RT \ln C_s. \tag{3.3}$$

Thus a gradient of chemical potential can be expressed as a gradient of concentration:

i.e.
$$\frac{\partial\mu_s}{\partial x} = \frac{\partial\mu_s}{\partial C_s} \cdot \frac{\partial C_s}{\partial x} = \frac{RT}{C_s} \cdot \frac{\partial C_s}{\partial x},$$

and (3.1) may be rewritten as:

$$\bar{v}_s = -\frac{1}{f_{sw}} \cdot \frac{RT}{C_s} \cdot \frac{\partial C_s}{\partial x}. \tag{3.4}$$

Across a plane of unit area of the solution, the total mass flow of solute, J_s, is equal to the product of the mean velocity of the solute molecules and their concentration in that plane:

$$J_s = \bar{v}_s C_s = -\frac{RT}{f_{sw}} \cdot \frac{\partial C_s}{\partial x}. \tag{3.5}$$

Equation (3.5) is identical with Fick's first law of diffusion which usually represents the term RT/f_{sw} as the diffusion coefficient, D_s, of the solute. An alternative way of writing (3.5) would be to make use of the fact that the product of RT and the concentration is equal to the osmotic pressure of the solution, so the mass flow by diffusion is related to the gradient of osmotic pressure:

i.e.
$$J_s = -\frac{1}{f_{sw}} \cdot \frac{\partial \pi_s}{\partial x}. \tag{3.6}$$

So far we have considered net diffusion in terms of the solute molecules moving through a stationary matrix of solvent and we have also thought of the total potential energy of the system as a force driving the solute. At first sight this may appear to be incorrect. The variations in solute concentration represent gradients of chemical potential for water which are equal and opposite to those of the solute. Instead of focussing our attention upon the solute it would be just as reasonable to consider diffusion in terms of the water moving from the less concentrated to the more concentrated regions of the solution.

In reality both movement of solute and movement of water occur but these movements are dependent upon one another. If the volume of the solution remains constant, the net displacement of a given volume of solvent in one direction is accompanied by the displacement of an equal volume of solvent in the opposite direction. The process of net diffusion is determined by the velocity of the solute "relative" to that of the solvent. By regarding the diffusion process as the movement of solute through a stationary framework of solvent, its velocity is equivalent to its velocity relative to that of the solvent and in this way diffusion in free solution may be thought of as movement of the solute alone.

B. Diffusion and Bulk Flow across Membranes

When a membrane divides two solutions of the same solute it is usual to regard flows across the membrane with reference to the membrane, and it is no longer valid to regard the solvent also as at rest.

A membrane can modify the transport of water and solutes by bulk flow and net diffusion: (i) by altering the cross sectional area through which flow can occur; (ii) by offering an additional but different resistance to the solute and the solvent molecules.

A coarse membrane (that is a membrane penetrated by pores whose dimensions are orders of magnitude greater than the solute and solvent molecules) affects diffusion and bulk flow entirely by changing the cross-sectional area of the system. Suitable constants describing this change of area may be incorporated into equations of bulk flow and diffusion in simple solution to describe passive transport across these membranes. But if a membrane hinders the movements of solute and solvent through it to differing extents, the processes of bulk flow and diffusion have to be re-examined.

Let us consider the case of a membrane which hinders the movement of solute more than the movement of solvent. If the membrane separates two solutions of the same solute which are initially at different concentrations, solute moves from the more concentrated to the less concentrated solution and solvent moves in the opposite direction. This diffusional flow, J_D, which may be defined as the velocity of the solute relative to that of the solvent, is proportional to the difference in osmotic pressure across the membrane, $\Delta\pi$. The constant of proportionality relating J_D and $\Delta\pi$ is a coefficient the nature of which is determined by the diffusibility of the solute and solvent within the membrane:

i.e.   Diffusional flow $= J_D = L_D \Delta\pi.$ (3.7)

Since the membrane impedes solute movement more than solvent movement, this is not the only flow occurring. Solvent crosses the membrane more rapidly than solute travels in the opposite direction. As a result of this, the volume of the more concentrated solution increases at the expense of the less concentrated solution and the net volume flow across the membrane is the osmotic flow. The magnitude of the osmotic flow is proportional to the gradient of osmotic pressure across the membrane through a coefficient, L_{PD}, which is determined by the relative conductivity of the membrane for solute and solvent:

i.e.   Osmotic flow $= J_v = L_{PD} \Delta\pi.$ (3.8)

Just as a concentration gradient across a membrane can give rise to net volume flow, so the bulk flow of a solution of uniform concentration through a membrane can give rise to a diffusional flow. Let us consider the membrane, which resists solute more than solvent flow, separating two dilute equi-molar solutions of the same solute. If a pressure gradient is applied across the membrane, the volume flow which results is almost equal to the solvent flow and is related to the pressure gradient through the conductivity of the membrane for the solvent (L_P):

i.e. $J_v = L_P \Delta P$ (3.9)

Because the membrane resists solute movement more than solvent movement, the solvent crosses it more rapidly, and the solution leaving the membrane has a lower concentration of solute than that entering it. This process of ultra-filtration may be thought of as a diffusional flow (i.e. flow of solute relative to that of solvent) proportional to the pressure gradient across the membrane through a coefficient, L_{DP}, which is determined by the relative conductivities of the membrane for solute and solvent.

i.e.   Flow of solute relative to that of solvent $= J_D = L_{DP} \Delta P.$ (3.10)

Equations (3.7), (3.8), (3.9) and (3.10) may be combined into two statements about volume flow and diffusional flow for a membrane separating solutions of different osmotic and hydrostatic pressures:

$$\text{Volume flow} = J_v = L_P \Delta P + L_{PD} \Delta \pi \tag{3.11}$$

$$\text{Diffusional flow} = J_D = L_{DP} \Delta P + L_D \Delta \pi. \tag{3.12}$$

The two flows, J_v and J_D, are linked to one another through the two forces responsible for them. This coupling of flows and forces represents an example of a more general set of relationships of irreversible thermodynamics. The theory of these relationships was explored by Onsager (1931a, b) who argued that the cross coefficients were identical with one another. In (3.11) and (3.12) this means that

$$L_{PD} = L_{DP}. \tag{3.13}$$

The equivalence of the coefficient of osmotic flow and the coefficient of ultrafiltration may be appreciated when it is remembered that both represent the difference between the volume flow of solvent and the volume flow of solute across the membrane.

The coefficient, L_P, represents the solvent conductivity of the membrane and since water is the solvent in biological systems it is also known as the hydraulic conductivity or filtration coefficient. In physical terms it represents the reciprocal of the coefficient of friction between the solvent molecules and the membrane (f_{wm}).

i.e.
$$L_P = \frac{1}{f_{wm}}. \tag{3.14}$$

It is often useful to think of L_{PD} and L_{DP} with reference to L_p. The osmotic pressure which can be measured across a membrane is the hydrostatic pressure which has to be applied to reduce the bulk flow across the membrane to zero. In terms of (3.11), when $J_v = 0$,

$$\text{Measured osmotic pressure} = \Delta P = -\frac{L_{PD}}{L_P} \Delta \pi. \tag{3.15}$$

If the membrane leaks solute then $-L_{PD}$ is less than L_P and the measured difference in osmotic pressure across the membrane is less than the difference in the osmotic pressure of the two solutions which are adjacent to it. The quotient $-L_{PD}/L_P$ has been called by Staverman (1951) the reflection coefficient and denoted by the symbol σ. From the foregoing we see that:

$$\sigma = -\frac{L_{PD}}{L_P} = \frac{v_w - v_s}{v_w} = 1 - \frac{v_s}{v_w}. \tag{3.16}$$

The reflection coefficient summarizes the selectivity of the membrane to solute and water and can be thought of as the fraction of solute "reflected" by the membrane during the bulk flow of a solution of uniform concentration. It can be incorporated into (3.11) which is then rewritten as:

$$J_v = L_P(\Delta P - \sigma \Delta \pi). \tag{3.17}$$

In most practical situations, we are concerned with the total mass flow of solute across a membrane rather than its volume flow relative to solvent. This total flow, J_s, may be readily calculated from (3.12) and (3.17) if the mean concentration of solute within the membrane ($\bar{C}_s$) is known, since:

$$J_s = (J_v + J_D)\bar{C}_s. \tag{3.18}$$

Substituting for J_v and J_D:

$$J_s = \{L_P(\Delta P - \sigma \Delta \pi) + (L_{PD} \Delta P + L_D \Delta \pi)\}\bar{C}_s.$$

From (3.17)

$$\Delta P = \frac{J_v}{L_P} + \sigma \Delta \pi$$

and remembering

$$\frac{L_{PD}}{L_P} = -\sigma$$

$$J_s = \{J_v + L_P \sigma \Delta \pi - L_P \sigma \Delta \pi - \sigma J_v + L_{PD} \sigma \Delta \pi + L_D \Delta \pi\}\bar{C}_s$$
$$= J_v(1-\sigma)\bar{C}_s + \Delta \pi (L_{PD} + L_D)\bar{C}_s. \tag{3.19}$$

When $J_v = 0$,

$$\frac{J_s}{\Delta \pi} = (L_{PD} - L_D)\bar{C}_s = \omega. \tag{3.20}$$

The quotient, $J_s/\Delta \pi$, when $J_v = 0$, represents the permeability of the membrane to solute and is for this reason given the separate symbol, ω; (3.19) may then be rewritten in more compact form as:

$$J_s = J_v(1-\sigma)\bar{C}_s + \omega \Delta \pi \tag{3.21}$$

and since

$$J_v = L_P(\Delta P - \sigma \Delta \pi) \tag{3.17}$$

$$J_s = L_P(\Delta P - \sigma \Delta \pi)(1-\sigma)\bar{C}_s + \omega \Delta \pi. \tag{3.22}$$

Equations (3.21) and (3.22) are general expressions for solute flow across a membrane in the presence of net volume flow and they reveal that even when the gradients of pressure and concentration across the membrane are known, three coefficients, L_P, σ and ω are necessary to describe total solute flow. Equations (3.17), (3.21) and (3.22) describe these flows when only one solute is present in the system, the simplest possible case. Furthermore they involve no assumptions about membrane structure.

Unfortunately only a few experiments on capillary permeability have been planned with these relationships in mind. In some cases, the conditions of the experiments allow calculation of one or two of the membrane coefficients and so are of use in a general description of the properties of the capillary wall.

C. FLOW THROUGH MEMBRANE PORES

Some years before Kedem and Katchalsky's (1958) formulation of the general principles governing flow across membranes, a more specific set of principles was proposed by Pappenheimer *et al.* (1951) to describe flow across membranes penetrated by water filled pores. These workers considered the flow of water and diffusion of solutes through membranes penetrated either by cylindrical pores or by rectangular slits. They suggested that bulk flow of water across such a membrane could be described by the Poiseuille's relationship

$$J_v = \frac{\pi r^4 n}{8 \eta \Delta x} \Delta P \qquad (3.23)$$

where r = pore radius; n = the number of pores per unit area of membrane; η = the viscosity of the fluid in the pores; Δx = thickness of the membrane.

Since the pore area (per unit area of membrane), A_p, is $\pi r^2 n$, (3.23) may be rewritten as:

$$J_v = \frac{r^2}{8\eta} \cdot \frac{A_p}{\Delta x} \cdot \Delta P. \qquad (3.24)$$

As an alternative to the model of flow through cylindrical pores, Pappenheimer *et al.* consider the case of a membrane penetrated by rectangular slits of width equal to w. For this case

$$J_v = \frac{(w/2)^2}{3\eta} \frac{A_p}{\Delta x} \Delta P \qquad (3.25)$$

In the absence of net solvent flow across the membrane, it is argued that the rate of diffusion of solute may be calculated from an application of Fick's law of diffusion to the pore channels.

$$J_s = -D_s \frac{A_s}{\Delta x} \Delta C_s \qquad (3.26)$$

where D_s = the free diffusion coefficient of the solute in water, A_s = the apparent area available for diffusion of the solute in the water-filled channels of the membrane, Δx = thickness of membrane = length of pores.

The authors were quick to point out that A_s could diverge considerably from A_p depending upon the relative sizes of the solute molecule and the pore. This difference would arise not only from the steric factors operating at the entrance of the pore—which might be different for the solute and for water, but also from the additional frictional forces between the solute molecules and the walls of the pore. Thus A_s is not the true area but rather it is a coefficient which when multiplied by the free diffusion coefficient yields a value for the mobility of the solute in the membrane.

Pappenheimer devised a simple method for calculating A_s taking into consideration the radius of the pore and the diffusion (or Stokes–Einstein) radius of the molecule. It was argued that for a pore which was circular in cross section, the target area available for a molecule at the entrance to the pore would be less than the total area if the molecule had to enter the pore without touching the rim. The target area available to the probe molecule relative to the total pore area is:

$$\frac{A_s}{A_p} = \frac{\pi r^2 - \pi a^2}{\pi r^2} = 1 - \left(\frac{a}{r}\right)^2 \tag{3.27}$$

where $a =$ the molecular radius. Once a molecule has entered the pore, the frictional forces between it and the walls of the pore may significantly reduce its velocity through the pore. Pappenheimer used the empirical formula of Ladenburg which expressed the viscous drag, f, on a particle in a cylindrical tube relative to the viscous drag in free solution, f_0, as

$$\frac{f}{f_0} = 1 + 2 \cdot 4 \left(\frac{a}{r}\right). \tag{3.28}$$

Equations (3.27) and (3.28) are combined to yield an expression predicting the extent to which the diffusion of a molecule in a pore will differ from its diffusion in free solution:

$$\frac{D_{\text{restricted}}}{D_{\text{free}}} = \frac{A_s}{A_p} = \frac{1 - (a/r)^2}{1 + 2 \cdot 4(a/r)}. \tag{3.29}$$

Pappenheimer *et al.* also considered the case of diffusion through rectangular slits. The target area for molecules entering the slits is:

$$\frac{A_s}{A_p} = 1 - \frac{a}{w/2} \tag{3.30}$$

where $w/2$ is the half width of the slit. The effect of viscous drag is calculated from the empirical formula of Westgren who studied sedimentation and diffusion between parallel plates:

$$\frac{f}{f_0} = 1 + 3 \cdot 4 \left(\frac{a}{w/2}\right)^2. \tag{3.31}$$

The overall restriction to diffusion through rectangular slits is

$$\frac{D_{\text{restricted}}}{D_{\text{free}}} = \frac{A_s}{A_p} = \frac{(1 - 2a/w)}{[1 + 3 \cdot 4/(2a/w)^2]}. \tag{3.32}$$

In a later treatment of diffusion and bulk flow across artificial membranes

Renkin (1954) preferred the theoretical formulation of Faxén (1922) to Ladenburg's empirical equation. Renkin's equation for restricted diffusion through cylindrical pores is:

$$\frac{A_s}{A_p} = \left(1 - \frac{a}{r}\right)^2 \left[1 - 2\cdot104\left(\frac{a}{r}\right) + 2\cdot09\left(\frac{a}{r}\right)^3 - 0\cdot95\left(\frac{a}{r}\right)^5\right]. \tag{3.33}$$

When net filtration is occurring through a cylindrical pore, the bulk flow increases the movement of solute in the direction of the flow. Renkin applied Ferry's (1936) formulation for the steric hindrance at the entrance to a pore and combined it with (3.33) to obtain

$$\left(\frac{A_s}{A_p}\right)_{filtration} = \left[2\left(1 - \frac{a}{r}\right)^2 - \left(1 - \frac{a}{r}\right)^4\right]$$

$$\times \left[1 - 2\cdot104\left(\frac{a}{r}\right)^3 - 0\cdot95\left(\frac{a}{r}\right)^5\right]. \tag{3.34}$$

Most recent workers have preferred to use (3.33) and (3.34) rather than (3.29).

The most important feature of these equations is that they make very specific predictions about deviations of permeability coefficients from the diffusion coefficients of molecules of different sizes, and that these deviations are dependent only on the size of the molecules and of the pores.

If the permeability coefficients are known for a series of molecules of known molecular dimensions, then (3.32). (3.33) and (3.34) allow the calculation of the pore dimensions.

Pappenheimer and his colleagues described total solute flows across a membrane in terms of a diffusion flow and a bulk flow term:

$$J_s = D_s \frac{A_s}{\Delta x} \Delta C + J_v \cdot \frac{A_s}{A_w} C_p. \tag{3.35}$$

(A_w = pore area available to water, C_p = concentration of solute on the upstream side of the membrane when J_v is positive). Equation (3.35) very clearly resembles (3.21) and leads us to suggest that

$$\frac{A_s}{A_w} \simeq 1 - \sigma \tag{3.36}$$

a conclusion arrived at using different reasoning by Durbin (1960).

The importance of the pore hypothesis lies not only in its very concrete predictions about membrane structure, but also in the very convenient description it provides of flows across membranes. From a knowledge of the pore radius and the total pore area in a membrane the flow of solvent and solute across the membrane can be predicted on the assumption that bulk flow can be described by Poiseuille's law and diffusion can be described by Fick's law of diffusion, with the free diffusion coefficients multiplying the area term in accordance with the theory of restricted diffusion.

12*

The more general thermodynamic relations offer no such unifying prediction about flows across membranes. This theory for the flow of a solute across a membrane demands, in addition to a coefficient describing hydraulic flow, a further two coefficients which describe the movement of that molecular species only. No simple relation between the reflection coefficient and the membrane permeability is proposed.

Relatively few experiments on capillary permeability have been designed with this background of theory in mind. The pore theory was proposed by Pappenheimer *et al.* (1951) and these workers supplied more information relevant to it than has been collected since. The difficulty of measuring a simple permeability term or a permeability surface area product is considerable and most workers have been content to measure this alone. Permeability used in this general sense will be denoted by the symbol M, and its relation to the other symbols used so far is

$$M_s = \frac{J_s}{A\Delta C} = \omega RT = D_s \frac{A_s}{\Delta x} \frac{1}{A} \tag{3.37}$$

where A = the total area of the capillary wall, and A_s = area available to the molecule s. However relatively more attempts have been made to measure the passage of water across the capillary wall and it is appropriate to consider these measurements first.

4. WATER FLOW ACROSS THE CAPILLARY WALL

In 1896 Starling proposed an hypothesis to account for the steady state distribution of water between the blood and the tissues. He suggested that the outward filtration of water, resulting from a higher hydrostatic pressure in the capillary lumen than in the extracapillary fluid, was balanced by re-absorption of fluid from the tissues into the blood down a gradient of osmotic pressure, resulting from the higher concentrations of protein in the plasma as compared with their concentrations in the interstitial fluid. Starling's hypothesis can be represented as:

$$J_{v_F}A = L_P A(\Delta P - \Delta \pi_p) \tag{4.1}$$

where

J_{v_F} = net filtration of water out of unit area of the capillary wall,

L_P = hydrostatic conductivity (or filtration coefficient) of the capillary wall,

A = area of capillary wall,

$\Delta P, \Delta \pi_p$ = mean gradients of hydrostatic pressure, and protein osmotic pressure across the capillary wall.

Starling suggested that there was normally a small excess of filtration over reabsorption and this accounted for the lymph flow from the tissues. Lymph flow is of considerable importance to the maintenance of the Starling balance, for although capillary walls are almost impermeable to plasma proteins the permeability is yet finite. If the interstitial fluid were a closed compartment, its protein concentration would slowly rise and so reduce and finally abolish the osmotic pressure gradient relative to the plasma. The steady filtration of water through the interstitial space dilutes any protein leaving the capillary and so maintains the protein concentration of the interstitial fluid at a low level.

Starling provided clear evidence for his belief that fluid could be absorbed directly from the tissues into the blood. He also made the first measurements of protein osmotic pressure, determining a value for the plasma proteins which he believed to be comparable with the mean capillary pressure. Thirty years elapsed between the publication of Starling's paper and the publication by Landis of the first reliable estimates of capillary pressure and of fluid movements across the capillary wall. Since then, an impressive body of experimental evidence has been obtained from studies on single capillaries and on whole capillary beds. Here we shall consider the experimental findings under the sub-headings of these two very different ways of approaching the problem.

A. STUDIES ON SINGLE CAPILLARIES

The first reliable estimates of capillary pressure were made in 1926 by Landis. Using a micromanipulator and a micropipette filled with a coloured solution and attached to a manometer system, he cannulated single capillaries in the transilluminated tissues of the frog mesentery. The pressure inside these vessels was measured by adjusting the pressure in the manometer system until the flow of coloured fluid through the tip of the micropipette was zero.

Landis (1927) also devised a most ingenious method for measuring the net movement of water across single capillaries. He observed that when he occluded a capillary with a microneedle, red cells would sometimes flow towards the occlusion and on other occasions would flow away from it. Landis argued that movement of a red cell towards the occlusion was the result of water being filtered from the column of plasma between the red cell and the point of occlusion. Reabsorption of fluid into such a column would cause the red cell to move away from the occlusion. Knowing the diameter of such a capillary and assuming that it was circular in cross section, Landis was able to convert the linear movements of the red cells (measured on a micrometer scale) into fluid flow. By measuring the pressure inside the capillary using his micropipette technique, he was able to define the relationship between the movement of fluid across the capillary walls and the pressure inside the vessels. This is shown in Fig. 4 and although there is a fair degree of scatter, the linear correlation, which is predicted by (4.1), is a good one. Furthermore the pressure range in which neither filtration nor reabsorption appeared to occur corresponded with the range of protein osmotic pressures determined by White (1924) for plasma of frogs of the same species. If the hydrostatic and protein osmotic pressures of the interstitial

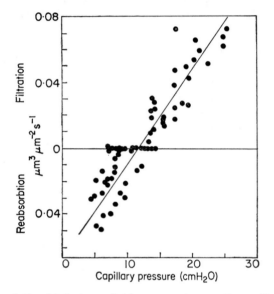

FIG. 4. The relationship between fluid movement across the capillary wall and the capillary pressure as determined by Landis (1927) in single capillaries of the frog mesentery.

fluid are close to zero, then Landis's data are direct evidence in favour of Starling's hypothesis. Landis determined the capillary pressure in the mesenteric vessels of the rat and the guinea-pig (Landis, 1930a) and also in the nail bed capillaries of man (Landis, 1930b). The mean values of such measurements agreed well with the mean values for the plasma colloidal osmotic pressure of these species.

From the slope of the regression line in Fig. 4 relating fluid movement and capillary pressure, Landis calculated a value for the filtration coefficient of frog mesenteric capillaries and obtained a value of $0 \cdot 0056 \ \mu m^3 \ \mu m^{-2}$ $(cmH_2O)^{-1} \ s^{-1}$. In later experiments he showed that this slope was considerably increased (while the pressure corresponding to zero flow across the capillary wall was also considerably reduced) when frog mesenteric capillaries were damaged by either alcohol or mercuric chloride or a combination of anoxia and circulatory arrest.

It is arguable that Landis's values for the filtration coefficient represent mean values for the capillary bed only if the scatter in his data results from random variations in the filtration coefficients, and the colloidal osmotic pressure gradients across the walls of the vessels he investigated, as well as variations introduced by the limitations of the method. An observation made a few years later suggested that the local pressure and the local filtration rate in a population of capillaries might be correlated. One might expect that those capillaries which have a high intraluminal pressure are closer to the arterial end of the capillary bed than those vessels having a lower ambient pressure. Using the readiness with which dyes were able to pass from the living circulation into the tissues as an index of capillary permeability, Rous et al. (1930) obtained strong evidence, in both frog and mammalian tissues, that the venous end of the capillary bed was more permeable than the arterial end. Later studies have confirmed these findings (Chambers and Zweifach, 1940) and it now appears that the arteriovenous gradient of permeability to dyes is mirrored by an arteriovenous gradient in the filtration coefficient. These findings imply that the filtration coefficient calculated from the regression line through Landis's data represents more closely the lower value of filtration coefficient found among vessels at the arterial end of the capillary bed. Evidence in favour of this idea has recently been put forward by Zweifach and Intaglietta (1968).

In recent years Zweifach and his colleagues have reported values for the filtration coefficients of capillaries in rabbit omentum and rat cremaster muscle. Their technique does not involve the cannulation of individual capillaries but requires the determination of the plasma colloidal osmotic pressure and the measurement of filtration rate (by a modernized version of the Landis method). Zweifach and Intaglietta (1968) have determined the filtration rate in single capillaries of rabbit omentum before and after the injection of an albumin solution into the blood. Expressing the two sets of values for filtration rate and plasma colloidal osmotic pressure in terms of two simultaneous equations of the form of (4.1), the two unknowns L_P and ΔP can be calculated providing one assumed that L_P, ΔP and the colloidal osmotic pressure of the interstitial fluid is the same when the two measurements of filtration rate are made. This assumption must blunt the precision of the method, particularly as the changes in plasma colloidal osmotic pressure are not large. Nevertheless, Zweifach and Intaglietta (1968) have been able to obtain a good correlation between fluid movement and plasma colloidal osmotic pressure and reproducible calculated values for ΔP in the same capillary which has given them confidence to investigate the variability of filtration coefficients in capillary beds. A further development of this method has been described by Smaje et al. (1970) in their work on the capillaries of rat cremaster muscle. In these studies the filtration rate was measured in a single capillary before and after a change in the colloid osmotic pressure of the extravascular fluid brought about by an alteration in the composition of the superfusate which washed the tissue. Capillary pressures calculated from filtration rates and filtration coefficients agreed well with values obtained by micropuncture.

Levick and Michel (1971) have perfused frog mesenteric capillaries with dye-protein solutions via a micropipette and then occluded the vessel some way downstream. They have applied step changes in pressure through the micropipette to the closed-off section of the vessel and measured the corresponding changes in filtration rate from the changes in optical density resulting from the concentration of dye in the capillary. In this way it has been possible to detect vessels which leaked protein and also to investigate the filtration coefficient at different capillary pressures. Their findings suggest that those capillaries that retain dye protein complex for several minutes have filtration coefficients which are slightly greater than the Landis value (i.e. $0 \cdot 009 \, \mu m^3 \, \mu m^{-2} \, (cmH_2O)^{-1} \, s^{-1}$ as opposed to Landis's $0 \cdot 0056 \, \mu m^3 \, \mu m^{-2} \, (cmH_2O)^{-1} \, s^{-1}$), though there is a considerable range of variation. This variation between capillaries appears to support the evidence of a gradient of permeability.

Within a given capillary, however, they have been able to demonstrate the linearity of (4.1) by showing that over the range of capillary pressure and colloid osmotic pressure from $15 \, cmH_2O$ to $35 \, cmH_2O$, the filtration coefficient is independent of hydrostatic and osmotic pressure.

B. MEAN CAPILLARY PRESSURE, FILTRATION RATES AND FILTRATION COEFFICIENTS IN CAPILLARY BEDS

A most ingenious method for estimating the mean capillary pressure in the isolated perfused hind limb of cats and dogs was described by Pappenheimer and Soto-Rivera in 1948. The weight of the limb was recorded throughout the perfusion and it was argued that when limb weight was constant, a condition referred to as the isogravimetric state, no net movement of fluid was occurring between the blood and the tissues. When the blood flow was varied and the limb held in the isogravimetric state by variations in venous pressure, then the mean capillary pressure should be related to the venous pressure through the blood flow and the post-capillary resistance, i.e.

$$\bar{P}_c = P_v + \rho_v \dot{Q} \qquad (4.2)$$

where

$\bar{P}_c$ = mean capillary pressure
P_v = the venous pressure
ρ_v = post capillary resistance
$\dot{Q}$ = blood flow through limb.

If the post-capillary resistance is independent of P_c, P_v and $\dot{Q}$, then with P_c constant (isogravimetric condition) rearrangement of (4.2) indicates a linear relationship between P_v and $\dot{Q}$ having a slope of ρ_v and an intercept at $Q = 0$ of $\bar{P}_c$. Pappenheimer and Soto-Rivera were able to show that this was indeed the case and $\bar{P}_c$ and ρ_v could be determined in this way (see Fig. 5).

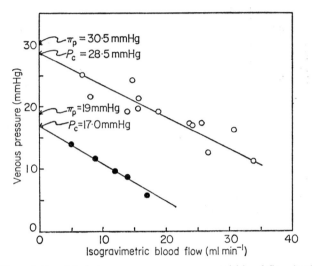

FIG. 5. The relationship between venous pressure and blood flow in the isolated perfused cat hind limb maintained in an isogravimetric state. The two lines represent determinations made at two different concentrations of circulating plasma protein. Note the close agreement between the plasma protein osmotic pressure (π_p) and the mean capillary pressure (P_c). From Pappenheimer and Soto-Rivera (1948).

A similar relation to (4.2) can be written in terms of the precapillary resistance and the arterial pressure, but the precapillary resistance varies with the flow (or pressure drop across it) and the extrapolation of the non-linear relation between arterial pressure and blood flow is less certain.

Pappenheimer and Soto-Rivera were able to show a close correlation between the protein osmotic pressure and the mean (isogravimetric) capillary pressure. Furthermore, having determined the value of ρ_v, they substituted this value in (4.1) to calculate the changes in P_c following a step change in venous pressure. Under these circumstances, the limb ceased to be isogravimetric and the movement of water from the blood into the tissues (or from the tissues into the blood) could be followed from the changes in the weight of the limb.

The relationship between increments in limb-weight and the calculated increments of capillary pressure was very linear (see Fig. 6) and had a slope of 0.002 g/100 g of tissue/mmHg min^{-1}. Assuming that the capillaries of the isolated perfused hind-limb are largely those of skeletal muscle and that surface area of the muscle capillary bed is 7000 cm^2/100 g muscle, Pappenheimer and Soto-Rivera calculated their results as a filtration coefficient of the muscle capillaries.

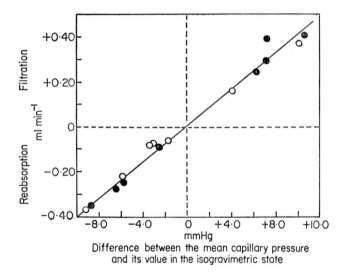

Difference between the mean capillary pressure
and its value in the isogravimetric state

FIG. 6. The relationship between transcapillary fluid movement and the mean capillary pressure in the isolated perfused hind limb of a cat (from Pappenheimer and Soto-Rivera, 1948). The results are expressed as the rate of filtration or reabsorption of fluid from the blood into the tissues of the hind limb following changes in the mean capillary pressure away from its isogravimetric value. The closed circles represent determinations made when the hind limb was perfused with normal plasma; the open circles represent determinations made when the protein concentration of the perfusate had been increased by the addition of bovine albumin.

Instead of using limb-weight to estimate fluid movement between the blood and the tissues one may also use limb volume. This idea was first tried by Krogh et al. (1932) who correlated the filtration of fluid (measured with a plethysmograph) with changes in venous pressure. Landis and Gibbon (1933) elaborated the technique and the results they obtained indicated a linear relation between fluid movement and venous pressure from which one may estimate a filtration coefficient if one is prepared to guess the post-capillary resistance.

A plethysmographic technique for measuring filtration coefficients has been developed in recent years by Mellander, Folkow and their colleagues (see Mellander, 1960). They have argued that the isovolumetric state is equivalent to an isogravimetric state, and if the plasma protein concentration is normal, the mean capillary pressure may be assumed to be 20 mmHg. If the total blood flow through the limb and the arterial and venous pressures are separately measured, then the ratio of pre- to post-capillary resistance can be estimated. Changes in capillary pressure may be calculated from changes

TABLE 1

Filtration coefficients of capillary walls as measured in single capillaries and in capillary beds

Tissue or organ	Filtration coefficient $\mu m(s\ cmH_2O)^{-1}$	Authors
Single capillaries		
Frog mesentery	$5 \cdot 6 \times 10^{-3}$	Landis, (1927)
Frog mesentery	$4 \cdot 0 – 16 \cdot 0 \times 10^{-3}$ (no protein leakage) $15 \cdot 0 – 50 \cdot 0 \times 10^{-3}$ (protein leakage)	Levick and Michel, (Unpublished observations).
Rabbit omentum	$2 – 8 \times 10^{-3}$ arterial capillaries $16 – 25 \times 10^{-3}$ venous capillaries	Zweifach and Intaglietta, (1968)
Rat cremaster	1×10^{-3}	Smaje et al., (1970)
Capillary beds†		
Human forearm	1×10^{-4}	Landis and Gibbon, (1933)
Cat, dog hind limb	$2 \cdot 5 \times 10^{-4}$	Pappenheimer and Soto-Rivera, (1948)
Cat hind limb	$3 \cdot 5 – 5 \cdot 2 \times 10^{-4}$	Mellander, (1960)
Rabbit heart	$8 \cdot 6 \times 10^{-4}$	Vargas and Johnson, (1964)
Dog lung	$2 \cdot 21 \times 10^{-5}$	Guyton and Lindsey, (1959)

†The following figures have been assumed for the area of capillary wall per 100 g of tissue: human forearm, $7 \cdot 10^3$ cm²; cat, dog hind limb, $7 \cdot 10^3$ cm²; rabbit heart, $5 \cdot 10^4$ cm²; dog lung, $4 \cdot 10^5$ cm².

in venous pressure, and the capillary filtration coefficient can be determined from these changes and the accompanying slow changes in limb volume. The figures obtained by Mellander for the filtration coefficient of dog and cat hindlimbs agrees very closely with the values obtained by Pappenheimer and Soto-Rivera (see Table 1).

Table 1 summarizes the values obtained for the filtration coefficients of different capillaries and capillary beds determined by workers using different methods. It is perhaps worth emphasizing that where filtration measurements are made on whole organs or tissues, a knowledge of the total area of capillary wall involved in the filtration process must be available before the figure derived for filtration coefficient can be related to the structures in the capillary wall which are providing the resistance to flow. Although very careful estimates of capillary surface area have been made for skeletal muscle of cats and dogs (Pappenheimer, 1953; Landis and Pappenheimer, 1963) and in heart muscle (Johnson and Simmonds, quoted by Schafer and Johnson, 1964) there is always some degree of approximation in the application of these figures to physiological measurements where the total number of open capillaries is unknown.

C. DISCUSSION OF THE DETERMINATION OF CAPILLARY FILTRATION
COEFFICIENTS

A study of Table 1 reveals that the values of the capillary filtration coefficient obtained for capillary beds are considerably less than those values obtained for single capillaries. It has already been pointed out that the values of capillary surface area can only be approximate as far as the capillary beds are concerned but it is unlikely that these estimates could be so erroneous as to account for this discrepancy. The measurements on single vessels all involve exposure and illumination of the tissue as well as occlusion of the capillaries with glass microneedles and although it might be supposed that all these procedures increase the permeability of the capillary wall the lower range of values obtained for frog mesenteric capillaries refer to vessels which do not appear to leak dye-stained protein when this is perfused through them for several minutes. Of course the single capillaries, whose filtration coefficients are known, do not belong to capillary beds whose filtration coefficients are known, and the discrepancy may be the result of a false comparison. It is nevertheless a very surprising one.

Recently Wiederhielm (1968) has questioned (4.1) as a description of fluid movements in a capillary bed. He has pointed out that because the surface area of capillary wall and the filtration coefficient (expressed in terms of unit area) are both greater at the venous than at the arterial end of the capillary bed, separate equations should be written for the filtration of water from the blood and its reabsorption from the tissues. Furthermore, he points out that the processes of filtration and reabsorption will modify the gradients of colloidal osmotic pressure across the capillary wall. In the presence of filtration, the extra-capillary concentration of protein will be low through dilution by the filtration stream, thus steepening the gradient of protein osmotic pressure and limiting the filtration rate, whereas in regions of reabsorption, the pericapillary protein concentration may be expected to rise and thus reduce the protein osmotic pressure gradient.

Wiederhielm (1968) has developed an analogue computer model which takes these factors into account and incorporates in addition the permeability of the capillary wall to protein and the flow of lymph out of the tissue. The model makes many interesting predictions and can account for the failure of tissues to become oedematous following moderate decrements in plasma protein concentration and moderate increments in venous pressure.

It would appear that Wiederhielm's model may yield values for the filtration coefficients of capillary beds which vary with changes in venous pressure and plasma osmotic pressure. Such a prediction is at variance with the findings of Pappenheimer and Soto-Rivera (1948) but Wiederhielm has argued that since these experiments were preceded by a period of prolonged filtration and since the plasma perfusing the limb in the control state had a low osmotic pressure, the hydrostatic and osmotic pressures of the interstitial fluid differed from those normally surrounding a capillary bed.

The values which Wiederhielm has used in his model for the capillary surface area, capillary pressure and interstitial fluid pressure are based on measurements made on the bat's wing, and the values for the arteriovenous gradient of filtration coefficient are from frog mesenteric capillaries. It is to be hoped that as more information about other capillary beds becomes available, Wiederhielm's model (or its offspring) will be applied to these other tissues.

At present the exact values of the hydrostatic pressure and the osmotic pressure of the interstitial fluid are very controversial subjects. Until ten years ago it was believed that the hydrostatic pressure of the interstitial fluid was equal to or was slightly greater than the atmospheric pressure, but measurements using an implanted capsule (Guyton, 1963) or an implanted wick (Scholander *et al.*, 1968) suggest that the interstitial fluid is several mm Hg less than atmospheric. The origin of this sub-atmospheric pressure is hotly disputed and the reader is referred to the review of Guyton (1969) and the paper of Stromberg and Wiederhielm (1970) for different points of view.

5. SOLUTE FLOW ACROSS THE CAPILLARY WALL

Although there are many experiments reported in the literature which describe the accumulation of solutes in tissues, relatively few attempts have been made to correlate solute flow with the gradient of concentration across the capillary wall and so express the results in terms of capillary permeability. Because the blood moves from the arterial to the venous end of a capillary while exchange is occurring, the concentration gradient and net volume flow across the capillary wall vary from point to point along the length of the vessel. So far it has not been possible to measure the concentration gradient at a single point along a vessel and attempts to measure capillary permeability have depended upon our estimate of the mean concentration gradient.

Shortly after radioactive isotopes were introduced into physiology it was thought that exchange between the blood and interstitial fluid could be analysed as exchange between two compartments. These analyses assumed that the concentration of solute in the blood compartment could be obtained from its arterial value. The error of this assumption may be considerable particularly for substances which equilibrate rapidly (as pointed out by Pappenheimer *et al.*, 1951) and although data obtained in this way may be empirically useful it yields little information about the exchange across the endothelial cell barrier. For slowly equilibrating molecules, the objections to compartmental analysis of exchange are less serious. But when such methods are used to estimate changes in capillary permeability, the results must again be examined with caution. A pharmacologist investigating the effect of a drug upon the accumulation of dye-stained protein in a tissue should account for changes in capillary blood flow and capillary pressure before he interprets an increased accumulation of the tracer in the tissues as a change in capillary permeability.

Mathematical models of exchange in the capillary bed are very complex (see for example Schmidt, 1952) and to be exact they require information on the extracapillary spaces which is rarely available. As the models attempt to incorporate more and more of the factors involved, so they become more formidable (e.g. Johnson and Wilson, 1966; Blum, 1960; Schmidt, 1952, 1953; Goresky *et al.*, 1970; Levitt, 1971). Nevertheless an attempt to apply Schmidt's model to experimental results has been made by Schafer and Johnson (1964). From experimental studies of the penetration of sucrose and inulin into the tissues of the perfused rabbit heart they calculated values of capillary permeability from the permeation times which were comparable with those obtained by other methods.

These other methods have involved rather simpler models of capillary exchange but before we consider them in more detail we shall examine some of the more elementary consequences of blood flow upon exchange.

If a substance is injected into the blood, its concentration along the length of a capillary falls as it leaves the plasma and enters the interstitial fluid. This is illustrated in Fig. 7 which depicts the fall in concentration with distance along a capillary or fall in concentration with the time the blood spends in the capillary. For substance A, equilibrium between the blood and the tissue is achieved after the blood has spent only a fraction of its total time in the exchange. For substance B equilibrium is achieved at the end of the vessel whereas substance C is not in the capillary long enough to equilibrate with its surroundings during a single transit. The amount of solute transferred is the product of the arteriovenous concentration difference and the blood flow and its value would be the same for A and B but it would be rather less for C.

If the blood flow were reduced so that the capillary transit time was increased, the uptake of A and B from the blood would be reduced in direct proportion to the blood flow (constant arteriovenous difference). The uptake of C might also be reduced, but the reduction would not be proportional

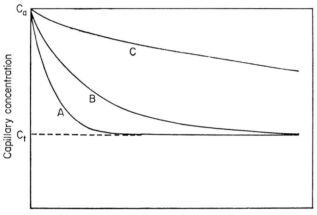

Distance along capillary or time spent in capillary

FIG. 7. The fall in blood concentration of three substances as they equilibrate with the tissues during their passage through a capillary. The capillary wall is more permeable to A than B, and more permeable to B than C. Because equilibrium is achieved for A and B before the blood leaves the capillary net movement of these substances from the blood into the tissues can only be increased by increasing the blood flow and the exchange of A and B is said to be flow limited. Substance C does not equilibrate completely during a single transit and its exchange is said to be diffusion limited.

to blood flow, for the longer residence time of the blood within the capillaries would lead to a widening of the arteriovenous difference. Increasing the blood flow would increase the uptake of all three substances, having a greater effect upon the uptake of A than of B, and of B than of C.

Since the exchange of A and B can only be increased by increasing the blood flow, the exchange of A and B is said to be "flow limited". Since C did not reach equilibrium in a single transit, the exchange of C across the capillary wall is said to be "diffusion limited".

Diffusion limited exchange and flow limited exchange can be defined in terms of the extraction of a test substance from the blood, If C_a, C_v and C_t

are the arterial, venous and tissue concentrations of the substance, then the extraction, E, is:

$$E = \frac{C_a - C_v}{C_a - C_t}. \tag{5.1}$$

For flow limited exchange extraction is unity and where diffusion limitation exists extraction is always less than one. When applying (5.1) in this way it is very important to know that there are no arteriovenous shunts across a capillary bed for they would give rise to arteriovenous differences indicative of diffusion limited exchange when in reality the exchange process might be severely flow limited.

It is perhaps worth pointing out that the net exchange of a diffusion limited substance is increased by increasing the blood flow except when diffusion limitation is so severe that the arteriovenous difference is negligible. It has also been argued that even the most diffusible substances are diffusion limited on the grounds that their rate of diffusion out of the blood is limited by the rate at which they can distribute themselves in the extravascular space (Hills, 1970). Such arguments merely point out that diffusion limitation and flow limitation are terms which do not withstand semantic analysis. Providing they are defined in accordance with Fig. 7 or (5.1), the terms are useful in describing the exchange process.

The importance of detecting flow limited exchange becomes apparent when one attempts to measure capillary permeability to substances such as A and B. If one attempts to calculate the mean concentration gradient across the capillary wall from the arterial and venous concentrations one would arrive at the same answer for both substances and thus ascribe to them similar values for capillary permeability. This sort of difficulty has meant that it has not been possible so far to obtain figures for the capillary permeability to highly diffusible substances such as small fat soluble molecules.

Most of the work carried out on solute flow across capillary walls has been concerned with lipid insoluble molecules and it is these measurements which are considered in more detail below. We shall describe the principles which have been used and the assumptions which they involve before discussing the results and their interpretation.

A. OSMOTIC TRANSIENT TECHNIQUE OF PAPPENHEIMER, RENKIN AND BORRERO

The quantitative study of solute flow across capillary walls dates from the monumental paper of Pappenheimer *et al.* (1951). Using the isolated perfused hind limb preparation of Pappenheimer and Soto-Rivera (1948) they estimated the net solute flow from the blood into the tissues from the product of the blood flow and the arteriovenous concentration difference and they estimated the mean concentration gradient across the capillary walls from the osmotic pressure which resulted from it.

The test solute was added to the perfusion system and when it reached the capillary bed the gradient of osmotic pressure across the capillary wall caused fluid to shift from the tissues into the blood. This fluid movement could be detected as a fall in the weight of the limb and it could be opposed by raising the hydrostatic pressure in the capillaries by raising venous pressure in the perfusion system. Since the relationship between venous pressure and capillary pressure could be determined for any given preparation, the changing transcapillary osmotic pressure could be followed.

To convert the osmotic pressure gradient to the mean concentration gradient, Pappenheimer *et al.* used van't Hoff's law of osmotic pressure,

i.e. $\Delta C = \Delta \pi / RT,$

and calculated the product of permeability and capillary surface area as

$$D_s \frac{A_s}{\Delta x} = \frac{J_s}{\Delta \pi_s / RT}. \qquad (5.2)$$

Using this technique, Pappenheimer and his colleagues obtained a value for capillary permeability to a wide range of lipid insoluble molecules. It was these results which led to the theory of restricted diffusion through pores and the proposal that the capillary wall was penetrated by pores of 3·0 to 3·5 nm in radius or by slits 3·7 nm in width.

The major criticism of this technique is the assumption that the concentration gradient can be calculated from the osmotic gradient without reference to the reflection coefficient. It is hardly surprising that Pappenheimer and his colleagues were prepared to make this assumption, for Staverman's work on the reflection coefficient had not been published when their paper went to press. Pappenheimer (1953) and Landis and Pappenheimer (1963) attempted to calculate the influence of the reflection coefficient. Using the rather intuitive definition of σ as

$$\sigma = 1 - D_s A_s / D_w A_w \qquad (5.3)$$

they obtained a modified set of values for permeability which altered the original conclusions only slightly.

A more formal derivation of σ in terms of restricted pore area has been made by Durbin (1960). At zero volume flow (the condition of the experiments of Pappenheimer *et al.*)

$$\sigma = 1 - A_s / A_w. \qquad (3.36)$$

It is possible to examine the original data of Pappenheimer *et al.* combining

(3.36) with the theory of restricted diffusion to find a consistent value for equivalent pore radius. The figure derived in this way differs considerably from Pappenheimer's earlier estimates, being of the order of 14 nm.

Equations (3.36) and (5.3) both assume that the sole pathway for water and solute molecules is a common one and Pappenheimer (1970a) has recently pointed out that if a significant fraction of total water flow across the capillary wall occurs by a route unavailable to solute (e.g. across the endothelial cells) then the mean reflection coefficient of the capillary wall would be considerably higher than that calculated from equations such as (3.36). Yudilevich and Alvarez (1967) have provided strong evidence that water can exchange across a much larger area of capillary wall than is available to Na^+ (allowing for restricted diffusion) and suggested that whereas small lipid insoluble molecules are confined to the intercellular regions, water can exchange across the total endothelial cell area. So far it has not been possible to estimate the hydraulic conductivity of endothelial cells but Lifson (1970) and Tosteson (1970) have shown that Pappenheimer's original estimate of equivalent pore radius will be numerically correct if half the total filtration flow occurs across the cells.

B. OSMOTIC TRANSIENT TECHNIQUE OF VARGAS AND JOHNSON

A rather different osmotic transient technique was described in 1964 by Vargas and Johnson in experiments on the reflection coefficient of rabbit heart capillaries to urea, sucrose, raffinose and inulin. An isolated rabbit heart was prepared by the Langendorff method with a high flow rate and it was weighed continuously. During the initial control period, the heart was perfused at constant weight with a Ringer Locke solution. The perfusate was abruptly changed to a Ringer Locke solution containing the test solute and the subsequent osmotic transient recorded. From the initial rate of weight change, a flow was calculated corresponding to the initial osmotic gradient across the capillary walls. It was assumed that when this initial osmotic gradient was set up, the mean concentration of test solute in the capillaries was equal to the inflow concentration, on the grounds that flow rate was very high, and that the extracapillary concentration of solute was zero. The hydraulic conductivity of the capillary bed was determined from a separate osmotic transient when test perfusate contained albumin (for which it was assumed $\sigma = 1$), the osmotic pressure of which had been separately determined.

The reflection coefficient of the capillary wall to the test solute was calculated from

$$\sigma_s = \frac{J_v^\circ}{L_P RT C^\circ} \tag{5.4}$$

where σ_s = the reflection coefficient of the test solute, J_v° = the initial osmotic flow caused by the test solute, L_P = the hydraulic conductivity of the whole capillary bed and C° = the concentration of test solute in the perfusate.

In a later paper Vargas and Johnson (1967) used these data to calculate the permeability of the capillary wall to the test substances. They argued that if the ratio of capillary surface to extracapillary volume of distribution (A/V) of the test solute is known, the permeability (M) can be calculated from the time constant of the osmotic transient ($\alpha = 0.69$/half time), i.e.

$$M = \frac{\alpha}{(A/V)}. \qquad (5.5)$$

Various corrections were made for flow limitations, heterogeneous distribution outside the capillary, changes in extracellular volume, lymph flow and the effects of solvent drag and the authors admitted that because of the many assumptions involved in the calculation of permeability, their figures could only be regarded as rough estimates.

Perhaps the most serious criticisms of the technique concerns the assumption that the mean concentration gradient across the capillary walls at zero time is equal to the inflowing concentration of test solute. While the calculated initial concentration profile (Johnson and Wilson, 1966) suggests that the mean capillary concentration differs only slightly from the inflowing concentration, the concentration gradient across the capillary wall (or across the pore system) may be substantially less than the capillary concentration (Pappenheimer, 1970b). For a rapidly penetrating solute such as urea, it would be reasonable to suppose that by the time the non-extracted molecules had reached the venous end of the capillary, the gradient across the arterial end of the capillary wall would be considerably below its initial value. For the gradient across the endothelial cells to deviate from its initial value, only a relatively small number of molecules need leave the capillary and enter the wider parts of the intercellular cleft beyond the tight region.

In spite of criticisms of their technique, Vargas and Johnson's experiments are the only studies which have attempted to examine permeability of the capillary wall to low molecular solutes according to the principles laid down by Kedem and Katchalsky in 1958. In the theoretical sections of their papers they have also provided a lucid analysis of osmotic transients which might be a useful guide to further work.

C. THE INDICATOR DILUTION METHOD FOR MEASURING CAPILLARY PERMEABILITY

A very elegant method for investigating blood-tissue exchange has been devised by Chinard and his colleagues (Chinard et al., 1955). The technique derives from the single-injection indicator-dilution method for measuring blood flow of Stewart and Hamilton. An indicator which is confined to the vascular system is injected into an artery along with a second indicator which is known to cross the endothelial barrier and samples are drawn in rapid succession from a vein draining the capillary bed. The concentrations of diffusible and indiffusible tracer in any sample of venous blood provide a figure for the fraction of diffusible indicator which has left the blood and entered the tissues. A penetrating analysis of the method has been provided by Zierler (1963).

Crone (1963) and Martin de Julián and Yudilevich (1964) have used the technique to estimate capillary permeability. They have examined the earliest stages of extraction and have argued that at these times the extravascular concentration of diffusible tracer is zero. Under these circumstances the concentration profile of the diffusible substance between the arterial and venous ends of a capillary should vary according to a simple exponential relation derived by Kety (1951) and Renkin (1959a) (and identical to the derivation of Bohr in his definition of pulmonary diffusing capacity)

$$C_v = C_a \exp\left(-MA/\dot{Q}\right) \tag{5.6}$$

or when the tissue concentration (C_t) is constant but not equal to zero

$$C_v - C_t = (C_a - C_t) \exp\left(-MA/\dot{Q}\right). \tag{5.7}$$

Equation (5.7) may be expressed in terms of extraction of the diffusible indicator and a convenient form for calculating permeability is

$$MA = -\dot{Q} \ln\left(1 - E\right). \tag{5.8}$$

C_a is calculated from the concentration of indiffusible tracer (usually labelled plasma protein): C_v is the venous concentration of diffusible tracer and E is defined by (5.1), $\dot{Q}$, the capillary blood flow, is assumed to be equal to the total blood flow through the tissues.

The method provides an intoxicating combination of experimental elegance and fascinating theory. The fact that it can be used to measure the permeability of a capillary bed when the circulation is intact, adds to its attractiveness and to the attention it will continue to receive.

The method is not free from difficulties. In calculating C_a from the concentration of non-exchanging tracer in the venous blood, it is assumed that the indiffusible tracer and those molecules of diffusible tracer which do not cross the capillary walls are dispersed to a similar extent in the vascular system. Renkin (1959b), Bate et al. (1969) and Lassen and Crone (1970) have pointed out that this is not true. Tracer molecules are dispersed within the vascular system to some extent according to their diffusion coefficients. Since the indiffusible tracer usually has a smaller diffusion coefficient than the diffusible tracer, its volume of distribution within the blood is smaller.

This phenomenon of dispersal by diffusion during bulk flow was first described by Taylor in 1954, and its importance to the indicator diffusion method is considerable as it can lead to low extractions being spuriously overestimated. The Taylor effect may be estimated by the method suggested by Perl (1970) or it may be circumvented by calculating the extraction from an arbitrary fraction of the total area under the curve (Lassen and Crone, 1970). Neither of these operations is entirely satisfactory. Perl's technique retains assumption which cannot be easily justified and the fractional area method compromises the simple analysis of unidirectional diffusion. As Pappenheimer (1970b) has emphasized, the gradient across the capillary wall can be greatly affected by the passage of a relatively small number of molecules and recent mathematical models of exchange (Bassingthwaighte et al., 1970) suggest that longitudinal and radial concentration gradients are present in the interstitial space even during the first passage of low molecular weight tracers.

A very serious assumption is that all the capillaries have similar extractions. This requires not only that they should be alike in their permeability properties but also that they should have equal values for the ratio of surface area to blood flow. In those tissues which can be visualized in the living state there is considerable variation in the length of capillaries and in the blood flow through them, the latter varying from moment to moment. Such non-uniformity in the capillary bed leads to under-estimates of permeability for substances of high permeability as the overall extraction is weighted towards vessels with low values of $A/\dot{Q}$ and the relation between extraction and $A/\dot{Q}$ is logarithmic (Renkin, 1968).

This is illustrated in Fig. 8 which shows the fall in concentration along the length of a capillary of uniform permeability (concentration profile). Two capillaries, each possessing the same diameter and blood flow but having lengths equal to OA and OB, have end capillary concentrations of C_x and C_y. The mean end capillary concentration is C_z, which taken with the mean capillary length (and thus the mean ratio of $A/\dot{Q}$) suggest a lower permeability to the substance than either capillary possesses. When ratios of extractions are used to estimate permeability ratios, the sort of error produced by this sort of non-uniformity becomes considerable (see, for example, Trap-Jensen and Lassen, 1971).

To minimize the effects of non-uniformity of $A/\dot{Q}$, very high flow rates are employed (Yudilevich and Alvarez, 1967; Alvarez and Yudilevich, 1969) and the extractions are calculated for the first part of the dilution curve. Evidence of a constant early extraction is taken to indicate that the Taylor effect is small and at the high flow rates it is hoped that the end capillary concentrations of diffusible tracer all lie on the steeper parts of the concentration profile curve so that the averaging of end capillary samples gives

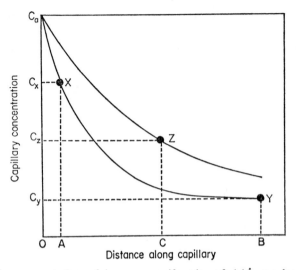

FIG. 8. A representation of how non-uniformity of $A/\dot{Q}$ can lead to under-estimates of permeability when permeability is calculated from the arteriovenous difference. The curve C_aXY represents the fall in concentration of a substance along the length of a capillary of uniform diameter. Two capillaries possessing the same value of permeability but having lengths equal to OA and OB yield end capillary concentrations of C_x and C_y. If both capillaries have equal blood flows, the mean capillary concentration is C_z and the mean value of $A/\dot{Q}$ corresponds to a mean capillary length, OC.

The point, Z, which results from plotting C_z against OC, lies on a curve C_aZ which represents a capillary permeability which is only 43 per cent of the value given by the curve C_aXY.

rise to only small errors. It is worth pointing out that Trap-Jensen and Lassen (1970) have studied the permeability of human forearm capillaries to low molecular weight solutes and did not find any evidence for restricted diffusion with a resting blood flow but clear evidence for restricted diffusion when the vessels were dilated by exercise or hyperaemia.

The indicator dilution method has been used by a large number of workers in recent years and extensive sets of data have been collected for the capillary bed of the perfused dog heart by Alvarez and Yudilevich (1969), and for the capillary bed of the human forearm by Trap-Jensen and Lassen (1970).

D. THE MEASUREMENT OF PERMEABILITY FROM LYMPH : PLASMA
CONCENTRATION RATIOS

When the volume of the cells in a tissue is unchanging, the volume of the interstitial fluid is held constant by a steady state balance between the excess filtration of water across the capillary wall and the flow of lymph out of the tissue. If the permeation of solute across the capillary wall occurs less rapidly than can be achieved by bulk flow in the same filtration stream, steady differences in concentration between the plasma and the interstitial fluid will be maintained, and these differences may be used to calculate the capillary permeability (Renkin, 1964).

For such a substance, the mass flow out of the capillary into the interstitial space should equal the mass flow out of the interstitial space into the lymph,

i.e.

$$MA(C_p - C_e) + J_{v_F}(1 - \sigma)\bar{C}_s = J_{v_L} C_l \qquad (5.9)$$

where J_{v_L} = the lymph flow rate, C_p = plasma concentration, C_e = interstitial space concentration, and C_l = lymph concentration.

In the steady state $J_{v_F} = J_{v_L}$, and

$$MA = J_{v_L} \frac{C_l - (1 - \sigma) C_s}{(C_p - C_e)}. \qquad (5.10)$$

On the grounds that σ is very close to unity for the molecules which may be investigated in this way, Renkin (1964) chose to neglect the bulk flow term across the capillary wall. Under this condition (5.10) becomes

$$MA = J_{v_L} \frac{C_l}{C_p - C_e}. \qquad (5.11)$$

Renkin also suggested that $C_e \simeq C_l$ whence

$$MA \simeq J_{v_L} \frac{C_l}{C_p - C_l}. \qquad (5.12)$$

The lymph : plasma concentration of substances of known free diffusion coefficient have been determined by Grotte (1956) for dextrans of molecular weight ranging between 10 000 and 70 000. Using a form of (5.12) to analyse Grotte's data, Renkin (1964) has been able to show that dextrans of mol. wt. between 10 000 and 25 000 appear to be distributed in hind limb lymph in accordance with an extrapolation of the findings of Pappenheimer et al. (1951).

For dextrans of free diffusion coefficients greater than albumin the value of permeability declined very much less than expected (or not at all) with increasing molecular size. These findings are discussed in the section concerned with the flow of large molecules across the capillary wall (vide infra).

Since Grotte's work, other sets of data have been obtained for the steady-state distribution of intermediate and large molecules between the plasma and the lymph or extracellular fluid (Mayerson et al., 1960; Boyd et al., 1969; Youlton, 1969; Garlick and Renkin, 1970).

The principle assumptions of the method are:

(i) that the bulk flow term in (5.10) is negligible;

(ii) that the concentration gradient between the capillary wall and the lymph is negligible for the molecules under consideration in the steady state;

(iii) that the concentration of macromolecules in the lymph is an average of their concentration in the steady state.

Renkin (1964) was immediately able to justify the first of these assumptions. Grotte had determined the distribution of dextrans between the plasma and the hind limb lymph of dogs under conditions of normal lymph flow and after the lymph flow had been doubled by venous congestion. The permeabilities calculated under these two conditions were the same, suggesting that the bulk flow term was negligible.

That the concentration gradient between the capillary wall and the lymph is negligible is less certain. An analysis of the values of MA calculated from the data of Grotte (1956) and Boyd et al. (1969) suggests such a concentration gradient might exist for very large molecules. It would be small and probably negligible for smaller molecules. This matter is discussed in greater detail below.

The assumption that the lymph is representative of the interstitial fluid can be more seriously questioned for large molecules than for smaller molecules. The flow of lymph from a given region is likely to be dominated by the flow of macromolecules and water from the most permeable capillaries. If a small number of capillaries in a capillary bed are excessively permeable to protein, then the local concentration of protein in the interstitial fluid is also likely to be high. A situation could arise where reabsorption or only a minute degree of filtration occurs across the majority of vessels, but in a small fraction, water and protein are leaking into the interstitial space at relatively high rate giving rise to a lymph which represents the ultrafiltrate of most permeable vessels.

E. OTHER METHODS OF ESTIMATING CAPILLARY PERMEABILITY TO SMALL LIPID INSOLUBLE MOLECULES

Although methods other than those already described have been devised to study capillary permeability, they have so far yielded little information; about the movement of solutes across the capillary wall. A quasi-steady state technique for examining blood-tissue exchange has been devised by Renkin (1959a) who has applied it very successfully to investigation of the control of the exchange. An elegant form of the tissue clearance method has been described by Lassen and Trap-Jensen (1968), Strandell and Shepherd (1968) and Gosselin (1967) and this may also be useful in providing information about blood-tissue exchange. The method consists of injecting into a small localized region a γ-emitting hydrophilic ion and an inert gas. It is assumed that the clearance of the gas is proportional to blood flow and the clearance of the test substance can be used to calculate its extraction from the tissue. Like the indicator diffusion technique this method assumes uniformity of the capillary bed and the absence of concentration gradients in the interstitial space. From the work of Crone and Garlick (1970) it seems likely that gradients do exist in the interstitial space when even relatively small molecules are being cleared by the blood. Using the isolated perfused gracilis preparation, these workers found that the fractional rate of escape of tracer from the tissue was not monoexponential as the theory of the tissue clearance method would demand.

A method for measuring the permeability of single capillaries to dye molecules has recently been reported by Michel and Levick (1971). A single capillary (of frog mesentery) is perfused via a micropipette with Ringer solutions containing dye, and the change in optical density of the tissue over and immediately surrounding a small section of the perfused vessel are examined. An initial step change in optical density occurs as the dye present moves through the capillary and this is followed by a steady increase in optical density as dye accumulates in the tissue. If the earliest accumulation of dye in the tissue occurs when the concentration gradient across the capillary wall is equal to the capillary concentration, the permeability can then be calculated from these optical density changes and the dimensions of the vessel.

F. DISCUSSION OF THE STUDIES ON CAPILLARY PERMEABILITY TO SMALL LIPID INSOLUBLE MOLECULES

Following the work of Pappenheimer et al. (1951) most discussions of capillary permeability values are in terms of the equivalent pore theory. There are, however, two fundamental assumptions underlying permeability studies which we shall consider first. These are: the independence of permeability on concentration and the effects of bulk solvent flow upon net exchange of small molecules.

The independence of permeability on the concentration gradient across the capillary wall is so fundamental an assumption of the indicator dilution method that this technique yields no information on the subject. Evidence for the belief that permeability is uninfluenced by the concentration, however, can be derived from the findings of Pappenheimer et al. (1951). During an osmotic transient these authors found that the value of $A_s/\Delta x$ was constant when it was calculated from the changing uptake of solute from the blood and the simultaneous osmotic pressure gradient across the capillary walls. One may argue that Pappenheimer et al. were calculating $A_s/\sigma\Delta x$ and that during an osmotic transient there could have been changes in A_s and σ_s which tended to cancel one another out. The latter is not very convincing, for if both A_s and σ_s varied with ΔC_s, they would be expected to vary in opposite directions and changes in $A_s/\sigma_s\Delta x$ would tend to maximize any concentration dependent changes in permeability. That the values of $A_s/\Delta x$ calculated by Pappenheimer et al. are constant suggests that both A_s and σ are independent of ΔC_s.

In the measurements of Pappenheimer et al. the bulk flow component of net solute flow across the capillary wall could be neglected because their experiments were carried out under conditions of zero net volume flow (the isogravimetric state). Having obtained capillary permeability values in the absence of net bulk flow, Pappenheimer et al. calculated the effects of net solvent flow upon solute movements. They concluded that this would be significant only for molecules of a size equal to or greater than inulin and they carried out experiments to show the effects of prolonged filtration upon inulin exchange. The assumption that bulk flow can be regarded as playing only a minor or negligible role in the net movements of small lipid insoluble molecules arises largely from the conclusions of Pappenheimer et al. In the indicator dilution technique, the molar concentrations of solutes are usually minute and they are unlikely to give rise to a significant bulk flow term and it is also assumed that during the course of these experiments net volume flow across the capillary wall is zero.

A direct attempt to investigate effects of bulk flow upon exchange was made by Hyman et al. (1952). These workers found the rate of clearance of ^{24}Na and ^{131}I from skin were not appreciably affected by concurrent oedema formation. More recently, Lundgren and Mellander (1967) have found that bulk flow may indeed influence net exchange but in a rather different manner from that predicted by (3.21) and (3.35). The clearance of ^{131}I, ^{24}Na, ^{56}Rb and ^{133}Xe from the hind limbs of cats was found to have a minimal value when the tissues were in a state of Starling balance. Both net filtration and net reabsorption of fluid across the capillary walls augmented the clearance of all the tracers, the effect being about the same for the clearance of ^{131}I, ^{24}Na and ^{56}Rb and rather less for the clearance of ^{133}Xe. This enhancement of solute transfer appeared to increase progressively with the rate of fluid movement and it was not related to changes in the area of the capillary bed. As noted earlier, Crone and Garlick (1970) have provided evidence for concentration gradients in the interstitial space of muscle, and it is possible the bulk flow is enhancing exchange by disrupting these gradients. Whatever the mechanism of the effect may prove to be, Lundgren and Mellander's findings must rank among the most interesting that have been obtained in recent years on the subject of transcapillary exchange, for they question an assumption which has become generally accepted. It is to be hoped their work will be extended to investigate, for example, its implications to the indicator dilution technique.

G. CAPILLARY PERMEABILITY VALUES FOR SMALL LIPID
INSOLUBLE MOLECULES AND THE EQUIVALENT PORE THEORY

The values which have been obtained for capillary permeabilities vary considerably depending upon the methods used, and the capillary beds which have been investigated. To minimize this variation we shall discuss the data obtained from one capillary bed separately from those obtained from another. Since the theory of restricted diffusion through equivalent pores or slits makes definite predictions about the variation of capillary permeability with molecular size, it is particularly convenient to interpret the results in this way and so examine the applicability of the theory.

(1) *Hind limb capillaries of cats and dogs*

Figure 9 shows the relationship between the logarithm of permeability-surface product (MA) per 100 g of tissue and the logarithm of the molecular (Stokes-Einsten) radius calculated from the data of Pappenheimer *et al.* (1951) and Grotte (1956). No attempt has been made to "correct" the data of Pappenheimer *et al.* for reflection coefficients. The data obtained by

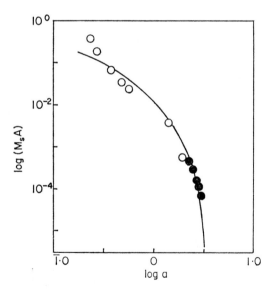

FIG. 9. The permeability of cat and dog hind limb capillaries to molecules of different molecular size. The logarithm of the permeability surface product has been plotted against the logarithm of the molecular (Stokes-Einstein) radius. The data of Pappenheimer *et al.* (1951) are shown as ○ and those of Grotte (1956) are shown as ●. The curve represents restricted diffusion through pores of 4 nm radius.

Grotte for the permeability of molecules larger than 3 nm in radius have been omitted and will be discussed in the section concerned with large molecules. The curve drawn through the data has been constructed from the theory of restricted diffusion for pores of radius 4 nm. The internal consistency between the two sets of data and the pore theory is very good.

In their original paper, Pappenheimer et al. used an additional method for calculating the equivalent pore radius. Plotting the relationship between $A_s/\Delta x$ (which is $M_s A/D_s$) against molecular size they obtained a value for $A_w/\Delta x$, the area per unit path length available to water molecules. Rearranging (3.24) and substituting for $A_w/\Delta x r$ could be obtained from:

$$r = [(8\eta J_v/\Delta P)/(A_w/\Delta x)]^{\frac{1}{2}}. \tag{5.13}$$

For the model of equivalent slits (3.25) gives

$$w = 2[(3\eta J_v/\Delta P)/(A_w/\Delta x)]^{\frac{1}{2}}. \tag{5.14}$$

The values of pore radius and slit width obtained from (5.13) and (5.14) are very close to those obtained from the theory of restricted diffusion.

Consistency is a very persuasive argument in physiology but the recent arguments of Pappenheimer (1970), Lifson (1970) and Tosteson (1970) on the importance of the reflection coefficient suggest that the agreement between the values of r calculated from the theory of restricted diffusion and the filtration coefficient implies that half the water crossing the capillary wall travels by a route unavailable to the solute molecules. It will be interesting to see if this original convincing agreement between the values of r calculated independently from restricted diffusion and filtration data are the result of two factors, reflection coefficients and the separate pathways for water, which cancel each other out.†

(2) *Human forearm capillaries*

Trap-Jensen and Lassen (1970) have reported a series of values for the permeability of human forearm capillaries obtained by the indicator dilution technique. The blood flow through the forearm was increased by exercise hyperaemia in order to reduce the effects of non-uniformity and flow limitation. Plotted as log $M_s A$ against log molecular radius, the results are shown in Fig. 10. There is strong evidence for restricted diffusion through pores of radii 3·5–4·0 nm or slits of width 4 nm. It is, however, worth pointing out that the absolute value of pore area per unit path length is about a tenth of the value obtained by Pappenheimer et al. (1951). There is evidence

---

†Perl (1971) has argued that the constricted nature of the interendothelial cleft gives an effective pathlength for filtration which is about one fifth of that for diffusion. Perl argues that the constriction effect is almost equal and opposite to the effect of reflection coefficients upon the Pappenheimer calculation of equivalent pore radius.

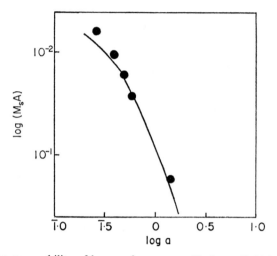

FIG. 10. The permeability of human forearm capillaries to lipid insoluble molecules of varying molecular size based on the data of Trap-Jensen and Lassen (1970). The logarithm of the permeability surface product has been plotted against the logarithm of the molecular (Stokes Einstein) radius. The curve represents restricted diffusion through cylindrical pores of 3·5 nm radius or through slits 4 nm in width.

that it should be less from values of the filtration coefficients of cat and dog hind limb capillaries and human forearm capillaries, but the difference is only two-fold.

(3) *Heart muscle capillaries*

Alvarez and Yudilevich (1969) have obtained values for the permeability of the capillary bed of the canine heart for a wide variety of substances of low molecular weight. It is interesting that they found little evidence for restricted diffusion. The sieving of dextrans between plasma and coronary lymph of dogs has been investigated by Areskog *et al.* (1964). When values of $M_s A$ calculated from these data and values of Alvarez and Yudilevich are plotted as log $(M_s A)$ against log a, they appear to be consistent with a pore radius of 9 nm (see Fig. 11). There is, however, a large extrapolation covering a range of molecular radii between 2 and 4 nm. The values obtained by Vargas and Johnson (1967) for the permeability of rabbit heart capillaries are also shown in Fig. 11, and the disagreement is perhaps not as great as might have been expected. This is partly the result of plotting the data on a logarithmic scale but if the permeability value for inulin is ignored then the data taken with that of Areskog *et al.* is consistent with pores of 9 nm radius.

Pores of 8–10 nm radius or slits of similar width are apparently not consistent with the electronmicroscopy of heart capillaries, but this should

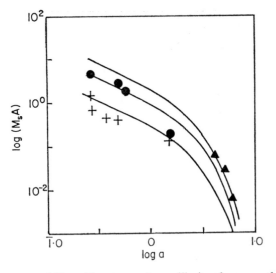

Fig. 11. The permeability of heart muscle capillaries shown as the relationship between the logarithm of the permeability surface product and logarithm of the molecular radius. The data of Alvarez and Yudilevich (1969) are shown as $+$; those of Vargas and Johnson (1967) as $\bullet$; and those of Areskog *et al.* (1964) as $\blacktriangle$. The curves are based on restricted diffusion through pores of 9 nm radius. The different curves represent different total pore areas.

not deter us from continuing to use equivalent pore radius in an operational sense. Furthermore, as argued in Section 2, it is quite possible that pathways for the diffusion of small molecules are electron-dense and electron-lucent regions need not be diffusion pathways.

6. Transport of Large Molecules across the Capillary Wall

Although it has been asserted from time to time that normal capillaries are impermeable to molecules equal to or greater than serum albumin in size, it is now generally accepted that such molecules are transported from the blood into the tissue fluid under the most physiological of conditions. The quantitative study of capillary permeability to large molecules owes much to the work of Grotte (1956). Using a series of dextrans, of known molecular weight and free diffusion coefficient, Grotte studied the steady state concentration of these probe molecules in the plasma and in the lymph from various parts of the body. Similar work was reported in 1960 by Mayerson *et al.*

In the hind limb of the anaesthetized dog, Grotte found a progressive fall in the lymph: plasma concentration ratio (C_l/C_p) with increasing molecular size for dextrans of Stokes-Einstein radii of up to 3 nm. This decline in permeability with increasing molecular size was in accordance with the predictions of Pappenheimer et al. (1951) for molecular sieving through cylindrical pores of 3·5–4·0 nm radius. For molecules of greater molecular dimensions, it appeared that C_1/C_p became constant and did not decrease with further increase in molecular size. Similar results were obtained by Mayerson et al. (1960) for C_1/C_p of cervical lymph. For hepatic and intestinal lymph, however, Mayerson et al. noted a difference in the relationship between permeability and molecular size for small molecules and large molecules, though here apparent permeability continued to decline with molecular size even for the largest dextrans.

To account for his findings Grotte (1956) proposed that in addition to the system of small pores in the capillary wall which provided a pathway for the transfer of small molecules, a very small number of large pores were also present. Although such large pores would also be available to small molecules, they would represent only a minute fraction of the total area available for the diffusion of the small molecules and their contribution to the total flow of water and low molecular substances would be negligible.

Grotte (1956) investigated the effects of increasing the net filtration rate (and hence the lymph flow) upon C_1/C_p. By comparing the changes in ratio for small molecules with those for large molecules, he calculated the relative number of large ($r = 15$–20 nm) to small (3.5 nm) pores and concluded that only one large pore was available for every 30 000 pores. In making these calculations Grotte assumed that the large molecules were carried across the capillary wall in a filtration stream and he was guided in estimating the maximum size of large pores, by his experiments with Juhlin and Sandberg (1960), where it was found that plastic microspheres of diameter 30–70 nm did not cross the endothelial barrier of the hind limb.

Mayerson et al. (1960) also regarded a small number of very large pores as a likely mechanism to account for the transcapillary transport of large molecules. As an alternative they suggested that large molecules might be carried across the endothelial cells by the pinocytotic vesicles which had received so much attention from the electromicroscopists, a mechanism which Moore and Ruska (1957) had called cytopempsis.

These two sets of data were discussed very fully by Renkin (1964) in his Bowditch lecture. Expressing the results in terms of permeability-surface area products he attempted to distinguish between transport via vesicles and transport via large pores by considering the relationship between the logarithm of the MA value and the logarithm of molecular weight. For dextran molecules, the diffusion coefficient declines with the square root of the molecular weight, so that on this plot a line of slope $-\frac{1}{2}$ represents a fall in permeability in strict accord with the decline of the diffusion coefficient. Renkin suggested that the flow of large molecules through large pores would be seen on his diagram as a fall in a line of slope $-\frac{1}{2}$ or, if restricted diffusion was occurring through the large pore, of slope greater than $-\frac{1}{2}$. If the large molecules were carried by the vesicles, then permeability

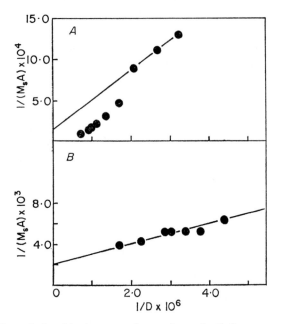

Fig. 12. The relationship between the reciprocal of the permeability-surface product and the reciprocal of the free diffusion coefficients for large molecules. A represents the data of Boyd *et al.* (1969) obtained from samples of pulmonary lymph in adult sheep. The points representing the three largest molecules (highest values of $1/M_sA$ and $1/D$) lie on a straight line and the lengthy back extrapolation yields a positive intercept in accordance with equation 5.1.

B is based on the data of Grotte (1956) for the steady state distribution of high molecular weight dextrans between plasma and the lymph of the dog hind limb. The data conform closely to a straight line with a positive intercept.

should be independent of molecular weight and the slope of the logarithmic relation should be zero.

The findings on hepatic and intestinal lymph suggested a decrease of log permeability with log molecular weight equal to or greater than $-\frac{1}{2}$. This strongly suggests the presence of large pores in these capillary beds and as we have seen, Clementi and Palade (1969a, b) have now produced strong electronmicrographic evidence that these large pores may be identified with the fenestrae. Thus both physiological measurement and ultrastructural appearances appear for once to agree.

Grotte's leg lymph data and the cervical lymph data of Mayerson *et al.*, however, suggested MA for large molecules was independent of molecular weight, but the scatter was sufficient for it to be possible to draw a line of $-\frac{1}{2}$ through the points without incurring too much error.

The electronmicroscope pictures provide no evidence for a large pore system in unfenestrated capillaries nor, as Karnovsky (1970) has pointed out, are they likely to be distinguished from artefacts if Grotte's estimate of the number of large pores in such capillaries is correct by an order of magnitude. As we have seen there is considerable evidence, however, for transport by vesicles across the endothelium of unfenestrated capillaries.

Apparently strong evidence for the existence of large pores in unfenestrated endothelium has been provided by Landis (1964) who has perfused single capillaries of the frog mesentery with Ringer solutions containing the dye T-1824 and albumin. The dye appeared to leave the capillaries rapidly at one or two sites only within the first few seconds of a perfusion. Only one or two highly permeable sites were seen on each capillary (there were more at the venous end than the arterial end of the vessels) and Landis suggested they might represent the large pore system. Levick and Michel (1969) while confirming these appearances have shown that when the concentration of dye and albumin in the perfusate is adjusted so that nearly all the dye is present as dye protein complex, no dye is seen to leave the vessels within the first minute of a perfusion. When the dye protein complex does leave the microcirculation it does so in a more uniform fashion. They suggest that the diffusion of dye described by Landis represents the movement of unbound dye and the variability of its passage, variation in the permeability of the capillary wall to small molecules.

On the evidence available at present it would appear that transfer of large molecules across continuous unfenestrated endothelia occurs by cytopempsis rather than through a large pore system. Attempts to distinguish between these two sorts of mechanism may have to be more subtle than those carried out so far. For example, the method of calculating capillary permeability from the lymph: plasma concentration ratio may be valid for molecules which equilibrate fairly rapidly between the extracapillary fluid and the lymph, but concentration gradients in the interstitial space may well exist for the larger molecules. The resistance to diffusion between the plasma and lymph could represent the sum of the resistance at the capillary wall and the resistance of the interstitial space. If the latter were inversely proportional to the free diffusion coefficient of the test molecules, a decline of apparent permeability (calculated from 5.8) should accompany increasing molecular weight even if transfer across the capillary wall is achieved by the vesicle system, i.e.

$$\begin{bmatrix}\text{Total resistance to} \\ \text{movement between} \\ \text{plasma and lymph}\end{bmatrix} = \begin{bmatrix}\text{Resistance at} \\ \text{the capillary} \\ \text{wall}\end{bmatrix} + \begin{bmatrix}\text{Resistance in} \\ \text{the interstitial} \\ \text{space}\end{bmatrix}$$

$$\frac{1}{(\overline{MA})} = \frac{1}{(MA)_c} + \frac{K}{D} \tag{6.1}$$

where D is the free diffusion coefficient of the molecule and K/D is the resistance of the interstitial space.

If (6.1) is a reasonable approximation, then for molecules carried entirely by the vesicle system, $1/(\overline{MA})$ should be linearly related to $1/D$. Such a linear relation does appear to describe some of the more recent studies on the distribution of large molecules between the lymph and the plasma.

Renkin (1964) used the permeability of hind limb capillaries to very large molecules and the available evidence from electronmicroscopy on the density of vesicles in endothelial cells, to calculate the mean transit times of vesicles. His figure of five minutes was reduced to twenty-five seconds by Bruns and Palade (1968) who had carried out an extensive quantitative study of the density of vesicles in endothelial cells. Both Renkin and Bruns and Palade assumed that all the vesicles crossed the endothelial cells but the more recent models of Shea *et al.* (1969) and Tomlin (1969) have suggested that the movement of vesicles is the result of Brownian motion; transfer across the endothelial cell could occur in a few milliseconds though only 4–5 per cent of the total number of vesicles actually make the journey. The majority would finish up on the side of the membrane from which they derived and would not contribute to net transfer.

As mentioned on page 280, Renkin found no evidence of an effect of changes in water filtration upon permeabilities calculated from the steady-state lymph–plasma ratios. This finding applies to the large molecules as well as the intermediate sized dextrans and is consistent with either cyto-pempsis or the large pore hypothesis. It may be worth adding that an increased filtration rate across the capillary wall will steepen the concentration gradient for large molecules and so increase the net transfer by cytopempsis as well as by molecular sieving. Increase in temperature may also be expected to increase transfer by a vesicle system as well as transfer via a pore system though one might anticipate a larger effect upon the vesicle system if the viscosity of endothelial cytoplasm is more temperature-sensitive than the viscosity of the extracellular fluid. These attempts to distinguish between vesicle transport and a large pore system by studying the effects of temperature or filtration rate upon net transfer of large molecules between the blood and the lymph (Renkin and Garlick, 1970) are unlikely to be successful until experiments are designed to give more clear-cut results than they have been so far.

As far as the transcapillary movements of large molecules are concerned we can summarize current opinion fairly succintly. There are two hypotheses: a small number of large pores or a system of vesicles. In fenestrated capillaries there is good evidence that fenestrae act as large pores. In unfenestrated capillaries, the evidence is not wholly clear-cut. At present it favours transfer via vesicles.

7. Conclusions

It would appear from physiological measurements that the flow of water and low molecular weight lipid insoluble solutes across the capillary wall occurs through a system of small pores or slits. It would also appear that the electron microscopists have identified a pathway in the intercellular regions of unfenestrated capillaries which has the dimensions predicted by the pore theory. Furthermore there is direct evidence *in vivo* that the exchange pathway for low molecular weight dye molecules is located in the intercellular clefts. At last, it may seem, there is agreement between the physiological measurements and ultrastructural appearances.

But before drawing a neat line underneath these satisfying conclusions let us examine one or two pieces of evidence which do not fit so satisfactorily into this general picture. It will be remembered that the data on the capillaries of heart muscle were consistent with pores of 9 nm radius (Fig. 11), an equivalent pore size which is considerably larger than that predicted for skeletal muscle capillaries. It is true that this conclusion required us to neglect the permeability of rabbit heart capillaries to inulin determined by Vargas and Johnson (1967) and such arbitrariness cannot be wholly justified. It might have been fairer to represent the data on rabbit heart capillaries separately from those on the canine heart but there can be little doubt that the latter are consistent with an equivalent pore radius of 9–10 nm rather than 3–4 nm.

The ultrastructural evidence for the 4 nm slit between the endothelial cells arose from work on cardiac capillaries. In this case the cardiac capillaries were those of the mouse and other studies on the rat heart suggested that the capillaries of this animal were similar in appearance. Furthermore it seems unlikely that the cardiac capillaries of rats are penetrated by pores of 9 nm radius for if they were present they would permit the rapid transendothelial passage of ferritin and Jennings and Florey (1967) showed clearly that there was no readily available pathway for this tracer. It is perhaps unwise to jump to conclusions about the permeability of cardiac capillaries until both physiological and ultrastructural studies have been carried out on capillary beds of the same species of animal.

Fortunately ultrastructural studies have been carried out on the capillary

13*

bed of cat skeletal muscle (Karnovsky, 1970) and there is agreement between the physiological predictions and electron micrographic appearances.

A second slightly awkward piece of information is also available to us from the electron microscopists. If the *caveoli intracellulares* on the luminal surface of the endothelial cell communicate freely with the capillary lumen, their contents would be expected to equilibrate rapidly with the capillary plasma. The dimensions of the vesicles are so small that even the largest molecules might be expected to equilibrate within 250 ms. This means that if an electron micrograph is a fair representation of the arrangement of vesicles at a particular moment in time, 20–30 per cent of the vesicles should be labelled with the largest molecules capable of entering them within one second. This is obviously not true. Jennings and Florey (1967) found only single ferritin particles in occasional endothelial vesicles when the perfusing blood had contained tracer for up to half-an-hour. Bruns and Palade (1968b) found labelled vesicles in rat diaphragm capillaries three minutes after the injection of ferritin but these labelled vesicles were (judging from their pictures) rather few and far between. Bruns and Palade (1968a) have drawn attention to an electron-dense "diaphragm" which does appear to cover the mouths of some vesicles and it could be that this structure greatly impedes free access to the vesicular cavity.

That the whole of the endothelial cell might be covered with a layer of mucopolysaccharide was mentioned in Section 2. A much older idea is that plasma proteins might be absorbed on to the surface of the capillary wall. This view is based on evidence familiar to all physiologists who perfuse tissues and organs with artificial perfusates. A trace of albumin appears to render the colloidal osmotic pressure of artificial colloids more effective. Following the pioneer experiments of Drinker (1927) and Danielli (1940) support for the belief that the plasma proteins were acting on the capillary wall was provided by Kinter and Pappenheimer (1963) who demonstrated an effect upon the capillary filtration coefficient. More recently Levick and Michel (1970) have shown an increase in the rate of passage of dyes perfused through single capillaries of frog mesentery when albumin is absent from the perfusing fluid. This increase cannot be accounted for by an alteration in the binding of dye to the protein, or to an alteration in the bulk flow component of transport. Unpublished experiments by Mason and Michel have shown the filtration coefficient of single capillaries may be reversibly increased at least five-fold by the removal of albumin from the plasma and that there appears to be little difference between the frog's own plasma and bovine albumin in restoring the filtration coefficient to its normal value.

The purpose of emphasizing this apparently small issue is that the albumin is having an effect which must be present under physiological conditions. If albumin is a component of the diffusion barrier it is unlikely to be seen with the electron microscope for the albumin molecule is electron lucent and there is indeed little difference in the ultrastructural appearance of normal capillaries and capillaries perfused with albumin-free solutions. It could well be that some components of the endothelial barrier are electron lucent and some electron-dense regions are permeable to the smaller molecules.

Sometimes in experimental science, when different lines of evidence on a particular phenomenon begin to agree, the few awkward pieces which do not fit together lead to a new level of understanding. It could be that the study of capillary permeability has reached this stage.

REFERENCES

Alvarez, O. A. and Yudilevich, D. L. (1969). Heart capillary permeability to lipid-insoluble molecules. *J. Physiol.* **202**, 45–58.
Areskog, N.-H., Arturson, G., Grotte, G. and Wallenius, G. (1964). Studies on heart lymph. II. Capillary permeability of the dog's heart using dextran as a test substance. *Acta Physiol. Scand.* **62**, 218–223.
Arnold, J. (1875). Cited by Florey, Lord. In "General Pathology" (Florey, Lord, ed.), 4th edition, pp. 84 and 102, Lloyd Luke, London.
Bassingthwaighte, J. B., Knopp, T. J. and Haselrig, J. B. (1970). A concurrent flow model for capillary-tissue exchanges. *In* "Capillary Permeability" (C. Crone and N. A. Lassen, eds.), pp. 60–80, Munksgaard, Copenhagen.
Bate, Hilary, Rowlands, S., Sirs, J. A. and Thomas, H. W. (1969). The influence of molecular diffusion on the dispersion of indicators in the circulation. *J. Physiol.* **202**, 38–39. P.
Blum, J. J. (1960). Concentration profiles in and around capillaries. *Amer. J. Physiol.* **197**, 991–998.
Boyd, R. D. H., Hill, June R., Humphreys, P. W., Normand, I. C. S., Reynolds, E. O. R. and Strang, L. B. (1969). Permeability of lung capillaries to macromolecules in foetal and new-born lambs and sheep. *J. Physiol.* **201**, 567–588.
Brightman, M. W., Reese, T. S. and Feder, N. (1970). Assessment with the electronmicroscope of the permeability to peroxidase of cerebral endothelium and epithelium in mice and sharks. *In* "Capillary Permeability" (Crone, C. and N. A. Lassen, eds.), pp. 468–476, Munksgaard, Copenhagen.
Bruns, R. R. and Palade, G. E. (1968a). Studies on blood capillaries. I. General organization of muscle capillaries. *J. Cell Biol.* **37**, 244–276.
Bruns, R. R. and Palade, G. E. (1968b). Studies on blood capillaries. II. Transport of ferritin molecules across the walls of muscle capillaries. *J. Cell. Biol.* **37**, 277–299.
Chambers, R. and Zweifach, B. W. (1940). Capillary endothelial cement in relation to permeability. *J. Cell. Comp. Physiol.* **15**, 255–272.
Chambers, R. and Zweifach, B. W. (1947). Intercellular cement and capillary permeability. *Physiol. Rev.* **27**, 436–463.
Chinard, F. P., Vosburgh, G. J. and Enns, T. (1955). Transcapillary exchange of water and other substances in certain organs of the dog. *Amer. J. Physiol.* **183**, 221–234.

Clementi, F. and Palade, G. E. (1969a). Intestinal capillaries. I. Permeability to peroxidase and ferritin. *J. Cell. Biol.* **41**, 33–58.

Clementi, F. and Palade, G. E. (1969b). Intestinal capillaries. II. Structural effects of EDTA and histamine. *J. Cell. Biol.* **42**, 706–714.

Collin, H. B. (1969). Ultrastructure of fenestrated blood capillaries in extra-ocular muscles. *Exp. Eye Res.* **8**, 16–20.

Crone, C. (1963). The permeability of capillaries in various organs as determined by use of the "indicator diffusion" method. *Acta Physiol. Scand.* **58**, 292–305.

Crone, C. and Garlick, D. (1970). The penetration of inulin, sucrose, mannitol and tritiated water from the interstitial space in muscle into the vascular system. *J. Physiol.* **210**, 387–404.

Danielli, J. F. (1940). Capillary permeability and oedema in the perfused frog. *J. Physiol.* **98**, 109–129.

Drinker, C. K. (1927). The permeability and diameter of the capillaries in the web of the brown frog (*Rana temporaria*) when perfused with solutions containing pituitary extract and horse serum. *J. Physiol.* **63**, 249–269.

Durbin, R. P. (1960). Osmotic flow of water across permeable cellulose membranes. *J. gen. Physiol.* **44**, 315–326.

Farquhar, M. G. and Palade, G. E. (1963). Junctional complexes in various epithelia. *J. Cell. Biol.* **17**, 375–412.

Faxén, H. (1922). Der Widerstand gegen Bewegung einer starren Kugel in einer zähen Flüssigkeit, die zwischen zwei parallelen ebenen Wanden eingeschlossen ist. *Ann. Physik.* **68**, 89–119.

Ferry, J. D. (1936). Statistical value of sieve constants in ultrafiltration. *J. gen. Physiol.* **20**, 95–104.

Florey, H. W. (1926). Capillary permeability. *J. Physiol.* **61**, i–iii.

Florey, H. W. (1964). The transport of materials across the capillary wall. *Quater. J. Exp. Physiol.* **49**, 117–128.

Garlick, D. and Renkin, E. M. (1970). Transport of large molecules from plasma to interstitial fluid and lymph in dogs. *Amer. J. Physiol.* **219**, 1595–1605.

Goresky, C. A., Ziegler, W. H. and Bach, G. C. (1970). Capillary exchange modeling: barrier limited and flow limited distribution. *Circulation Res.* **27**, 739–764.

Gosselin, R. E. (1967). Blood tissue exchanges of radioactive solutes in cardiac and skeletal muscle. Influences of isoproterenol, methacholine and Nitroglycerine. *Fed. Proc.* **26**, 398.

Grotte, G. (1956). Passage of dextran molecules across the blood lymph barrier. *Acta Chir. Scand.* Suppl. **211**, 1–84.

Grotte, G., Juhlin, L. and Sandberg, N. (1960). Passage of solid spherical particles across the blood lymph barrier. *Acta Physiol. Scand.* **50**, 287–293.

Guyton, A. C. (1963). Concept of negative interstitial pressure based on pressures in implanted perforated capsules. *Circulation Res.* **12**, 399–414.

Guyton, A. C. (1969). Interstitial fluid pressure-volume relationships and their regulation. *In* "Circulatory and Respiratory Mass Transport" (G. E. Wolstenholme and J. E. Knight, eds.), pp. 4–20, J. and A. Churchill, London.

Guyton, A. C. and Lindsey, A. W. (1959). Effects of elevated left atrial pressure and decreased plasma protein concentration on the development of pulmonary oedema. *Circulation Res.* **7**, 647–657.

Hills, B. A. (1970). An assessment of the expression $C = \dot{Q}[1 - \exp(-PS/\dot{Q})]$ for estimating capillary peremeabilities. *Phys. Med. Biol.* **15**, 705–713.

Hyman, C., Rapaport, I., Saul, A. M. and Morton, M. E. (1952). Independence of capillary filtration and tissue clearance. *Amer. J. Physiol.* **168**, 674–679.

Jennings, M. A. and Florey, Lord (1967). An investigation of some properties of endothelium related to capillary permeability. *Proc. Roy. Soc. B.* **167**, 39–63.

Johnson, J. A. and Wilson, T. A. (1966). A model for capillary exchange. *Amer. J. Physiol.* **210**, 1299–1303.

Johnson, J. A. (1970). Reflection coefficients of non electrolytes in the myocardium *In* "Capillary Permeability" (C. Crone and N. A. Lassen, eds.), pp. 219–292, Munksgaard, Copenhagen.

Katchalsky, A. and Curran, P. F. (1965). "Non-equilibrium thermodynamics in Biophysics. Harvard University Press, Cambridge, Mass.

Karnovsky, M. J. (1967). The ultrastructural basis of capillary permeability studied with peroxidase as a tracer. *J. Cell. Biol.* **35**, 213–236.

Karnovsky, M. J. (1970). Morphology of capillaries with special reference to muscle capillaries. *In* "Capillary Permeability" (C. A. Crone and N. A. Lassen, eds.), pp. 341–350, Munksgaard, Copenhagen.

Kedem, O. and Katchalsky, A. (1958). Thermodynamic analysis of the permeability of biological membranes to non electrolytes. *Biochim. Biophys. Acta* **27**, 229–236.

Kedem, O. and Katchalsky, A. (1961). A physical interpretation of the phenomenological coefficients of membrane permeability. *J. Gen. Physiol.* **45**, 143–179.

Kety, S. S. (1951). The theory and applications of the exchange of inert gas at the lungs and tissues. *Pharmacol. Rev.* **3**, 1–41.

Kinter, W. B. and Pappenheimer, J. R. (1963). Unpublished observations quoted by Landis, E. M. and Pappenheimer, J. R. Exchanges of substances through the capillary walls. *In* "Handbook of Physiology", Section 2, Circulation, Vol. II (W. F. Hamilton and P. Dow, eds.), p. 994, American Physiological Society, Washington, D.C.

Krogh, A., Landis, E. M. and Turner, A. H. (1932). The movement of fluid through the human capillary wall in relation to venous pressure and to the colloid osmotic pressure of the blood. *J. Clin. Invest.* **11**, 63–95.

Landis, E. M. (1926). The capillary pressure in frog mesentery as determined by microinjection. *Amer. J. Physiol.* **75**, 548–570.

Landis, E. M. (1927). Microinjection studies of capillary permeability. II. The relation between capillary pressure and the rate at which fluid passes through the walls of single capillaries. *Amer. J. Physiol.* **82**, 217–238.

Landis, E. M. (1930a). The capillary blood pressure in mammalian mesentery as determined by the microinjection method. *Amer. J. Physiol.* **93**, 353–362.

Landis, E. M. (1930b). Microinjection studies of capillary blood pressure in human skin. *Heart* **15**, 209–228.

Landis, E. M. (1964). Heteroporosity of the capillary wall as indicated by cinematographic analysis of the passage of dyes. *Ann. N.Y. Acad. Sci.* **116**, 765–773.

Landis, E. M. and Gibbon, J. H. (1933). The effects of temperature and of tissue pressure on the movement of fluid through the human capillary wall. *J. Clin. Invest.* **12**, 105–138.

Landis, E. M. and Pappenheimer, J. R. (1963). Exchange of substances through the capillary walls. *In* "Handbook of Physiology", Section 2, Circulation, Vol. II (W. F. Hamilton and P. Dow, eds.), pp. 961–1034, American Physiological Society, Washington, D.C.

Lassen, N. A. and Trap-Jensen, J. (1968). Theoretical considerations on measurements of capillary diffusion capacity in skeletal muscle by the local clearance method. *Scand. J. Clin. Lab. Invest.* **21**, 108–115.

Lassen, N. A. and Crone, C. (1970). The extraction fraction of a capillary bed to hydrophilic molecules: theoretical considerations regarding the single injection technique with a discussion of the role of diffusion between laminar streams (Taylor's effect). *In* "Capillary Permeability" (C. Crone and N. A. Lassen, eds.), pp. 302–305, Munksgaard, Copenhagen.

Levick, J. R. and Michel, C. C. (1969). The passage of T 1824-albumin out of individually perfused capillaries of the frog mesentery. *J. Physiol.* **202**, 114–115. P.

Levick, J. R. and Michel, C. C. (1970). The effect of bovine albumin on the permeability of frog mesenteric capillaries. *J. Physiol.* **210**, 36–37. P.

Levick, J. R. and Michel, C. C. (1971). A densitometric method for estimating the filtration coefficient of frog mesenteric capillaries. *J. Physiol.* **218**, 25–26. P.

Levitt, D. G. (1971). Evaluation of the early extraction method of determining capillary permeability by theoretical capillary and organ models. *Circulation Res.* **27**, 81–96.

Lifson, N. (1970). Revised equation for the osmotic transient method. *In* "Capillary Permeability" (C. Crone and N. A. Lassen, eds.), pp. 302–305, Munksgaard, Copenhagen.

Loewenstein, W. R. (1966). Permeability of membrane junctions. *Ann. N. Y. Acad. Sci.* **137**, 441–472.

Luft, J. H. (1965). The ultrastructural basis of capillary permeability. *In* "The Inflammatory Process (B. W. Zweifach, L. Grant and R. McCluskey, eds.), pp. 121–159, Academic Press, New York and London.

Lundgren, O. and Mellander, S. (1967). Augmentation of tissue blood transfer of solutes by transcapillary filtration and absorption. *Acta Physiol. Scand.* **70**, 26–41.

Majno, G. (1965). Ultrastructure of the vascular membrane. *In* "Handbook of Physiology", Section 3, Circulation, Vol. II (W. F. Hamilton and P. Dow, eds.), pp. 2293–2375, American Physiological Society, Washington, D.C.

Martín de Julián, P. and Yudilevich, D. L. (1964). A theory for the quantification of transcapillary exchange by tracer dilution curves. *Amer. J. Physiol.* **207**, 162–168.

Mayerson, H. S., Wolfram, C. G., Shirley, H. H., Jr. and Wasserman, K. (1960). Regional differences in capillary permeability. *Amer. J. Physiol.* **198**, 155–160.

Mellander, S. (1960). Comparative studies on the adrenergic neurohumoral control of resistance and capacitance blood vessels in the cat. *Acta Physiol. Scand.* **50**, Suppl. 176, 1–86.

Mende, T. J. and Chambers, E. L. (1958). Studies on solute transfer in vascular endothelium. *J. Biophys. Biochem. Cytol.* **4**, 319–322.

Michel, C. C. (1969). The passage of a low molecular weight dye molecule (Patent Blue V) out of individually perfused capillaries of the frog mesentery. *J. Physiol.* **204**, 62–63. P.

Michel, C. C. (1970). Direct observations of sites of permeability for ions and small molecules in mesothelium and endothelium. *In* "Capillary Permeability" (C. Crone and N. A. Lassen, eds.), pp. 628–642, Munksgaard, Copenhagen.

Michel, C. C. and Levick, J. R. (1971). Measurement of permeability of single capillaries of frog mesentery to dyes. *Proc. XXV Int. Congr. Physiol. Sci. Munich*, Vol. IX, p. 389.

Moore, D. H. and Ruska, H. (1957). The fine structure of capillaries and small arteries. *J. Biophys. Biochem. Cytol.* **3**, 457–462.

Muir, A. R. and Peters, A. (1962). Quintuple layered membrane junctions at terminal bars between endothelial cells. *J. Cell. Biol.* **12**, 443–448.

Onsager, L. (1931a). Reciprocal relations in irreversible processes. I. *Physiol. Rev.* **37**, 405–426.

Onsager, L. (1931b). Reciprocal relations in irreversible processes. II. *Physiol. Rev.* **38**, 2265–2279.

Palade, G. E. (1953). Fine structure of blood capillaries. *J. appl. Phys.* **24**, 1423.

Palade, G. E. (1960). Transport in quanta across the endothelium of blood capillaries. *Anat. Rec.* **136**, 254.

Pappenheimer, J. R. (1953). Passage of molecules through capillary walls. *Physiol. Rev.* **33**, 387–423.

Pappenheimer, J. R. (1970a). Osmotic reflection coefficients in capillary membranes. *In* "Capillary Permeability" (C. Crone and N. A. Lassen, eds.), pp. 278–286, Munksgaard, Copenhagen.

Pappenheimer, J. R. (1970b). Discussion of paper by J. A. Johnson. *In* "Capillary Permeability" (C. Crone and N. A. Lassen, eds.), pp. 293–295, Munksgaard, Copenhagen.

Pappenheimer, J. R. and Soto-Rivera, A. (1948). Effective osmotic pressure of the plasma proteins and other quantities associated with the capillary circulation in the hind limb of cats and dogs. *Amer. J. Physiol.* **152**, 471–491.

Pappenheimer, J. R., Renkin, E. M. and Borrero, L. M. (1951). Filtration, diffusion and molecular sieving through peripheral capillary membranes. *Amer. J. Physiol.* **167**, 13–46.

Perl, W. (1970). An interpolation model for evaluating permeability from indicator dilution curves. *In* "Capillary Permeability (C. Crone and N. A. Lassen, eds.), pp. 185–201, Munksgaard, Copenhagen.

Perl, W. (1971). Modified filtration-permeability model of transcapillary transport —a solution of the Pappenheimer pore puzzle? *Microvasc. Res.* **3**, 233–251.

Reese, T. S. and Karnovsky, M. J. (1967). Fine structural localization of a blood-brain barrier to exogenous peroxidase. *J. Cell. Biol.* **34**, 207–217.

Renkin, E. M. (1954). Filtration, diffusion and molecular sieving through porous cellulose membranes. *J. Gen. Physiol.* **38**, 225–243.

Renkin, E. M. (1959a). Transport of potassium 42 from blood to tissue in isolated mammalian skeletal muscles. *Amer. J. Physiol.* **197**, 1205–1210.

Renkin, E. M. (1959b). Separation of solutes in washout of cylindrical tubes. *Fed. Proc.* **18**(1), 127.

Renkin, E. M. (1964). Transport of large molecules across capillary walls. *Physiologist* **7**, 13–28.

Renkin, E. M. (1968). Transcapillary exchange in relation to the capillary circulation. *J. Gen. Physiol.* **52**, 965–1085.

Renkin, E. M. and Garlick, D. G. (1970). Transcapillary exchange of large molecules between plasma and lymph. *In* "Capillary Permeability" (C. Crone and N. A. Lassen, eds.), pp. 551–559, Munksgaard, Copenhagen.

Rous, P., Gilding, H. P. and Smith, F. (1930). The gradient of vascular permeability. *J. Exp. Med.* **51**, 807–830.

Schafer, D. E. and Johnson, J. A. (1964). Permeability of mammalian heart capillaries to sucrose and inulin. *Amer. J. Physiol.* **206**, 985–991.

Schmidt, G. W. (1952). A mathematical theory of capillary exchange as a function of tissue structure. *Bull. Math. Biophys.* **14**, 229–263.

298 C. C. MICHEL

Schmidt, G. W. (1953). The time course of capillary exchange. *Bull. Math. Biophys.* **15**, 477–488.

Scholander, P. F., Hargens, A. R. and Miller, S. L. (1968). Negative pressure in the interstitial fluid of animals. *Science, N.Y.* **161**, 321–328.

Shea, S. M., Karnovsky, M. J. and Bossert, W. H. (1969). Vesicle transport across endothelium. Simulation of a diffusion model. *J. Theor. Biol.* **24**, 30–42.

Smaje, L., Zweifach, B. W. and Intaglietta, M. (1970). Micropuncture and capillary filtration coefficients in single vessels of the cremaster muscle of the rat. *Microvasc. Res.* **2**, 96–110.

Starling, E. H. (1896). On the absorption of fluids from the connective tissue spaces. *J. Physiol.* **19**, 312–326.

Staverman, A. J. (1951). The theory of measurement of osmotic pressure. *Rec. Trav. Chim.* **70**, 344–352.

Strandell, T. and Shepherd, J. T. (1968). The effects in humans of exercise on relationship between simultaneously measured ^{133}Xe and ^{24}Na clearances. *Scand. J. Clin. Lab. Invest.* **21**, 99–107.

Stromberg, D. D. and Wiederhielm, C. A. (1970). Effects of oncotic gradients and enzymes on negative pressures in implanted capsules. *Amer. J. Physiol.* **219**, 928–932.

Taylor, G. I. (1954). The dispersion of soluble matter in solvent flowing slowly through a tube. *Proc. Roy. Soc. A.* **219**, 186–203.

Tomlin, S. G. (1969). Vesicular transport across endothelial cells. *Biochim. Biophys. Acta* **183**, 559–564.

Tosteson, D. C. (1970). Closing Discussion. *In* "Capillary Permeability" (C. Crone and N. A. Lassen, eds.), pp. 658–662, Munksgaard, Copenhagen.

Trap-Jensen, J. and Lassen, N. A. (1970). Capillary permeability for smaller hydrophilic tracers in exercising skeletal muscle in normal men and in patients with long term diabetes mellitus. *In* "Capillary Permeability" (C. Crone and N. A. Lassen, eds.), pp. 135–152, Munksgaard, Copenhagen.

Trap-Jensen, J. and Lassen, N. A. (1971). Restricted diffusion in skeletal muscle capillaries in man. *Amer. J. Physiol.* **220**, 371–376.

Vargas, F. and Johnson, J. A. (1964). An estimate of reflection coefficients from rabbit heart capillaries. *J. Gen. Physiol.* **47**, 667–677.

Vargas, F. and Johnson, J. A. (1967). Permeability of rabbit heart capillaries to non-electrolytes. *Amer. J. Physiol.* **213**, 87–93.

Wiederhielm, C. A. (1968). Dynamics of transcapillary fluid exchange. *J. Gen. Physiol.* **52**, 295–615.

White, H. (1924). On glomerular filtration. *Amer. J. Physiol.* **68**, 523–529.

Youlton, L. J. F. (1969). The permeability to human serum albumin (HSA) and polyvinylpyrrolidone (PVP) of skeletal (rat cremaster) blood vessel walls. *J. Physiol.* **204**, 112–113.

Yudilevich, D. L. and Alvarez, O. (1967). Water, sodium and thiourea transcapillary diffusion in the dog heart. *Amer. J. Physiol.* **213**, 308–314.

Zierler, K. L. (1962). Theoretical basis of indicator dilution methods for measuring flow and volume. *Circulation Res.* **10**, 393–407.

Zweifach, B. W. and Intaglietta, M. (1968). Mechanics of fluid movement across single capillaries in the rabbit. *Microvasc. Res.* **1**, 83–101.

Chapter 18

Pulmonary Hemodynamics

WILLIAM R. MILNOR

*Department of Physiology,
The Johns Hopkins University School of Medicine,
725 North Wolfe Street, Baltimore,
Maryland, U.S.A.*

1. INTRODUCTION

The pulmonary circulation is in some respects an ideal system with which to illustrate the application of mechanical principles to vascular beds in general. Not the least of its qualifications is the diversity of the disciplines that have been used to study it, for investigators in physiology, clinical medicine and engineering have all found problems to interest them in the pulmonary bed. The major vessels are relatively accessible in man as well as in animals by virtue of the modern techniques of cardiovascular catheterization, so that the sources of experimental data range from human subjects to isolated segments of pulmonary vessels. The pulmonary bed has also generated, for some reason, more than its share of models—electrical, mechanical and mathematical—which has encouraged a quantitative and analytic approach to pulmonary hemodynamics.

The characteristics of the pulmonary circulation most fundamental to fluid dynamics are the dimensions, numbers and visco-elastic properties of its component vessels, and the architectural pattern in which they are combined. These qualities, the substrate on which hemodynamic principles operate in any vascular bed, will be considered first, followed by a section outlining the normal levels of pressure, flow, wave-velocity, impedance and transmission in the pulmonary vessels. Subsequent sections are concerned with the external forces that act on pulmonary vessels, some of which are unique to the pulmonary bed, and the hydraulic energies associated with pulmonary blood flow. We have limited our discussion almost exclusively to the normal resting state, with only a brief indication of the responses to exercise and to vascular occlusion in the last part of the chapter.

In keeping with the general theme of this volume we have touched only superficially on neural control of the pulmonary circulation, and have omitted completely the respiratory function of the lung and the effects of oxygen, carbon dioxide, or pharmacologic agents. Equations have not been included because the appropriate expressions for impedance, reflection coefficients, and other functions appear elsewhere (Chapter 10). In citing references, preference has been given to relatively recent papers and monographs in which more complete special bibliographies may be found. Unless otherwise specified, quantitative statements apply to the adult human pulmonary vascular bed.

2. PHYSICAL PROPERTIES OF THE SYSTEM

Students of hemodynamics soon discover that all too little is known about the mechanical properties and even the anatomy of specific vessels and vascular beds, and this is no less true of the pulmonary bed than of other parts of the circulation. Reliable data on the dimensions and physical properties of the main pulmonary artery and its early branches are available (Attinger, 1963; Patel et al., 1960; Frasher and Sobin, 1960; Patel et al., 1962; Harris et al., 1965) and the structure of the pulmonary microcirculation has been studied in some detail (e.g. Staub, 1961; Weibel, 1963; Lauweryns, 1964). Much less information on the intermediate vessels 0·1 to 3·0 mm in diameter is available, although the recent work of Cumming et al. (1969) goes far to remedy this situation as far as the arterial tree is concerned.

The pulmonary artery has almost the same cross-sectional area as the aorta, but differs radically from it in length. The aorta continues for perhaps half a meter as a large trunk giving off right-angled branches to various organs, while the main pulmonary artery extends only 4 or 5 cm before dividing into right and left main branches. The subsequent branchings of the pulmonary artery do not, of course, follow a precise geometric pattern, but they approximate an "irregular" dichotomy in which each artery divides into two daughter branches of unequal cross-section until the capillaries are reached. The pulmonary capillaries form a complex network investing each of the pulmonary alveoli, and eventually drain into a venous tree whose converging branches resemble the arterial tree in reverse. The length of the average arterial path from pulmonic valve to capillaries is approximately 15 cm in man, with individual path lengths ranging from 8 to 20 cm (Cumming et al., 1969). The length of the average intravascular path from pulmonic valve to the junction of the pulmonic veins with the left atrium is therefore about 30 cm in man, or about 20 cm in the dog. The length of each arterial-segment, from one point of branching to the next, tends to decrease distally. Few measurements of this dimensional sequence are available and the range *in vivo* is doubtless quite wide, but a ratio of 0·8 (length of daughter vessels equals 80 per cent of length of parent vessels) approximates Attinger's (1963) data on the larger arteries, and gives a reasonable fit in models of the whole pulmonary bed (Wiener et al., 1966).

The change in cross-sectional area at points of vascular branching is usually described by a "branching coefficient" (k_B), defined as the ratio of the combined areas of the daughter vessels to that of the parent vessel. Throughout most of the pulmonary arterial tree the total cross-sectional area increases as we move toward the capillaries so that $k_B > 1\cdot0$. The principal exception to this rule is the division of the main trunk into right and left main branches, where k_B is about 0·8 (Patel et al., 1960; Attinger, 1963). In subsequent arterial branching the coefficient probably increases gradually toward the periphery. Although it is often said that $k_B = 1\cdot2$ or more (Engleberg and Du Bois, 1959; Caro and Saffman, 1965; Wiener et al., 1966), the data provided by Attinger (1963) show an average branching coefficient of only 1·08 for the first six arterial generations in the dog, and the measurements of Cumming et al. (1969) on human lungs suggest coefficients between 1·10 and 1·20, since these co-workers found that the cross-sectional area of the bed increased by a factor of 5·6 between the main pulmonary artery and vessels about 75 μm in diameter, which must include something between 15 and 25 dichotomous generations.

In the precapillary region (vessels less than 50 μm in diameter) the proliferation of branches can no longer be represented by simple dichotomy, and the branching coefficient presumably reaches much larger values. The pulmonary capillaries are arranged in a kind of mesh surrounding each alveolus, a pattern quite different from the somewhat longer, though freely-anastomosing, tubular capillaries found in most parts of the systemic circulation. Weibel (1963) likens this bed to a pattern of contiguous hexagons made up of capillary segments approximately 12 μm long and 8 μm in diameter. Each segment is shared by two of the hexagons, and the whole network forms a single sheet between two adjacent alveoli. Although the capillary pattern *in vivo* is obviously less regular than this geometric abstraction, the hexagonal model is a good approximation, and the measurements made by Weibel on five human lungs constitute one of the most detailed and quantitative studies yet made of any part of the circulation. Fung and Sobin (1969) have derived a theory of "sheet flow" that is particularly appropriate to this kind of network, but the nature of blood itself remains the major problem in analyzing blood flow through these and other capillaries, since the diameter of the undeformed red cell is approximately the same as that of the capillary lumen. The branching pattern and coefficients of the pulmonary venous tree have not been described in any detail, though it seems safe to assume that the total cross-section diminishes steadily from capillaries to the veno-atrial junctions. A secondary path of blood flow in the lungs exists in the bronchial arteries and veins, though the flow through these channels amounts to only about one per cent of the total pulmonary blood flow. The distribution of these vessels and their anastomoses with the pulmonary arterial and venous beds have been described in detail by Daly and Hebb (1966).

The larger pulmonary arteries are elliptical in cross-section, rather than circular. According to Attinger (1963), the ratio of major to minor diameters is about 1·25 in the main pulmonary artery of the dog, and ranges from 1·91 to 1·07 in the next five generations of arteries, approaching more closely to a circular cross-section in each successive generation. Small degrees of ellipticity are in general of little hemodynamic significance (see Caro and Saffman, 1965), but the rather marked departure from a circular cross-section in the initial arterial branches may be important in theoretic treatments of pressure and flow in these vessels.

The volume of blood contained in the pulmonary vessels and its distribution among the various kinds of vessels are summarized in Table 1. The major physiologic significance of these volumes lies in the relation between systemic and pulmonic blood volumes and the shifts that can occur between them under certain circumstances (McGaff *et al.*, 1963; Yu, 1969). Since the volume of any vessel depends on its unstressed dimensions, compliance, and transmural pressure or other mechanical stresses applied to its walls, it follows that changes in pulmonary blood volume are the result of changes in these variables, not the primary cause of any hemodynamic event. Methods that determine separately the volume of the arterial, capillary and

TABLE 1

Typical hemodynamic conditions in the pulmonary circulation

	Man (75 kg; 1·85 m²)		Dog (20 kg)	
	Mean	Peak/ minimum	Mean	Peak/ minimum
Heart rate, (s⁻¹)	1·20		1·50	
Radius, PA, (cm)	1·40		0·75	
Pressure, PA, (mm Hg)	15	25/10	17	26/11
„ PC, (mm Hg)	10	12/9	10	12/9
„ PV, (mm Hg)	7	8/6	7	8/6
Blood flow, PA, (cm³ s⁻¹)	100	500/0	42	170/0
„ „ PC, (cm³ s⁻¹)	100	280/40	42	95/15
„ „ PV, (cm³ s⁻¹)	100	200/50	42	70/20
Blood velocity, PA, (cm s⁻¹)	16	80/0	24	96/0
Blood acceleration, PA (max), (cm s⁻²)	1010		1800	
Pulmonary vascular resistance, (dyne s cm⁻⁵)	106		318	
Characteristic input impedance, (dyne s cm⁻⁵)	22	(30/16)†	180	(245/130)†
Wave velocity, (cm s⁻¹)	180		270	
Pulse transmission time, PA–PC, (s)	0·120		0·085	
„ „ PA–PV, (s)	0·180		0·110	
Blood volume, arterial,(cm³)	130		60	
„ „ capillary, (cm³)	150		68	
„ „ venous, (cm³)	160		72	
„ „ total, (cm³)	440		200	

†Maximum/minimum between 2 and 12 Hz.
PA: pulmonary artery, main trunk; PC: pulmonary capillaries; PV: pulmonary veins at veno-atrial junction.

venous compartments provide an indirect guide to the numbers and dimensions of different classes of vessels (Engleberg and Du Bois, 1959; Feisal et al., 1962; Wiener et al., 1966), though there are occasional difficulties in reconciling morphologic data with the volumes estimated.

Turning to the viscoelastic properties of the pulmonary vessels, it is again the main pulmonary artery that has been most frequently studied, in the dog (Frasher and Sobin, 1960; Patel et al., 1960, 1962; Patel et al., 1964; Caro and Saffman, 1965; Bargainer, 1967) and in man (Patel et al., 1964; Harris et al., 1965; Milnor et al., 1969).

Experimentally, vascular elasticity may be determined by direct measurements of compliance, or by measuring wave velocity, either of these parameters being theoretically predictable from the other (see McDonald, 1960). The results of these two different approaches to the elasticity of the main pulmonary artery do not entirely agree, though they at least give answers of the same order of magnitude. The relative volume compliance $(dV/V_0 dP)$ of this artery in the dog has been reported as about 2·4 per cent cmH_2O^{-1} (Patel et al., 1962; Frasher and Sobin, 1960). Other experiments in which the "pressure-strain elastic modulus" was measured imply somewhat a smaller volume compliance, about 2·0 per cent cmH_2O^{-1} for the canine and 1·3 to 2·0 per cent cmH_2O^{-1} for the human pulmonary artery (our calculations from the data of Patel et al., 1964; and Harris et al., 1965), perhaps because these observations related the total pressure pulse to the full excursion of the wall with each cardiac cycle. Indirect estimates of the absolute compliance of the pulmonary arterial tree as a whole in the dog (Engleberg and Du Bois, 1959) and in man (Shaw, 1963), are not inconsistent with these values, but such data are not strictly comparable to measurements of compliance of the main pulmonary artery alone.

The wave velocities reported in man suggest compliances somewhat higher than any of these values. Our own data (Milnor et al., 1969) and those of Caro and Harrison (1962) give an average of 175 cm s^{-1} in the main pulmonary artery of normal human subjects, which would correspond to a compliance of about 4 per cent cmH_2O^{-1}. Wave velocities of 275 cm s^{-1} have been reported for the dog (Bargainer, 1967) and 85 cm s^{-1} for the rabbit (Caro and McDonald, 1961). In each case, the distance from pulmonary artery to capillaries is consequently about one-tenth wave length for the fundamental harmonic, at the resting heart rate. The elastic moduli of the arterial wall (Young's modulus) computed from these velocities range from $0·48 \times 10^6$ dyne cm^{-2} in man to $1·19 \times 10^6$ dyne cm^{-2} for the dog. For the present, it seems wisest to attribute this wide spread of values to the technical difficulties involved in measuring compliance and wave velocity, rather than to true species differences.

All these observations demonstrate a much larger compliance in the pulmonary artery than in the systemic arteries. Wave velocity in the ascending aorta is at least three times that in the pulmonary artery, and increases rapidly in the distal aorta and its branches. Because of this higher compliance, the characteristic impedance of the pulmonary artery is much lower than that of the aorta, just as the vascular resistance is much lower in the pulmonic bed than in the systemic because of the relative numbers and dimensions of their vessels.

The elasticity of vessels beyond the main artery has been less completely explored. There is abundant evidence (see Bergel, 1964) that the stiffness of the systemic arteries increases distally, and the same is apparently true in the pulmonary arterial tree (Harris and Heath, 1962). The observations of Caro and Saffman (1965), based on radiographic measurements of pulmonary vessels in isolated rabbit lungs, show that large arteries are more distensible than either small arteries or large veins. The smallest vessels in this study were approximately 0·8 mm in diameter. Their results are reported in the form of "circumferential extensibilities", but calculations based on their graphs indicate that the volume compliance of small arteries is perhaps half that of the large arteries, and that wave velocity in the distal arteries is some 40 per cent higher than that in the main trunk. The observations of Maloney and Castle (1969) on the distensibility of pulmonary vessels *in vivo* in the frog are consistent with these conclusions. The large veins appear to be the least compliant vessels in the pulmonary bed, while small veins may be even more compliant than the large arteries (Caro and Saffman, 1965).

The compliance of pulmonary capillaries presents special problems, both conceptually and experimentally. Capillaries are usually considered to have very little compliance because of their small diameter, acting as almost rigid tubes when open, or collapsing completely when their transmural pressure falls to zero. Evidence that true distension of capillaries can occur dictates some modification of this view (Glazier *et al.*, 1969), but it seems likely that the total capillary volume depends principally on the number of vessels open rather than on such distension. The marked increase in total pulmonary capillary volume that occurs with exercise, for example, is probably largely the result of recruitment, or opening of capillaries previously closed. Under these circumstances the transmural pressure-volume relationship of the capillaries has a significance quite different from the compliance of other vessels. Wave velocity in the capillaries is probably quite high, yet large changes in capillary volume may occur in response to small changes in pressure at critical levels, giving an apparently high "compliance".

The sequence of compliances through the bed is of considerable theoretic importance, being a major determinant of the vascular impedances and reflections. The best composite picture that can be drawn for the human pulmonary vessels appears to be relative volume compliances of 4 per cent cmH_2O^{-1} for the main pulmonary artery, 2 per cent for the small arteries, 5 per cent for the small veins, and 1·8 per cent for the large veins. This set of values must be regarded only as a tentative and approximate working hypothesis until further data are available. It must be further stipulated that these are intended as estimates of the compliances when pressures are normal, and when the lung is inflated only to its normal expiratory volume, since pulmonary vascular compliance varies with the degree of inflation of the lung and is also a function of transmural pressure.

Complete specification of the visco-elastic properties of the pulmonary vessels should include the effects of wall viscosity, which can be expressed as the phase lag between changes in pressure and changes in vessel diameter. This lag is quite small in the systemic arteries, amounting to a phase angle of about $0\cdot1$ radian in the thoracic aorta (Learoyd and Taylor, 1966; Bergel, 1964), and probably no more than that in the main pulmonary artery (Patel et al., 1964). This is not to say that the viscous behaviour of pulmonary arteries is negligible, however, for even small amounts of viscosity in the vascular wall can have appreciable effects on wave transmission (Taylor, 1966b).

3. NORMAL DYNAMICS

A. PRESSURE, FLOW, VELOCITY

Information on intravascular pressure and flow in the pulmonary circulation ranges from well-documented direct measurements in some vessels to little more than educated guesses in others. Typical observations at the inlet and outlet of the bed are shown in Fig. 1.

Countless measurements of pressure in the main pulmonary artery have been made in man and a variety of other animals, and under normal resting conditions the mean pressure usually lies between 10 and 20 mmHg. Indeed, one of the most remarkable observations in comparative physiology is the similarity in magnitude of pulmonary arterial pressures in animals of widely varying size. The same constancy is found within species at different stages of growth, once the immediate postnatal period is past. The principal changes in vascular length during the period of growth are in the larger, low-resistance, vessels, which clearly contributes to this constancy (Ferencz, 1969).

Pulmonary capillary pressure has been measured only rarely and in most cases by very indirect methods involving "wedged" catheters (see Fishman, 1963) or the movement of fluids through the capillary wall (e.g. Agostini and Piiper, 1962). In mid-capillary the average pressure in vessels at the same hydrostatic level as the pulmonic valve is probably in the neighborhood of 9 or 10 mmHg, a value significantly lower than the 24 mmHg reported in systemic capillaries (see Landis and Pappenheimer, 1963). Near the pulmonary veno-atrial junctions the mean venous pressure ordinarily ranges from 5 to 10 mmHg. The total pressure-drop across the pulmonary bed is thus relatively small, perhaps one sixth that in the systemic circuit, and the drop across the arterial portion of the pulmonary bed is not much greater than that across the veins. In measuring such small pressures the technical problem of defining a "zero reference level" becomes critical, and this doubtless accounts in part for the wide range of absolute values reported in the literature. Although little is known about the drop in pressure in the intervening vessels, it is possible, using the pulmonary arterial, capillary, and left atrial pressures

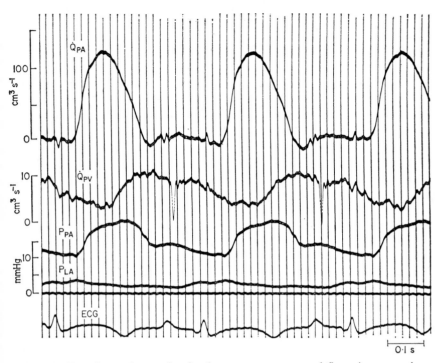

FIG. 1. Experimental records of pulmonary pressures and flows in a conscious dog, at rest. Symbols: Q̇, blood flow; P, pressure; PA, pulmonary artery; PV, pulmonary vein, within 2 cm of the left atrium; LA, left atrium; ECG, electro-cardiogram, lead I. Sharp downward spikes in the pulmonary venous flow tracing and smaller spikes in the pulmonary arterial flow during diastole are electro-cardiographic signals. Timing lines appear at intervals of 0·02 s.

as benchmarks and relying on the vascular dimensions discussed earlier, to arrive at the kind of "pressure profile" shown in Fig. 2. Pulse-pressure in the main pulmonary artery is ordinarily 8 to 20 mmHg; the transmission of this pulse through the bed will be considered in a later section.

Total pulmonary blood flow is equivalent to the cardiac output, and mean flow is the same at all cross-sections of the bed, though the flow pulsations are not. Because the cross-section of the arterial tree increases distally, blood moves more slowly as it advances toward the capillary bed, then speeds up again as the veins converge and vascular cross-section diminishes. The mean velocity gradually changes in this way from about 15 cm s^{-1} in the main pulmonary artery to perhaps 0·05 cm s^{-1} in the capillaries, and back to almost its original speed at the venous termination of the bed. One consequence of this changing velocity is the conversion of kinetic energy into

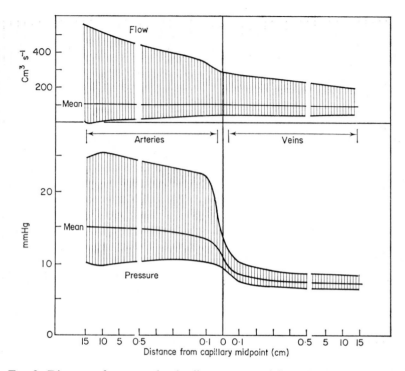

FIG. 2. Diagram of mean and pulsatile pressure and flow along an average path through the human pulmonary vascular bed. Abscissa represents distance from the capillary mid-point. Note changes of scale at 0·5 cm. Based on references cited in text.

pressure in the arterial bed, and the reverse in the veins. The pressures observed at any point are influenced by such interconversion, but the effect is so small with normal basal flows as to be negligible. When pulmonary blood flow increases two- or three-fold, however, as in exercise, this phenomenon may be of physiologic significance. Flow is presumably laminar in most of the pulmonary vessels because of the low velocities and relatively small diameters. In the main pulmonary artery in man, peak Reynolds numbers are 5000 to 8000, well above the level at which transition from laminar flow to turbulence is expected. Only a few observations of the velocity profile in the pulmonary artery have been made, but the measurements of Schultz and his co-workers indicate that the profile is relatively flat under normal conditions, with no gross evidence of turbulence. In a patient with congenital stenosis of the pulmonic valve, however, they recorded highly turbulent flow throughout most of systole (Schultz et al., 1969).

The ratio of pulmonary arterial cross-section to cardiac output appears to be of the same order of magnitude in a number of different species of animals. Though the evidence on this point is rather meager, it suggests that the mean velocity of flow in the pulmonary artery tends to be relatively constant, regardless of body size. Estimates of the mean velocity in the human pulmonary artery are, nevertheless, lower than those in the dog (see Table 1). This may be a real difference, or it may only reflect the fact that it is easier to induce the low cardiac output of a basal state in man than in the dog.

The pulsations of blood flow in the pulmonary artery have been studied frequently in the dog, usually with electromagnetic flowmeters (e.g. Patel *et al.*, 1963; Elliott *et al.*, 1963; Morkin *et al.*, 1965a; Bergel and Milnor, 1965; Morgan *et al.*, 1966a; Karatzas *et al.*, 1970), but in some instances ultrasonic instruments (Franklin *et al.*, 1962; Fricke *et al.*, 1970) or other devices (Pieper, 1963). Instantaneous velocity in the pulmonary arteries of conscious human subjects has also been measured (Gabe *et al.*, 1969). The contour of the pulmonary arterial flow pulse shows a slightly lower, more rounded peak than that in the ascending aorta (Figs. 1 and 3) though the area under these two instantaneous flow curves must be identical when the stroke volumes of the two ventricles are exactly equal. The period of forward flow is also slightly longer in the main pulmonary artery than at the aortic root, since the pulmonic valve opens a few milliseconds before the aortic, and closes after it. The amplitude of the flow pulse, like the pressure pulse, tends to diminish as it moves through the pulmonary bed, but pulsations persist into the large pulmonary veins. The venous pulse (see Fig. 1) lags behind, and falls more slowly than the pulmonary arterial flow wave, and may or may not reach zero between pulsations (Morkin *et al.*, 1965a).

The wave-form of pressure and flow pulsations can be judged qualitatively from records like those in Fig. 1, and the measurement of systolic and diastolic values is a step toward more exact description of these pulses, but the most complete quantitative approach for many purposes is that of harmonic analysis (see McDonald, 1960).

B. HARMONIC CONTENT OF PRESSURE AND FLOW PULSATIONS

Most of the characteristic features of the pulmonary arterial pressure and flow pulsations, and more than 95 per cent of their energy is contained in the first six harmonics (Bergel and Milnor, 1965). Measurable components extend up to the 11th harmonic (Patel *et al.*, 1963), but beyond that level the signal-to-noise ratio becomes too small for reliable determinations. The fundamental harmonic corresponds to the heart rate, which usually lies between 1 and 2 Hz, so that the frequency range from 0 to 12 Hz is the region of interest for most investigation *in vivo*.

The results of Fourier analysis, or what might be called the "harmonic content" of pulmonary arterial pressure and flow waves, can be described as follows (Patel *et al.*, 1963; Attinger, 1963; Bergel and Milnor, 1965; Patel *et al.*, 1965; Caro *et al.*, 1967a; Karatzas *et al.*, 1970).

In both pressure and flow the first harmonic or fundamental has the

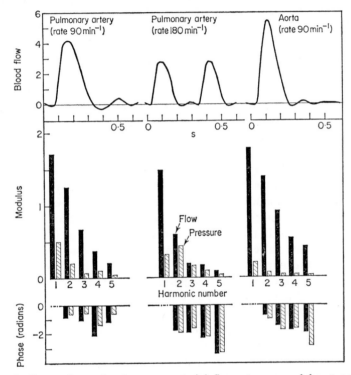

FIG. 3. Comparison of pulmonary arterial flow at a normal heart rate (left) with that at a faster rate (center), and with aortic flow (right). The corresponding pressure and flow harmonics are shown below the flow pulses in each case. Ordinates for flow and for the harmonic moduli are expressed as proportions of mean flow (mean flow = 1·0). Phase lag between harmonics is plotted in relation to the timing of the first harmonic (phase = 0·0). Impedance phase (relation between pressure and flow phases) is not shown (see Fig. 4).

largest modulus, while the subsequent harmonics become progressively smaller (Fig. 3). The second harmonic ordinarily lags the first in phase by at least 0·5 radians and the higher harmonics tend to lag still further behind the first. The relations between harmonics of the flow pulse (and to lesser extent the pressure pulse) is a function of heart rate because of the character of right ventricular ejection (Milnor *et al.*, 1966). As heart rate increases, the length of the cardiac cycle shortens principally by a reduction in the period of zero diastolic flow (Fig. 3). Systolic duration also decreases, but the shape of the systolic flow pulse changes very little. The harmonic equivalent of these alterations is a decrease in the modulus of the second and higher harmonics as compared with the first, and at very fast heart rates the higher harmonics become so small that the flow pulse more and more resembles a simple sinusoidal wave. As a rule, the phase lag between flow harmonics becomes greater as heart rate increases. The ratio of the first flow harmonic modulus to mean flow usually lies between 1·5 and 2·0, tending toward the lower part of this range with faster heart rates. In many experimental records the contrast between the sharply-peaked aortic flow pulse and the more rounded pulmonary arterial flow wave is obvious, yet the differences in harmonic structure are rather subtle (see Fig. 3). All harmonics of aortic flow are larger in proportion to mean flow than are the corresponding pulmonary arterial harmonics, but this in itself would only increase the amplitude of the excursion around the mean, not change the shape of the flow wave. The other differences in shape can be attributed only to a slightly greater relative prominence of the third to fifth harmonics in aortic flow, and slight differences in the phase relations between harmonics.

Fourier series like those represented in Fig. 3 are simply numerical descriptions of the shape of pulsations, but their great usefulness in cardiovascular physiology has been amply demonstrated by studies of pressure-flow relationships (e.g. Caro and McDonald, 1961; Patel et al., 1963; Bergel and Milnor, 1965), and wave transmission (Attinger, 1963; Caro et al., 1967a; Caro et al., 1967b; Karatzas et al., 1970) in the pulmonary circulation, and in theoretical hemodynamics (McDonald, 1960; Wiener et al., 1966). Spectral analysis by correlation, applied to a continuous train of pulses, is another method of examining frequency content. In combination with random pacing of the heart by an external stimulus (Taylor, 1966c) this technique gives a more detailed picture of the impedance spectrum than does the Fourier series.

C. RESISTANCE

The concept of vascular impedance (McDonald, 1960) is a general one that includes the ratio of sinusoidal pressures and flows at all frequencies including zero, but the "D.C. component" or "resistance" is often considered separately. The term "resistance" is employed in cardiovascular physiology in at least two different senses, and failure to distinguish between the two leads to confusion. Sometimes it is used to denote in a very general sense the energy-dissipating properties of a vascular system, while at other times it signifies a specific pressure/flow ratio analogous to electrical resistance.

Throughout this chapter, the phrase "pulmonary vascular resistance" denotes the value obtained by dividing cardiac output into the difference between mean pulmonary arterial and mean left atrial pressures. This operational definition has been profitably used in experimental work and clinical medicine, in spite of a tendency to over-simplify the interpretation of the resulting values (see below).

In normal adult human subjects the average pulmonary vascular resistance is in the neighborhood of 100 dyne s cm^{-5}, ranging from perhaps 50 to 200 dyne s cm^{-5}. Comparison with values in other species emphasizes the point that vascular resistance varies inversely with the size of the animal, a logical relationship if resistance depends in part on the number of parallel channels available to carry the total pulmonary blood flow. Total pulmonary vascular resistance in the unanesthetized dog at rest averages 300 to 600 dyne s cm^{-5} in our laboratory, the total pressure-drop across the lung being about the same as in man, but the cardiac output lower. Because of the relatively low pressures involved and the limitations of accuracy with which pressure and flow can be measured, changes in pulmonary resistance less than ± 20 per cent in a given individual can rarely be considered significant.

The distribution of resistance within the pulmonary bed cannot be stated with any precision, in spite of many experimental efforts to identify separately at least the arterial, capillary, and venous contributions. The problem has been attacked with a variety of different methods, including the insertion of very small catheters in the venous tree (Caro *et al.*, 1967a), measurement of transudation of fluid from pulmonary capillaries (Agostoni and Piiper, 1962), determination of regional transit times and pressure changes after injection of a low viscosity solution (Brody *et al.*, 1968), and the interpretation of perfusion data by the assumption of sluice-like behavior in collapsible vessels (Fowler *et al.*, 1966; McDonald and Butler, 1967), not to mention observation of the pressures recorded by "wedged" arterial or venous catheters. Leaving aside data obtained by this last method because one cannot be sure exactly where the pressure being measured exists, the results generally agree in demonstrating that the resistance of the arterial bed as a whole is only slightly greater than that of the venous bed. Several different methods lead to the conclusion that resistance is distributed in almost equal portions between "arteries, capillaries and veins", but these compartments are defined functionally rather than anatomically. The numbers and dimensions of the arteries and veins are such that under normal conditions (assuming laminar flow and dichotomy) the mean pressure-difference between the main trunks and vessels 0·5 mm in diameter must be less than 1·0 mmHg, implying that the major part of the total resistance lies in the most central part of the bed, within a few mm of the capillaries. The resistance of the capillaries, using that term in its strict anatomic sense, is not known, although estimates ranging from 5 to 50 per cent of the total pulmonary vascular resistance have been reported. The various indirect methods used to determine the distribution of resistance probably tend to overestimate the capillary component because they lump an indeterminate part of the small arteries or veins along with the true capillaries. Such techniques can sometimes provide information of functional importance, nevertheless, as witness the demonstration by Fowler *et al.* (1966) that the small vessels subjected to alveolar pressure on their outer surface have a total resistance greater than the more distal or more proximal regions. The only direct measurements of the pressure drop from arteriolar to venular end of the pulmonary capillaries, to our knowledge, are those made by Maloney and Castle (1970) on the frog lung, where they found that 15 to 28 per cent of the total pressure-drop from pulmonary artery to left atrium occurred between pre-capillary vessels 80 μm in diameter and post-capillaries of the same size.

It is difficult at present to postulate with any confidence a model that would predict the pressure-drop across the pulmonary capillary bed. The theory of "sheet flow" proposed by Fung and Sobin (1969) and applied by them to models of the pulmonary capillaries is a new and promising approach, much more appropriate to this complex network than analyses based on Poiseuille's law. Not enough is known, however, about the dimensions of the capillary bed as a whole to warrant theoretic predictions of its resistance. Weibel's investigation did not include a systematic study of the average distance from entrance to exit of the capillary bed, which is a critical point in this context, though he did cite preliminary data indicating that the number of precapillaries was 200 to 300 $\times$ 10^6 (Weibel, 1963).

Assume, for example, that the pulmonary capillary bed consists of one "capillary network unit" (Weibel, 1963) for each one of 200 $\times$ 10^6 precapillaries, and that each unit consists of a hollow "sheet" 300 μm long, 300 μm wide and 8 μm thick, with regularly recurring discontinuities ("posts" in the Sobin–Fung model) occupying 25 per cent of the sheet volume. The total pulmonary capillary resistance would then amount to 42·7 dyne s cm^{-5} (our calculations from the equations given by Fung and Sobin, 1969, not allowing for distensibility of the sheet), which would give a pressure-drop of 3·2 mmHg across the capillaries, if the flow were 100 cm^3 s^{-1}. Although the dimensions, blood volume (108 cm^3), and transit time (1·1 s for total flow of 100 cm^3 s^{-1}) of this pulmonary capillary model are not inconsistent with experimental data, the choice of other equally reasonable lengths, widths, or size of discontinuities could readily alter the resistance by a factor of two in either direction. Since these are precisely the variables on which we have least accurate information, such calculations are of limited value.

D. IMPEDANCE

Pulmonary vascular input has been studied in a number of different laboratories with consistent results in the dog (Caro and McDonald, 1961; Patel *et al.*, 1963; Bergel and Milnor, 1965) and in man (Milnor *et al.*, 1969). The impedance spectrum (impedance moduli and phases plotted against frequency) shows more-or-less orderly oscillations with frequency (see Fig. 4) similar to those produced by reflections in a transmission line

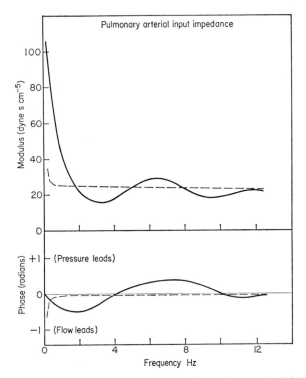

FIG. 4. Typical pulmonary arterial input impedance in man (solid line). Broken line indicates the theoretic input impedance for an elastic tube 2·8 cm in diameter, with a wave-velocity of 120 cm s^{-1}, ending in a perfectly-matched termination. Pulmonary vascular resistance is plotted at frequency = 0.

(McDonald, 1960; Taylor, 1966a). Under normal conditions the largest moduli of impedance are found at frequencies below 1 Hz, and the moduli decline with frequency to a minimum between 2 and 4 Hz, then rise to a maximum between 6 and 8 Hz. Above 10 Hz the impedance moduli remain almost constant as frequency increases. Impedance phase is negative (i.e. flow leads pressure) at low frequencies, becoming less negative as frequency rises; the phase changes from negative to positive ("zero crossing") at about the same frequency as the minimum modulus. A positive maximum of phase usually appears between 6 and 8 Hz, followed by a return toward zero at higher frequencies. The range of phase values recorded experimentally between 1 and 12 Hz is ordinarily $\pm 1 \cdot 0$ radian. In at least one respect, the phase of pulmonary input impedance seems not to resemble that in a transmission line: the frequencies at which the phase angle is zero do not exactly match the minima and maxima of impedance modulus (see Fig. 4). Because it is difficult to get accurate measurements of impedance phase experimentally, especially at higher frequencies, more data are needed before firm conclusions can be reached on this point. Figure 4 also shows the theoretic input impedance, calculated from Womersley's equations, for an elastic tube with the same diameter as the average human pulmonary artery and a wave velocity of 120 cm s^{-1}, ending in a perfectly-matched termination so that reflections do not occur. The correspondence between this theoretic characteristic impedance and the approximate average of the impedances observed demonstrates at least some consistency between theory and observations, though it is necessary to assume a wave velocity somewhat lower than the average of those reported so far.

The value usually plotted for the impedance modulus at a "frequency" of zero is that of the pulmonary vascular resistance. It can be argued that the mean pulmonary arterial pressure alone, rather than the pressure-drop across the bed, is the appropriate numerator in calculating the zero-frequency impedance, or "input resistance", inasmuch as the other impedance moduli are calculated from the pulmonary arterial pressures and flows without regard for the pulsations at the terminus of the bed. The choice between these two alternatives is unimportant, however, as long as it is clearly specified Experimentally, we have noted that impedance moduli at low frequencies almost never exceed the "input resistance", but occasionally do exceed the pulmonary vascular resistance.

The average of the moduli between 2 and 10 Hz is a useful value in describing impedance spectra, and can be regarded as an estimate of "characteristic impedance" if the differences between a vascular system and a simple elastic tube are kept in mind. The minimum and maximum moduli can then be expressed as proportions of this average impedance. In 10 to 30 kg dogs the characteristic impedance so calculated is usually 100 to 250 dyne s cm^{-5}, in both anesthetized, open-chest dogs and in unanesthetized, unrestrained, resting animals (Patel et al., 1963; Bergel and Milnor, 1965; Milnor et al., 1966). The first minimum and maximum amount to excursions of about ± 20 per cent of the characteristic impedance on the average. We have occasionally noted unusually high maxima at 6 to 8 Hz, approaching the resistance value, in moduli derived by Fourier analysis of single beats, but the non-reproducibility of these peaks in adjacent beats and their absence in moduli derived by cross-correlation lead us to regard these as artefacts.

To facilitate comparison of data from animals of differing size, Patel *et al.* (1963) normalized their impedance moduli by comparing them to the resistance, but the correlation between these variables is low (McDonald, 1964) and may become insignificant under certain experimental conditions or pharmacological influences. Relating the moduli to body weight would seem to be a better alternative, using blood flow per unit weight to calculate the moduli of impedance. Logical as weight-normalization seems, considering that the cardiac output unquestionably varies with body size, it does little to narrow the wide range of values observed in the dog. In 25 anesthetized dogs we found characteristic impedances ranging from 99 to 245 dyne s cm^{-5}, with an average of 168 dyne s cm^{-5}. After adjustment for body weight the range was 1600 to 4000 dyne s kg cm^{-5}. Whether weight-adjustment was employed or not, in other words, the range was approximately 50 to 140 per cent of the mean.

The moral appears to be that raw data are the best form for presentation of experimentally-measured impedances. Among different species, however, pulmonary vascular impedance clearly varies inversely with the size of the animal. The characteristic impedance is much higher in the dog than in man, and higher still in the rabbit. The average value in three relatively normal human subjects we studied was 23 dyne s cm^{-5} (Milnor *et al.*, 1969) and Caro and McDonald's (1961) data on the perfused rabbit lung indicate a characteristic impedance of about 1100 dyne s cm^{-5}. The corresponding weight-adjusted averages are approximately 1600 dyne s kg cm^{-5} for man, 3000 for the dog, and 3800 for the rabbit, so here too the differences cannot be accounted for by weight alone.

The usefulness of the impedance spectrum lies in the fact that it summarizes the effects of the properties of the vascular bed on pressure-flow relationships at the input. If the system is linear, these relationships will apply to any input signal. Given an appropriate model of the pulmonary vascular bed, the impedance spectrum should also allow the interpretation of experimental results in terms of the properties of specific parts of the bed.

Since it is probable that no relationship in the real world is perfectly linear, the important question here is: "How non-linear is the relationship between pressure, flow and physical properties in the pulmonary vascular bed?" or alternatively, "How large an error is introduced by treating it as a linear system?"

Using the artificially-paced heart as the source of a wide range of frequencies and amplitudes, Bergel and Milnor (1965) found that the pulmonary bed in the dog did resemble a linear system at the input, at least within the limits of their measurements. The observations of Maloney *et al.* (1968b) in the isolated lung confirm this conclusion. The non-linearity of the fundamental Navier–Stokes equations and of vascular elasticity virtually guarantee some degree of non-linearity in pressure-flow relationships, but the experimental detection of small deviations from linearity would be difficult. Even with careful attention to technique, measurements *in vivo* entail random uncertainties of at least ±5 per cent in flow and independent errors of the same magnitude in pressure, so that errors no less than ±10 per cent are to be expected in impedance data. Non-linearity that produced inconsistencies of less than 15 per cent in calculated impedance moduli (e.g. caused the impedance moduli to vary no more than ±15 per cent as a function of pressure amplitude) would probably be undetectable in most experiments. Conversely, the pulsatile pressure-flow relationships in the pulmonary artery are linear to this degree of accuracy. Whether the pulmonary vascular bed can be treated as a linear system without serious error depends, then, on the purpose of the investigator. For investigations of impedance the assumption of linearity is usually quite acceptable; some vasomotor drugs and pathologic situations, for example, alter the input impedance moduli by a factor of two or more (Bergel and Milnor, 1965; Milnor *et al.*, 1969), producing changes that far exceed the possible influence of non-linearities. For detailed studies of the elastic behaviour of individual vessels, on the other hand, investigation of relatively small non-linearities may be essential.

Although the characteristic, minimum and maximum impedances in a simple elastic tube bear a definite theoretic relationship to the properties of the tube and its termination (see Chapter 10, and McDonald, 1960), their significance in a system like the pulmonary vascular bed is more complicated. In a uniform tube with a "closed" end the first minimum of impedance occurs at that frequency for which the distance to the termination is one-quarter wave-length. Given the wave velocity and the input impedance spectrum of such a tube, one can predict the distance to the reflecting site. This computation has sometimes been applied to experimental data obtained *in vivo* (Caro and McDonald, 1961; Bergel and Milnor, 1965), but the single tube is certainly not the most suitable model for a branching, non-uniform system.

Reflecting sites in a vascular bed are both multiple and widely dispersed, and the longitudinally non-uniform elasticity of the arteries causes wave velocity to increase distally. The consequences of these properties are evident in appropriate models (Taylor, 1966a, b; Wiener *et al.*, 1966; Pollack *et al.*, 1968). Moreover, the impedance minimum falls at one-quarter wave-length from the reflecting site only if the reflection involves no phase shift, and mathematical models of the pulmonary circulation developed in our laboratory indicate that the waves reflected at each branch point differ considerably in phase as well as amplitude from the incident waves. The pressure reflection coefficients in our model are rarely close to 0° or 180° (the typical phase angles for "closed" and "open" ends, respectively), but have intermediate values. Under these conditions impedance minima can appear at distances quite different from one-quarter wave-length.

Only an optimist could hope to deduce much about the properties of the vascular bed from the input impedance spectrum under such circumstances, yet there is some evidence that optimism is warranted. Our models suggest, for example, that the modulus of the apparent reflection coefficient observed in the main pulmonary artery is determined principally by reflections in the most distal part of the arterial tree, while the transit time to these reflecting sites and back is dominated by the elasticity of the larger arteries. Changes in the amplitude of the minimum and maximum impedance moduli may therefore be attributed to changes in the distal part of the bed, while alterations of the frequency of the impedance minimum and maximum (or of the phase zero-crossings) suggest alterations in the elasticity of the larger arteries. This encourages the conclusion that it may be possible with further study to make useful deductions about the distributed properties of the pulmonary vessels from the input impedance spectrum.

E. TRANSMISSION OF PRESSURE AND FLOW PULSATIONS

As pressure waves travel through the pulmonary circulation they are modified in two different ways. The effects of viscosity tend to damp the amplitude of the wave, while reflections increase its amplitude in some regions and diminish it in others. Apparent phase velocity as well as amplitude is affected, and flow pulsations are altered at the same time. One consequence of these interactions is that a comparison of waves recorded simultaneously at two fairly-widely-separated sites in the pulmonary circulation may present the initially surprising finding that the downstream pulsation is the larger. Pressure in the main pulmonary artery and its primary branches exhibits this phenomenon, some harmonics increasing by 25 per cent or more in the first few cm (Attinger, 1963; Milnor et al., 1969), and similar effects on both flow and pressure may be present in more distal regions (Caro et al., 1967b; Wiener et al., 1966).

Experimental measurements of "transmission", the ratio of the amplitude of pulsations at some cross-section of the bed to that at the origin, thus include the effects of both viscosity and reflection. Experimental methods have been devised to distinguish between these effects (see McDonald, 1968) so as to measure the attenuation (the real part of the complex propagation constant), but no data on pulmonary vessels are yet available. Theoretic calculations on our models indicate attenuations for the first harmonic of about 0·2 per cent cm^{-1} in the main pulmonary artery, increasing to 6 per cent cm^{-1} in arteries 500 μm in diameter, and to still higher values in smaller vessels.

Direct measurements in the rabbit (Rappaport, Bloch and Irwin, 1959) and frog (Maloney and Castle, 1970) show that 50 to 60 per cent of the pulmonary arterial pressure pulse is transmitted to arterioles less than 100 μm in diameter. Experiments on the isolated dog lung by Maloney *et al.* (1968a, 1968b) show pressure transmission to "collapsible" vessels of about 20 per cent for sinusoidal waves at a frequency of 2 Hz. As these authors point out, their method measures not only transmission to the microcirculation but also a kind of "critical opening pressure" for closed vessels. While this lends an important functional significance to their results, it limits the conclusions that may be drawn about arterial transmission. In addition, the "collapsible vessels" and the capillary bed are not necessarily coextensive, and one cannot be certain whether or not their transmission values apply to the venular end of the capillaries, and hence include the effects of the capillary bed itself.

Caro *et al.* (1967b) report an average pressure transmission to pulmonary veins of 33 per cent at 1 to 2 Hz in human subjects. Reports of pressure transmission from main artery to the largest pulmonary veins in animals range from 28 per cent down to less than 10 per cent, if we include comparisons of overall pulse pressures as well as Fourier analyses of harmonics (Caro and McDonald, 1961; Bergel and Milnor, 1965; Wiener *et al.*, 1966; Caro *et al.*, 1967a; Pinkerson, 1967; Szidon *et al.*, 1968). The lowest of these values were observed in our laboratory in dogs (Bergel and Milnor, 1965) in veins temporarily ligated at the veno-atrial junction to eliminate the effects of atrial contraction. We assumed that the abnormal reflections under these conditions would produce venous pressure pulsations higher than those transmitted when the junction was normally open, but the weight of subsequent evidence suggests that our estimates were too low, and that transmission of 15 to 20 per cent is a reasonable estimate. This is not to say that the pressure amplitude may not change between capillaries and large veins, since it may well be altered by reflections in the intervening bed. Pressure transmission to the veins appears to be frequency-dependent, falling sharply as frequency rises from 0·05 to 2·00 Hz (Maloney *et al.*, 1968b) and less steeply at higher frequencies (Bergel and Milnor, 1965; Caro *et al.*, 1967a, b).

The time required for pressure and flow pulses to travel from pulmonary artery to the end of the pulmonary veins averages about 0·11 s in the dog, ranging from 0·08 to 0·16 s (Pinkerson, 1967; Szidon *et al.*, 1968). Transmission from main pulmonary artery to the capillary bed accounts for about two-thirds of this time (Morkin *et al.*, 1965a). These are "foot-to-foot" values; a few measurements of harmonic components in our laboratory fall within this range for the fundamental and suggest shorter times for the higher harmonics.

The understanding of flow transmission in the pulmonary bed has been greatly advanced by application of the nitrous oxide-plethysmographic method of measuring pulmonary capillary flow in man (Rigatto et al., 1961; Linderholm et al., 1962; Wasserman et al., 1966; Kaplan and Kimbel, 1970; Karatzas and Lee, 1970), and in the dog (Morkin et al., 1965b) and also by simultaneous measurement of pulmonary arterial and pulmonary venous flow with electromagnetic flowmeters in the dog (Maloney et al., 1968b; Szidon et al., 1968).

Peak flow in the pulmonary capillaries of the dog is approximately one-half that in the pulmonary artery, and harmonic analysis of these pulses shows transmission to the capillaries of about 50 per cent for the first harmonic (Karatzas et al., 1970). This is consistent with observations in man, where the peak/mean capillary flow ratios average 2·5, with a range of about 1·5 to 3·5), (Wasserman et al., 1966; Kaplan and Kimbel, 1970), or roughly half the peak/mean ratio usually found in the pulmonary artery. Other factors being equal, the amplitude of both arterial and capillary flow waves varies directly with stroke volume and inversely with heart rate, which means that both these factors must be taken into account before attributing a change in the amplitude of capillary flow to a change in transmission. It seems probable that transmission to the capillaries decreases with frequency for the first few harmonics (Wiener et al., 1966; Karatzas et al., 1970) but this has not been confirmed experimentally.

Estimates of flow transmission to the pulmonary veins are less consistent. Most published records of simultaneous arterial and venous flows show pulmonary venous pulses that are about 35 per cent of the arterial pulses in amplitude (e.g., Szidon et al., 1968; Morgan et al., 1966b). Our own measurements of pulmonary artery to vein transmission in four anesthetized, open-chest dogs average to 46 per cent (range 19 to 52 per cent) for the fundamental harmonic (2·2 to 2·8 Hz). Maloney and his colleagues (1968b), on the other hand, found in perfusing dog lungs with sinusoidal flows at relatively low frequencies that transmission from artery to vein fell from about 50 per cent at 0·1 Hz to only 10 per cent at 1·0 Hz. It is conceivable that transmission to the veins reaches a minimum at 1·0 Hz in accordance with the data of Maloney et al., then rises at higher frequencies to values consistent with the in vivo observations, but the records of Szidon et al. (1968) show that transmission to the veins, as judged by comparing simultaneous arterial and venous flow pulses in vivo, falls appreciably as the fundamental frequency (heart rate) rises from 1·0 to 2·0 Hz (their Fig. 5). Further experimentation is needed to resolve this apparent conflict.

4. FACTORS THAT INFLUENCE PRESSURE AND FLOW

Having considered the intrinsic properties of the pulmonary vascular bed, and normal levels of the most important hemodynamic variables to the extent these are known, it is appropriate to examine the forces that control and modify the pulmonary vascular pressure and flow relationships. These can somewhat arbitrarily be divided into two groups: neuromuscular factors and external forces.

A. NEUROMUSCULAR FACTORS

The neuromuscular elements of control include vascular smooth muscle, the autonomic nervous system that supplies it, the receptors of the pulmonary vascular bed, and the reflex arcs that involve pulmonary vessels. Important as these topics are, they must be regarded as peripheral to the central theme of the present volume, and will be treated only briefly here.

Smooth muscle fibers in the walls of all pulmonary vessels except capillaries (and perhaps the smallest venules) (Fishman, 1963; Daly and Hebb, 1966) are the means by which the caliber and distensibility of the vessels are controlled. The behavior of vascular smooth muscle in general is not yet fully understood (see Bergel, 1964; Bohr and Uchida, 1969 and Chapter 12). Activation of smooth muscle in the wall of a vessel tends to reduce the mean diameter of the vessel and decrease its compliance, as one might expect; the changes in caliber being most apparent in small vessels and the altered compliance most notable in large ones, but quantitative analysis of this response in terms of smooth muscle length and tension presents certain difficulties.

Neural control of blood vessels is less prominent in the pulmonary than in the systemic circulation, but this may be only because pressures and resistances are so much lower in the pulmonary bed. The concentration of smooth muscle in pulmonary vessels is lower than in systemic vessels of comparable size, a fact sometimes offered as evidence that the pulmonary bed is incapable of strong vasomotor reactions. Rather marked species differences also exist with respect to the amount of smooth muscle in the pulmonary vasculature (Ferencz, 1969) particularly in vessels less than 100 µm in diameter (Daly and Hebb, 1966). There is little doubt that a mechanism for active neural control of the pulmonary bed exists, for experiments have shown that efferent impulses through autonomic nerves to the pulmonary vessels can produce definite changes in their caliber and compliance (Daly and Hebb, 1966; Ingram et al., 1968). Such control can even be selective in its action, as demonstrated by an increase in the moduli of input impedance with no consistent change in pulmonary vascular resistance (implying a stiffening of larger pulmonary arteries with no change in smaller vessels) when pulmonary sympathetic nerves are stimulated (Ingram *et al.*, 1968). Work in our laboratory shows that thoracic sympathectomy in the dog produces just the opposite effect on impedance moduli, which fall to values significantly lower than in the control state. In addition, clinical investigation reveals many pathologic examples of active pulmonary vasoconstriction. It seems clear, therefore, that active autonomic nervous control of the pulmonary circulation over a fairly wide range of response is potentially available. The question that remains unanswered is the degree to which this control is actually utilized in normal adjustments of the circulation.

Receptors sensitive to stretching exist in the major pulmonary arterial branches, and perhaps in pulmonary veins. The reflexes that regulate the operation of the cardiovascular system as a whole involve the pulmonary bed, in many instances, and reflexes that originate in the pulmonary bed as well as others that impinge on it, have been described (see Daly and Hebb, 1966). The phenomenon of "autoregulation", whereby the resistance in many systemic beds is adjusted by some intrinsic mechanism to keep flow constant over a certain range of input pressure, does not appear in the pulmonary circulation, nor have "myogenic responses" involving an increase in wall tension in response to stretch, been demonstrated in pulmonary vessels. The intriguing possibility of a kind of intrapulmonary reflex mechanism is suggested, however, by reports of pulmonary vasoconstriction caused by pulmonary arterial distention (Hyman, 1968).

B. EXTERNAL FORCES

Factors that influence pulmonary pressures and flows but have their origin outside the pulmonary bed include the extravascular components of transmural pressure, the effects of respiratory inflation of the lung, the nature of the input signal generated by the right ventricle, and the influence of the left atrium as the termination of the bed.

(1) *Transmural pressures*

Although blood vessels are often thought of as distensible tubes that resume some finite diameter when transmural pressure is zero, the fact that they are compressible, or "collapsible", is of equal importance. Not only can the active tension of vascular smooth muscle reduce the circumference of a small vessel until its lumen is obliterated, in spite of a positive distending pressure, but the very thin-walled vessels that contain no smooth muscle may collapse completely at zero transmural pressure. The latter possibility is especially relevant in the pulmonary capillaries. The external pressure on these capillaries, and on adjacent parts of the microcirculation as well, is the pressure in the pericapillary tissue space (meager though that is), which depends to a large extent on intra-alveolar pressure. Extravascular pressure on other vessels within the lung is a function of interstitial pressures that may be negative (i.e. sub-atmospheric) (Howell *et al.*, 1961; West, 1969), while the large pulmonary vessels outside the parenchyma of the lung, like the heart itself, are subjected to intrapleural pressure.

The intravascular pressures produced in the pulmonary vessels by right ventricular ejection are relatively low, not only in comparison to systemic pressures but in relation to the hydrostatic pressure differences in the lung. In an erect human subject the weight of a column of blood extending vertically from the pulmonic valve to the top of the lung is equivalent to a hydrostatic pressure that approximately equals mean pulmonary arterial pressure, $20 \, cmH_2O$ for example. Since the mean arterial pressure is diminished in transmission to the capillaries, it follows that in the uppermost parts of the lung the intravascular pressures would be even lower than the atmospheric pressure in the alveoli, the capillaries would tend to collapse, and no perfusion would occur in this region. These expectations have been fully confirmed experimentally (West *et al.*, 1964). The importance of these interacting forces has given rise to an empiric distinction (see West, 1969) between "alveolar vessels" (those subject to alveolar pressure) and "extra-alveolar vessels" (all the rest), a functional dichotomy that comes naturally to respiratory physiologists. In studies of regional blood flow in the lung, the relation between intravascular, extravascular, and hydrostatic pressures has been used to identify three hemodynamically-different zones (West *et al.*, 1964):

Zone I: arterial < alveolar > venous pressures
Zone II: arterial > alveolar > venous pressures
Zone III: arterial > alveolar < venous pressures

The arterial and venous pressures referred to in this scheme are those in the terminal vessels, taking hydrostatic pressure into account. In the erect posture, these zones correspond roughly to the upper, middle, and lower parts of the lung, and blood flow is distributed accordingly.

The potentialities for capillary collapse complicate the relation of pulmonary arteriolar and venular pressure to capillary volume, resistance, and transmural pressure. A rigorous analysis of the dynamics of collapsible tubes is not readily available, and could probably not be put to use at this stage of our knowledge in any case, but Permutt, Riley and their associates have suggested a simple and attractive alternative (Permutt *et al.*, 1962; Permutt and Riley, 1963). Their proposal is that the pulmonary capillary be regarded as a thin-walled, collapsible tube (a "Starling resistor"), surrounded by a chamber that provides the "extravascular" pressure. The arteries and veins in this model are usually considered to have a low, constant resistance and

14*

compliance, though these assumptions are not crucial. The most important feature of the model appears when venous pressure is less, and arterial pressure greater, than "alveolar" (extracapillary) pressure (West's "Zone II" conditions). Flow then becomes a function of arterial and alveolar pressures, rather than arterial and venous pressures. The reason lies in partial collapse of the capillary tube, so that its distal end is almost completely closed. In this almost-occluded region the intravascular pressure is presumably just equal to the extra-vascular pressure, so that the lumen is not quite obliterated. Flow in the model under these conditions is virtually independent of venous pressure so long as venous pressure remains less than extracapillary pressure. The "capillary" thus acts like a sluice-gate, servo-controlled, as it were, by opposing signals from arterial and extracapillary pressure.

An extraordinary amount of fruitful investigation and re-interpretation has been stimulated by this proposal. Although the possibility that alveolar pressures, which are atmospheric on the average, might be higher than venous pressures may seem unrealistic on first thought, the consideration of hydrostatic pressure effects reminds us that venular pressures can indeed be subatmospheric in the upper parts of the lung. The obvious relevance of this concept to the transmission of pressure and flow through the capillaries has been exploited in a variety of experiments (e.g. Maloney et al., 1968a, 1968b; McDonald and Butler, 1967; West et al., 1964; West and Dollery, 1965)

Re-evaluation of pulmonary hemodynamics from this new point of view has led, among other things, to the suggestion that the conventional pulmonary vascular resistance equation has no useful significance unless alveolar pressure is substituted for left atrial pressure. While the latter procedure would be appropriate for calculating a resistance value for the arterial tree (plus some undetermined proximal part of the capillary bed) under "Zone II" conditions, the term "alveolar pressure" tends to obscure the fact that it is the intracapillary pressure (assumed to be equal to the alveolar) that is dynamically significant; blood flow still depends on the pressure gradient within the lumen and the geometric configuration of the channel. There is no reason, moreover, to modify the interpretation of the pulmonary vascular resistance as it is usually calculated and applied in vivo. Given constant blood viscosity, constant vessel lengths, and laminar flow, a change in pulmonary vascular resistance should be interpreted as evidence of a change in total vascular cross-section somewhere in the bed, as Poiseuille's law implies. The cause and site of this change in cross-section cannot be learned from measurements of pulmonary vascular resistance, whether or not collapsible vessels are part of the system. The assumption that pulmonary vascular resistance is predominantly an index of pulmonary arteriolar caliber was never warranted by theory, though it has played an empirically useful part in many investigations. Under "Zone II" conditions, the drop in pressure at the junction of the amost-collapsed capillaries with their venules must be very abrupt, and could be far greater than the drop across the arterioles. Looked at in another way, the mean pressure-gradient from pulmonary artery to left atrium is also a measure of the potential energy lost in the bed in relation to blood flow. The potential energy per unit time at any point is equal to the product of pressure and flow, so that the energy lost in the pulmonary bed (omitting pulsatile and kinetic terms) equals pulmonary vascular resistance times the square of the mean flow. The observation in the collapsible tube model under "Zone II" conditions that flow is not altered by changing venous pressure means, therefore, that more and more energy is dissipated in the model as venous pressure is lowered under these conditions. This increased energy loss may be the result of very small changes in lumen at the end of the tube, or of turbulence.

The theoretic basis for the conventional calculation of pulmonary vascular resistance, in short, is no less applicable in the presence of collapsible vessels than otherwise. The investigator must simply avoid bringing to the calculation a mental image of cylindrical tubes and the fourth power of their radii, and must look on the final result as a number related to the bed as a whole. When studying just one part of the lung, on the other hand, the concept of "zones" determined by alveolar and venous pressures is essential.

The action of transmural pressures on pulmonary vascular resistance depends strongly on the properties of the microcirculation. Many investigators have shown that resistance can be lowered by raising pulmonary arterial or venous pressures, but the mechanism for this effect is uncertain, and interpretation of the data depends on the model of the pulmonary bed that one adopts. The relationship is non-linear, as is that between perfusing pressure and pulmonary blood volume. Arteries and veins must participate to some extent in alterations of pulmonary blood volume, but the greater part of the change appears to take place in vessels that can be influenced by alveolar pressure, i.e. in the micro-circulation (Permutt et al., 1969). Whether increases in volume represent the opening of vessels previously closed (recruitment), actual distention of capillaries, or both, is still a moot point (see Permutt et al., 1969, and discussion following that paper). Either mechanism could decrease the resistance and so explain the fall in pulmonary vascular resistance as perfusing pressures are raised.

(2) *Pulmonary inflation*

The volume, resistance, and compliance of the pulmonary bed changes rhythmically with normal inspiration and expiration. Because inflation and deflation of the lung can be brought about only by changes in trans-pulmonary pressure (the difference between pressure in the alveoli, and that in the intrapleural space or its experimental analogue), it is not easy to distinguish between the direct mechanical effects of inflation and those of transmural pressure. It now appears that the mechanical effects act mainly on the larger vessels, through stretching or compression of the interstitial tissues or the vessels themselves, while the transmural pressures act principally on the compressible vessels of the micro-circulation. Other factors being equal, inflation decreases the volume of small vessels and increases the volume of larger ones (Howell et al., 1961). The relation between pulmonary vascular resistance and degree of inflation is "U-shaped", the minimum resistance corresponding to normal resting levels of transpulmonary pressure.

One other force involved in the interactions between transpulmonary pressure, degree of inflation, and capillary transmural pressure is the surface tension of the fluid film that normally lines the alveoli. The presence of this fluid of "surfactant" (see Pattle, 1966) lowers this surface tension, making the transpulmonary (and hence alveolar) pressures needed for normal inflation less than they would otherwise be. At the same time, the intervention of this low-tension film between the alveolar gases and the capillaries may tend to make pericapillary pressures lower than those in the alveolus. In these circumstances it could be predicted that the presence of surfactant would act to keep capillaries open even when their intraluminal pressure is lower than alveolar pressure, and the experiments of Bruderman et al. (1964) support this prediction. The data reported by West et al. (1964) seem to contradict this conclusion, for they state that capillaries are perfused only if the arterial pressure (including hydrostatic pressure) is at least equal to alveolar pressure. Bruderman and his colleagues found this to be true when the alveoli had been filled with fluid to abolish the normal air-liquid interface in the alveoli, but in the normally-inflated lung they found that flow could be produced by arterial pressures about 3 mmHg lower than alveolar pressure. If the surfactant effect is this small, the apparent conflict may arise only from differences in experimental methods.

The total effect of respiration on pulmonary hemodynamics involves changes in venous return to the right heart as well as the mechanical and pressure effects on the pulmonary vessels. Respiratory changes in total pulmonary blood flow are relatively small, but early studies with the bristle flowmeter showed that pulmonary arterial flow increased with inspiration (Brecher and Hubay, 1955). Subsequent work has not only confirmed this observation but also defined the concomitant changes in pulmonary venous flow and left ventricular output (Franklin et al., 1962; Morkin et al., 1965a; Morgan et al., 1966a,b). These reports indicate that in the dog right ventricular stroke volume and peak pulmonary arterial flow increase in the heartbeat immediately following the onset of inspiration, and that pulmonary venous and aortic flows increase promptly and proportionately, usually in the next beat. Increased outflow from the lungs thus lags the inflow only by the expected pulse-transmission time, about 0·1 s. Ventricular output and heart rate act together to produce this result; sometimes the stroke volume does not increase with inspiration, but a slight rise in heart rate ensures that mean pulmonary arterial flow does increase (Morgan *et al.*, 1966a). Recent observations in man (Gabe *et al.*, 1969) show a greater lag between right and left ventricular outputs, perhaps because deep inspirations were studied. Their pulmonary arterial flows increased with inspiration as expected, but left ventricular stroke volume fell steadily during inspiration and rose only toward the end of expiration, a lag of 3 or 4 s. Until further data are available, it seems probable that the difference between these observations in man and those in animals are related only to rate and depth of respiration.

Because pulmonary arterial and left atrial pressures are usually measured with respect to atmospheric pressure, recordings of these variables *in vivo* show a fall with inspiration that corresponds in time and magnitude to the increasing negativity of intrapleural pressure. Changes in pulmonary vascular resistance with normal respiration are extremely small, but there appears to be a slight increase with inspiration. In a few observations in dogs in our laboratory, we were unable to detect any respiratory change in pulmonary vascular impedance.

C. INPUT FROM THE RIGHT VENTRICLE

The characteristics of the pulsatile input from the right ventricle are as important as the properties of the pulmonary vascular bed in determining pressure and flow. Conversely, the function of the right ventricle *in vivo* depends in part on the "load" presented to it by the pulmonary vessels. From both points of view this relation deserves more attention than it has so far received, though a few studies on the left ventricle and aorta have been reported (e.g. Wilcken *et al.*, 1964). The influence on ventricular function of the "load", or opposition to flow, offered by the aorta and systemic circuit becomes evident when this load is changed. Reducing the aortic and systemic resistance leads to an increase in left ventricular stroke volume, peak flow, and maximum acceleration (though the latter changes relatively little), while increasing the outflow resistance has just the opposite effects (Wilcken *et al.*, 1964).

Qualitatively, the right and left ventricular ejection patterns are similar, reaching maximum acceleration early in systole, but maximum acceleration in the pulmonary artery is only about half that in the aorta and the pulmonary arterial flow has a lower, more rounded peak. The pressure gradient across the pulmonic valve probably reverses at about the time of peak flow, as in the left side of the heart, so that the lateral pressure in the ventricle becomes lower than in the pulmonary artery and the momentum already imparted to the blood becomes the dominant force, but this phenomenon is much less marked on the right side of the heart than on the left. The pulmonary vascular input impedance constitutes the load for the right ventricle, and when impedance is increased, the pulmonary arterial flow pulse changes in contour, assuming the more sharply-peaked, almost triangular shape of the aortic flow pulse. This effect can be produced by partial collapse of the lung (Franklin *et al.*, 1962) and we observed it in our experiments on the pulmonary vasoconstriction induced by serotonin (Bergel and Milnor, 1965). It is our impression that slowing of both acceleration and deceleration underlies this change in pulse contour, but this merits systematic investigation. Now that instantaneous flow measurements are feasible as part of ordinary diagnostic procedures in man (Gabe *et al.*, 1969) it will be interesting to see whether similar changes in the pulmonary arterial flow wave are found in clinical pulmonary hypertension.

Whether the ventricle should be regarded as a "flow source" or a "pressure source" is a question that inevitably faces those who would devise models of the circulation, but the phenomena observed *in vivo* hint that the answer need not lie in either of those alternatives. Rushmer has proposed an image of the ventricles as "impulse" generators, "impulse" being the product of force and time and thus a quantity that can readily be related to the velocity or acceleration of blood (Rushmer, 1964). An equally plausible case can be made for the heart as an energy source, imparting energy to the blood which is then manifested as pressure and flow in proportions dictated by the vascular impedance. The important practical point is that the pressures and flows measured experimentally under ordinary conditions contain the effects of the ventricular input as well as of the vascular properties. Relationships between pressure and flow (e.g. impedance) can be used to study the vascular properties *per se*, but the absolute values and time course of pressure or flow are determined by the character of the input as well as the state of the vessels.

D. THE LEFT ATRIAL TERMINATION

The left atrium represents the "terminal impedance" of the pulmonary bed, and is also a potential source of retrograde pressure and flow signals. Ordinarily the pressure-gradient across the veno-atrial junction is too small to be measured accurately, and the pressure pulsations at the end of the lobar veins are virtually the same as those in the left atrium. The influence of the left atrial and ventricular contractions on pulmonary venous pulsations is a matter of controversy. Szidon *et al.* (1968) found that when a lung was isolated and a reservoir substituted for the left atrium the pulmonary venous flow waves were the same in form, magnitude and transmission time as those *in vivo*, which argues strongly that the normal venous pulses are predominantly transmitted from the pulmonary artery. Morgan and his associates disagree, attributing the venous flow pulsations to the mechanical action of the left heart (Morgan *et al.*, 1966a,b). The presence of a small backflow from atrium to veins at the time of atrial systole, especially when heart rate is slow (Morgan *et al.*, 1966a), and the demonstration that some flow pulsations appear in the pulmonary veins even when pulmonary arterial flow is non-pulsatile (Morgan *et al.*, 1966b) provide evidence that some retrograde effects do occur. Their magnitude in relation to the effects of forward transmission is not clear, however. The relatively large size of the flow as opposed to the pressure pulsations in the veins is not in itself incompatible with forward transmission (see Wiener *et al.*, 1966), and is to be expected if the input impedance to the left atrium is relatively small. Considering all the evidence, it seems probable that the greater part of the pulmonary venous pulsation is transmitted from the pulmonary artery, but no more quantitative statement can be made at present.

5. HYDRAULIC ENERGY AND POWER

Modern flowmeters make it relatively easy to measure the hydraulic energy associated with blood flow, and concepts of hemodynamics in terms of energy distribution and dissipation should find a useful place in circulatory physiology. The energies associated with pulmonary arterial flow, for example, can be computed "on-line" to give continuous records of hydraulic power (energy per unit time as a function of time) (Fig. 5), or can be derived from harmonic analysis. In either case, the energies can be expressed as instantaneous hydraulic power, as energy per cardiac cycle, or as time-average power. The last of these, referred to simply as "hydraulic power", will be used here. Estimates of hydraulic power based on mean pressure and flow alone underestimate the actual energies in most situations, and even the "mean systolic" values of pressure and flow that were long used to calculate the external work of the heart are highly unreliable (Milnor *et al.*, 1966).

Two kinds of energy must be considered. The first, which represents energy stored in the vessel walls, and is equal to the product of pressure and the volume of blood in which that pressure obtains, may be called in the present context "potential" energy. The second, kinetic energy, is a function of blood velocity in accordance with the standard formula (kinetic energy equals one-half mass times the square of velocity). The rate of change of potential energy per unit time, or "potential power" is the product of pressure and flow, and the "kinetic power" is the kinetic energy per unit

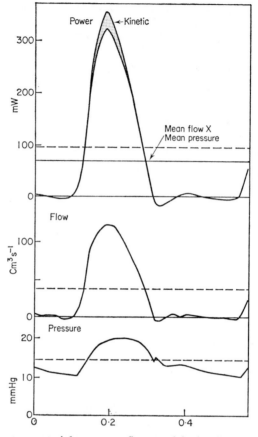

Fig. 5. Pulmonary arterial pressure, flow, and hydraulic power, derived from observations on the dog whose records appear in Fig. 1. Pulses in solid lines represent pressure, flow, and their instantaneous product (potential energy per unit time, or power). Broken lines indicate the averages of these pulses over one cardiac cycle. The product of mean flow and mean pressure, or average "steady-flow component", is shown in the upper section for comparison with the total average power. The difference between the two is the power associated with pulsations. Shaded area represent kinetic energy per unit time, which is too small to be visible on the graph except near peak flow.

volume of blood multiplied by the volume flow per unit time. Gravitational energy, or "potential energy of position" conferred on a unit of blood by virtue of its height above some reference level, is usually omitted in these calculations. Although of crucial importance in considerations of regional blood flow in the lung, as noted earlier, it can reasonably be ignored in considering hydraulic energy in the pulmonary bed as a whole, inasmuch as the arterial inlet and venous outlet of the bed are at nearly the same hydrostatic level.

By harmonic analysis it is possible to separate two components of these energies, one associated with the mean terms of pressure and flow, the other with the pulsations around these means. The first expresses the energy that would be required to produce a steady non-pulsatile flow under the observed conditions, while the second is a kind of "extra" energy entailed in the pulsations. The technical procedures and equations for applying this kind of analysis to experimental data have been reported elsewhere (Milnor *et al.*, 1966).

Typical values of the hydraulic power delivered to the pulmonary artery by the right ventricle, the power dissipated in the pulmonary vascular bed, and that appearing at the venous end of the bed, are listed in Table 2. The

TABLE 2

Hydraulic power associated with pulmonary blood flow.
Typical values in man and in the dog.

	Man (75 kg; 1·85 m²)			Dog (20 kg)		
	Input (mW)	Output (mW)	Dissipated (%)	Input (mW)	Output (mW)	Dissipated (%)
Potential power						
Mean terms	200	93	54	95	45	53
Pulsatile	88	4	95	35	1	97
Combined	288	97	66	130	46	65
Kinetic power						
Mean terms	1	1	0	1	1	0
Pulsatile	20	5	75	14	3	79
Combined	21	6	71	15	4	73
Total power						
Mean terms	201	94	53	96	46	52
Pulsatile	108	9	92	49	4	92
Combined	309	103	67	145	50	66
Proportions at input:						
Total pulsatile/ total combined		35%			34%	
Combined kinetic/ combined total		7%			10%	

values given, which are derived from our own observations, are significantly higher than those in the model reported by Skalak *et al.* (1966), perhaps because they assumed a heart rate (120 min^{-1}) faster than that in the resting conscious dog, and because their hypothetical animal appears to be relatively small, perhaps 12 kg. At rest, in both man and the dog, the power associated with pulsations in the pulmonary artery is about half the "steady-flow" component, or one-third the total energy input. This is much larger than the proportion in the aorta, where the ratio of pulsatile/steady-flow power is approximately 0·1, a difference that might be predicted from the relatively smaller ratio of pulse/mean pressure in the aorta. Observations in the dog indicate that 60 to 80 per cent of the energy that enters the pulmonary artery is dissipated in the pulmonary vessels (Milnor *et al.*, 1966; Skalak *et al.*, 1966). The pulsatile energy output at the venous end of the bed has not been measured in human subjects, but there is no reason to suppose that the proportions are significantly different.

The kinetic energy in the pulmonary artery is by no means negligible, though a calculation based only on mean velocity might suggest that conclusion. Kinetic energy contributes at least 6 per cent of the total input power in man (Milnor *et al.*, 1969) and 10 to 20 per cent in the unanesthetized dog (Milnor *et al.*, 1966, and subsequent unpublished data). The pulsatile wave-form of flow is particularly critical in determining the kinetic energy because kinetic power is in effect a function of the cube of flow. As is evident in Table 2, the pulsatile kinetic term is much larger than the steady-flow component.

The direct measurements needed to calculate energies are readily accessible only at the inlet and outlet of the bed, but Skalak and his associates have successfully combined experimental data, reasonable assumptions, and a mathematical model to describe the distribution of energies within the pulmonary bed (see Chapter 19 and Skalak *et al.*, 1966). The results define the dissipation of energy within the bed, the work done on vessel walls, and the interconversion of kinetic and potential energies as blood travels through the lung. This approach, which has also been used to treat the transmission of waves through the bed (Wiener *et al.*, 1966) throws new light on earlier data and suggests new experiments—surely the most desirable goals of model-making.

The energy associated with blood flow is important for both theoretic and empiric reasons. The energy needed to move blood into the pulmonary artery is, by definition, the external work demanded of the right ventricle, but there are other less obvious ways in which hydraulic energy may be useful in the interpretation of hemodynamics. The distinction between pulsatile and steady-flow components of energy, for example, can be regarded in a general way as a distinction between the effects of large arteries and those of the microcirculation. The properties of the proximal arterial tree are the major determinant of pulsatile energy components (though reflections from distal vessels also make a significant contribution), while the resistance of the microcirculation dominates the steady-flow energy (Milnor et al., 1966).

The relation between pulmonary arterial input power and heart rate also illustrates the empiric usefulness of energy and impedance calculations. The impedance spectrum of the pulmonary artery (Fig. 4) suggests that the input of potential energy per unit time should be inversely related to heart rate, up to about 180 beats min^{-1} (3 Hz), and this expectation has been confirmed experimentally (Milnor et al., 1966). One consequence of this relationship is that mean flow can be increased with less energy by raising heart rate than by increasing stroke volume.

The dissipation of energy as the blood moves through the bed depends on the same properties that are involved in the concepts of resistance and impedance. Skalak and his associates (1966), adapting this view of opposition to flow as an energy-dissipating phenomenon, have introduced the concept of "effective resistance", which is essentially the value of a constant resistance that would give the observed dissipation of energy (including kinetic) at the observed mean flow. One virtue of this "effective resistance" is its emphasis of the point that terms representing pulsatile and kinetic factors are not included in the conventional pulmonary vascular resistance. Closely related ideas are contained in the "pressure power coefficient" (Milnor et al., 1966), and the concept of "energy equivalent pressure", or "potential energy per unit flow volume" (see McDonald, 1968). Behind all these terms lies the search for a broadly-generalized statement of the energy-dissipating properties of the pulmonary bed, valid for one particular state of the bed regardless of heart rate or input wave-form. At present we are inclined to let the pulmonary vascular input impedance serve this purpose, since the impedance spectrum is in fact this kind of generalized statement about the bed, requires about the same amount of computation as the indices mentioned, and can be used to derive energies, given an input signal. A supplementary description of the termination is needed before the actual dissipation within the bed can be calculated from input impedance, but this is true in any case.

6. ADAPTIVE RESPONSES

In the course of applying the analytic method to one aspect or another of pulmonary vascular function one must not lose sight of the ultimate goal of such investigation—an understanding of the ways in which the whole organism adapts itself to varying circumstances. Among the most important and most extensively studied adjustments of this kind in the pulmonary circulation are the responses to exercise and to increased pulmonary vascular impedance.

A. EXERCISE

Physical exertion, including in this term all degrees of muscular and ambulatory activity from the basal state up to heavy exercise, is a fundamental physiologic stress that demands an increase in cardiac output and pulmonary blood flow. The best-known characteristic of the pulmonary vascular response to exercise is that mean pulmonary arterial pressure rises proportionately less than cardiac output (Fishman, 1963; Harris and Heath, 1962). The simultaneous changes in left atrial pressures are relatively small, and the arterial-to-left atrial pressure difference, like the mean pulmonary arterial pressure, rises less than blood flow, so that pulmonary vascular resistance falls. Direct measurements of left atrial pressure in exercise are surprisingly scarce in either man or the dog, partly because of an unjustified reliance on "wedged" pulmonary arterial pressures as an index of left atrial pressure. In general, however, left atrial pressure tends to decrease slightly as cardiac output increases in man, and our own observations in dogs running on a treadmill usually show a fall of 1 to 3 mmHg at levels of exercise that double the cardiac output. Whether this decreased resistance is brought about by active vasomotion, passive distention, or recruitment of previously closed capillaries is not known, and it is quite possible that all three are involved.

Pulmonary capillary flow pulsations and total capillary blood volume increase significantly with exercise (Yu, 1969; Johnson et al., 1960), and resistance to flow through the capillaries presumably falls. The transmission of pressure and flow waves to the veins has not been systematically studied, but one would guess that transmission is improved. Increased rate and depth of breathing is a prominent feature of exercise, and the oscillations of intrapleural pressure with inspiration and expiration are much greater than in the resting state. These exaggerated swings of pressure within the thorax, which we have found to be as high as 20 mmHg in the exercising dog, doubtless have an influence on venous return to the right heart, but their role in the total pulmonary hemodynamic response to exercise remains to be evaluated.

The net effect is an increase in the hydraulic energy dissipated in the pulmonary bed, though not so great an increase as would occur if no change in the pulmonary vessels accompanied exercise. Experiments in our laboratory show that a degree of exercise sufficient in the dog to double the cardiac output raises the total hydraulic energy dissipated in the pulmonary bed per unit time by a factor of about three. If the pulmonary resistance and impedance were the same during exercise as at rest, the energy dissipated would increase with the square of the flow, or four-fold. This saving of energy, which can be looked on as an improved efficiency in the transport of blood during exercise, depends on at least three different things: (1) the frequency-dependent characteristics of the pulmonary vascular input impedance spectrum; (2) the reduction of input pulse amplitudes that accompanies tachycardia; (3) an increase in total vascular cross-section, probably in the microcirculation.

B. VASOCONSTRICTION AND VASCULAR OBSTRUCTION

Obstruction of large or small vessels in the pulmonary bed is often encountered in clinical medicine, the most frequent causes being emboli brought to the lung from the systemic veins, or pathologic thickening of vascular walls. Active vasoconstriction of the smaller arteries and veins is also fairly common and can be produced by hypoxemia or vasomotor drugs as well as certain diseases. Pathologic states in which pulmonary blood flow or intravascular pressures remain at abnormally high levels for long periods of time (e.g. mitral stenosis, congenital left-to-right shunts) frequently lead to an obstruction of the pulmonary bed that involves both structural changes and functional vasoconstriction. (see Harris and Heath, 1962; Fishman, 1963).

The hemodynamic consequences of such abnormalities depend in part on how much of the pulmonary arteriolar bed is involved. Complete occlusion of the right or left main branch of the pulmonary artery in a healthy individual merely diverts the total cardiac output through one lung with little change in mean arterial pressure, the vascular resistance of one lung decreasing to accommodate the new flow. The effects of disease processes that obstruct the small vessels of any large part of the lung or of general arteriolar constriction are quite different, for then the pulmonary vascular resistance rises, and may reach levels more than five times the normal value. If ventricular function is normal, the heart maintains its output in the face of this increased load at first, and mean pulmonary arterial pressure rises. Karatzas and Lee (1970) report that the transmission of pulsatile flow to the pulmonary capillaries is diminished in patients with high pulmonary vascular resistance, which one might expect, but they also found that elevated pulmonary arterial pressures were associated with decreased transmission even when the pulmonary vascular resistance was normal. The pulsations of pulmonary arterial pressure depend on the input impedance, which in most conditions of this kind is elevated. An increase in impedance is to be expected, for elevation of the mean pulmonary arterial pressure would in itself tend to distend and stiffen the arterial tree, raising the characteristic input impedance, increasing wave velocity, and moving the impedance minimum to higher frequencies. Increased reflection from the affected small vessels would, in addition, exaggerate the oscillations of impedance with frequency, yielding high values in the low frequency range. Impedance spectra and wave velocities that conform closely to this description have been observed in some clinical cases of pulmonary hypertension (Milnor et al., 1969). It is not yet possible to say whether the increased characteristic impedance and wave velocity in such patients are the result of the high arterial transmural pressure, structural changes in the arterial wall, or increased active tension in the arterial smooth muscle.

REFERENCES

Agostoni, E. and Piiper, J. (1962). Capillary pressure and distribution of resistance in isolated lung. Amer. J. Physiol. 202, 1033–1036.
Attinger, E. O. (1963). Pressure transmission in pulmonary arteries related to frequency and geometry. Circulation Res. 12, 623–641.
Bargainer, J. D. (1967). Pulse wave velocity in the main pulmonary artery of the dog. Circulation Res. 20, 630–637.
Bergel, D. H. (1964). Arterial viscoelasticity. In Pulsatile Blood Flow" (E. O. Attinger, ed.), McGraw-Hill, New York.
Bergel, D. H. and Milnor, W. R. (1965). Pulmonary vascular impedance in the dog. Circulation Res. 16, 401–415.
Brecher, G. A. and Hubay, C. A. (1955). Pulmonary blood flow and venous return during spontaneous respiration. Circulation Res. 3, 210–214.
Bohr, D. F. and Uchida, E. (1969). Activation of vascular smooth muscle. In The Pulmonary Circulation and Interstitial Space" (A. P. Fishman and H. H. Hecht, eds.), University of Chicago Press, Chicago.
Brody, J. S., Stemmler, E. J. and duBois, A. B. (1968). Longitudinal distribution of vascular resistance in the pulmonary arteries, capillaries, and veins. J. Clin. Invest. 47, 783–784.
Bruderman, I., Somers, K., Hamilton, W. K., Tooley, W. H. and Butler, J. (1964). Effect of surface tension on circulation in the excised lungs of dogs. J. Appl. Physiol. 19, 707–712.
Caro, C. G., Bergel, D. H. and Seed, W. A. (1967a). Forward and backward transmission of pressure waves in the pulmonary vascular bed of the dog. Circulation Res. 20, 185–193.
Caro, C. G. and Harrison, G. K. (1962). Observations on pulse wave velocity and pulsatile blood pressure in the human pulmonary circulation. Clin. Sci. 23, 317–329.
Caro, C. G., Harrison, G. K. and Mognoni, P. (1967b). Pressure wave transmission in the human pulmonary circulation. Cardiovasc. Res. 1, 91–100.
Caro, C. G. and McDonald, D. A. (1961). The relation of pulsatile pressure and flow in the pulmonary vascular bed. J. Physiol. 157, 426–453.
Caro, C. G. and Saffman, P. G. (1965). Extensibility of blood vessels in isolated rabbit lungs. J. Physiol. 178, 193–210.
Cumming, G., Henderson, R., Horsfield, K. and Singhal, S. S. (1969). The functional morphology of the pulmonary circulation. In "The Pulmonary Circulation and

Interstitial Space" (A. P. Fishman and H. H. Hecht, eds.), University of Chicago Press, Chicago.

Daly, I. deB. and Hebb, C. (1966). "Pulmonary and Bronchial Vascular Systems." Williams and Wilkins, Baltimore.

Elliott, S. E., Hoffman, J. I. E. and Guz, A. (1963). An electromagnetic flowmeter for simultaneous measurements of pulmonary arterial and aortic blood flows in the conscious animal. *Med. Electron. Biol. Eng.* **1**, 323–331.

Engelberg, J. and DuBois, A. B. (1959). Mechanics of pulmonary circulation in isolated rabbit lungs, *Amer. J. Physiol.* **196**, 401–414.

Feisal, K. A., Soni, J. and DuBois, A. B. (1962). Pulmonary arterial circulation time, pulmonary arterial volume, and the ratio of gas to tissue volume in the lungs of dogs. *J. Clin. Invest.* **41**, 390–400.

Ferencz, C. (1969). Pulmonary arterial design in animals. Morphologic variation and physiologic constancy. *Johns Hopkins Med. J.* **125**, 207–224.

Fishman, A. P. (1963). Dynamics of the pulmonary circulation. *In* "Handbook of Physiology", Section 2, Vol. II (W. H. Hamilton and P. Dow, eds.), pp. 1667–1743, American Physiological Soc., Washington, D.C.

Fowler, K. T., West, J. B. and Pain, M. C. F. (1966). Pressure-flow characteristics of horizontal lung preparations of minimal height. *Resp. Physiol.* **1**, 88–98.

Franklin, D. L., Van Cilters, R. L. and Rushmer, R. F. (1962). Balance between right and left ventricular output. *Circulation Res.* **10**, 17–26.

Frasher, W. H. and Sobin, S. S. (1960). Distensible behaviour of pulmonary artery. *Amer. J. Physiol.* **199**, 472–480.

Fricke, G., Studer, U. and Scheu, H. D. (1970). Pulsatile velocity in the pulmonary artery of dogs: measurements by an ultrasound gauge. *Cardiovasc. Res.* **4**, 371–379.

Fung, Y. C. and Sobin, S. S. (1969). Theory of sheet flow in lung alveoli. *J. Appl. Physiol.* **26**, 472–488.

Gabe, I. T., Gault, J. H., Ross, J. Jr., Mason, D. T., Mills, C. J., Shillingford, J. P. and Braunwald, E. (1969). Measurement of instantaneous blood flow velocity and pressure in conscious man with a catheter-tip velocity probe. *Circulation* **40**, 603–614.

Glazier, J. B., Hughes, J. M. B., Maloney, J. E. and West, J. B. (1969). Measurements of capillary dimensions and blood volume in rapidly frozen lungs. *J. Appl. Physiol.* **26**, 65–76.

Harris, P. and Heath, D. (1962). "The Human Pulmonary Circulation". Williams and Wilkins, Baltimore.

Harris, P., Heath, D. and Apostolopoulos, A. (1965). Extensibility of the human pulmonary trunk. *Brit. Heart J.* **27**, 651–659.

Howell, J. B., Permutt, S., Proctor, D. F. and Riley, R. L. (1961). Effect of inflation of the lung on different parts of pulmonary vascular bed. *J. Appl. Physiol.* **16**, 71–76.

Hyman, A. L. (1968). Pulmonary vasoconstriction due to non-occlusive distention of large pulmonary arteries in the dog. *Circulation Res.* **23**, 401–414.

Ingram, R. H., Szidon, J. P., Skalak, R. and Fishman, A. P. (1968). Effects of sympathetic nerve stimulation on the pulmonary arterial tree of the isolated lobe perfused *in situ. Circulation Res.* **22**, 801–815.

Johnson, R. L., Jr., Spicer, W. S., Bishop, J. M. and Forster, R. E. (1960). Pulmonary capillary blood flow, volume, and diffusing capacity during exercise. *J. Appl. Physiol.* **15**, 893–902.

338   W. R. MILNOR

Kaplan, A. S. and Kimbel, P. (1970). Pulmonary capillary blood flow waves in subjects with abnormal pulmonary hemodynamics. *J. Appl. Physiol.* **28,** 793–801.

Karatzas, N. B. and Lee, D. de J. (1970). Instantaneous lung capillary blood flow in patients with heart disease. *Cardiovasc. Res.* **4,** 265–273.

Karatzas, N. B., Noble, M. I. M., Saunders, K. B. and McIlroy, M. B. (1970). Transmission of the blood flow pulse through the pulmonary arterial tree. *Circulation Res.* **27,** 1–9.

Landis, E. M. and Pappenheimer, J. R. (1963). Exchange of substances through the capillary walls. *In* "Handbook of Physiology", Section 2, Vol. II, (W. F. Hamilton and P. Dow, eds.), pp. 961–1034, American Physiological Society, Washington, D.C.

Lauweryns, J. (1964). L'angioarchitecture du poumon. *Arch. Biol.* **75,** suppl., 771–811.

Learoyd, B. M. and Taylor, M. G. (1966). Alterations with age in the viscoelastic properties of human arterial walls. *Circulation Res.* **18,** 278–292.

Linderholm, H., Kimbel, P., Lewis, D. and duBois, A. B. (1962). Pulmonary capillary blood flow during cardiac catheterization. *J. Appl. Physiol.* **17,** 135–141.

Maloney, J. E., Bergel, D. H., Glazier, J. B., Hughes, J. M. B., and West, J. B. (1968a). Effect of pulsatile pulmonary artery pressure on distribution of blood flow in isolated lung. *Resp. Physiol.* **4,** 154–167.

Maloney, J. E., Bergel, D. H., Glazier, J. B., Hughes, J. M. B. and West, J. B. (1968b). Transmission of pulsatile blood pressure and flow through the isolated lung. *Circulation Res.* **23,** 11–24.

Maloney, J. E. and Castle, B. L. (1969). Pressure-diameter of capillaries and small blood vessels in frog lung. *Resp. Physiol.* **7,** 150–162.

Maloney, J. E. and Castle, B. L. (1970). Dynamic intravascular pressures in the microvessels of the frog lung. *Resp. Physiol.* **10,** 51–63.

McDonald, D. A. (1960). "Blood Flow in Arteries." Williams and Wilkins, Baltimore.

McDonald, D. A. (1964). Frequency dependence of vascular impedance. *In* "Pulsatile Blood Flow" (E. O. Attinger, ed.), McGraw-Hill, New York.

McDonald, D. A. (1968). Hemodynamics. *Annu. Rev. Physiol.* **30,** 535–556.

McDonald, I. G. and Butler, J. (1967). Distribution of vascular resistance in the isolated perfused dogs lung. *J. Appl. Physiol.* **23,** 463–474.

McGaff, C. J., Roveti, G. C., Glassman, E. and Milnor, W. R. (1963). The pulmonary blood volume in rheumatic heart disease and its alteration by isoproterenol. *Circulation* **27,** 77–84.

Milnor, W. R., Bergel, D. H. and Bargainer, J. D. (1966). Hydraulic power associated with pulmonary blood flow and its relation to heart rate. *Circulation Res.* **19,** 467–480.

Milnor, W. R., Conti, C. R., Lewis, K. B. and O'Rourke, M. F. (1969). Pulmonary arterial pulse wave velocity and impedance in man. *Circulation Res.* **25,** 637–649.

Morgan, B. C., Abel, F. L., Mullins, G. L. and Guntheroth, W. G. (1966a). Flow patterns in cavae, pulmonary artery, pulmonary vein, and aorta in intact dogs. *Amer. J. Physiol.* **210,** 903–909.

Morgan, B. C., Dillard, D. H. and Guntheroth, W. G. (1966b). Effect of cardiac and respiratory cycle on pulmonary vein flow, pressure, and diameter. *J. Appl. Physiol.* **21,** 1276–1280.

Morkin, E., Collins, J. A., Goldman, H. S. and Fishman, A. P. (1965a). Pattern of blood flow in the pulmonary veins of the dog. *J. Appl. Physiol.* **20,** 1118–1128.

Morkin, E., Levine, O. R. and Fishman, A. P. (1965b). Pulmonary capillary flow pulse and the site of pulmonary vasoconstriction in the dog. *Circulation Res.* **15**, 146–160.

Patel, D. J., de Freitas, F. M. and Fry, D. L. (1963). Hydraulic input impedance to aorta and pulmonary artery in dogs. *J. Appl. Physiol.* **18**, 134–140.

Patel, D. J., de Freitas, F. M. and Mallos, A. J. (1962). Mechanical function of the main pulmonary artery. *J. Appl. Physiol.* **17**, 205–208.

Patel, D. J., Greenfield, J. C. and Fry, D. L. (1964). *In vivo* pressure-length-radius relationship of certain blood vessels in man and dog. *In* "Pulsatile Blood Flow" (E. O. Attinger, ed.), McGraw-Hill, New York.

Patel, D. J., Mason, D. T., Ross, J. and Braunwald, E. (1965). Harmonic analysis of pressure pulses obtained from the heart and great vessels of man. *Amer. Heart J.* **69**, 785–794.

Patel, D. J., Schilder, D. P. and Mallos, A. J. (1960). Mechanical properties and dimensions of the major pulmonary arteries. *J. Appl. Physiol.* **15**, 92–96.

Pattle, R. E. (1966). Surface tension and the lining of the lung alveoli. *In* "Advances in Respiratory Physiology" (C. G. Caro, ed.), Williams and Wilkins, Baltimore.

Permutt, S., Caldini, P., Maseri, A., Palmer, W. H., Sasamori, T. and Zierler, K. (1969). Recruitment versus distensibility in the pulmonary vascular bed. *In* "The Pulmonary Circulation and Interstitial Space" (A. P. Fishman and H. H. Hecht, eds.), University of Chicago Press, Chicago.

Permutt, S. and Riley, R. L. (1963). Hemodynamics of collapsible vessels with tone: the vascular waterfall. *J. Appl. Physiol.* **18**, 924–932.

Permutt, S., Bromberger-Barnea, B. and Bane, H. N. (1962). Alveolar pressure, pulmonary venous pressure and the vascular waterfall. *Med. Thoracalis* **19**, 239–260.

Pieper, H. P. (1963). Catheter-tip blood flowmeter for measurement of pulmonary arterial blood flow in closed-chest dogs. *Rev. Sci. Instrum.* **34**, 908–910.

Pinkerson, A. L. (1967). Pulse wave propagation through the vascular bed of dogs. *Amer. J. Physiol.* **213**, 450–454.

Pollack, G. H., Reddy, R. V. and Noordergraaf, A. (1968). Input impedance, wave travel, and reflections in the human pulmonary arterial tree: studies using an electrical analog. *I.E.E.E. Trans. Biomed. Eng.* **BME-15**, 151–164.

Rappaport, M. B., Bloch, E. H. and Irwin, J. W. (1959). A manometer for measuring dynamic pressures in the microvascular system. *J. Appl. Physiol.* **14**, 651–655.

Rigatto, M., Turino, G. M. and Fishman, A. P. (1961). Determination of the pulmonary capillary blood flow in man. *Circulation Res.* **9**, 945–962.

Rushmer, R. F. (1964). Origins of pulsatile flow: the ventricular impulse generators. *In* "Pulsatile Blood Flow" (E. O. Attinger, ed.), McGraw-Hill, New York.

Schultz, D. L., Tunstall-Pedoe, D. S., Lee, G. de J., Gunning, A. J. and Bellhouse, B. J. (1969). Velocity distribution and transition in the arterial system. *In* "Circulatory and Respiratory Mass Transport" (G. E. W. Wolstenholme and J. Knight, eds.), Little and Brown, Boston.

Shaw, D. B. (1963). Compliance and inertance in the pulmonary arterial system. *Clin. Sci.* **25**, 181–193.

Skalak, R., Wiener, F., Morkin, E. and Fishman, A. P. (1966). The energy distribution in the pulmonary circulation. II. Experiments. *Phys. Med. Biol.* **11**, 437–449.

Staub, N. C. (1961). Microcirculation of the lung utilizing very rapid freezing. *Angiology* **12,** 469–472.

Szidon, J. P., Ingram, R. H. and Fishman, A. P. (1968). Origin of the pulmonary venous flow pulse. *Amer. J. Physiol.* **214,** 10–14.

Taylor, M. G. (1966a). The input impedance of an assembly of randomly branching elastic tubes. *Biophys. J.* **6,** 29–51.

Taylor, M. G. (1966b). Wave transmission through an assembly of randomly branching elastic tubes. *Biophys. J.* **6,** 697–716.

Taylor, M. G. (1966c). Use of random excitation and spectral analysis in the study of frequency-dependent parameters of the cardiovascular system. *Circulation Res.* **18,** 585–595.

Wasserman, K., Butler, J. and van Kessel, A. (1966). Factors affecting the pulmonary capillary flow pulse in man. *J. Appl. Physiol.* **21,** 890–900.

Weibel, E. R. (1963). "Morphometry of the Human Lung." Springer-Verlag, Berlin.

West, J. B. (1969). Effects of interstitial pressure. *In* "The Pulmonary Circulation and Interstitial Space" (A. P. Fishman and H. H. Hecht, eds.), University of Chicago Press, Chicago.

West, J. B. and Dollery, C. T. (1965). Distribution of blood flow and the pressure-flow relations of the whole lung. *J. Appl. Physiol.* **20,** 175–183.

West, J. B., Dollery, C. T. and Naimark, A. (1964). Distribution of blood flow in isolated lung: relation to vascular and alveolar pressures. *J. Appl. Physiol.* **19,** 713–724.

Wiener, F., Morkin, E., Skalak, R. and Fishman, A. P. (1966). Wave propagation in the pulmonary circulation. *Circulation Res.* **19,** 834–850.

Wilcken, D. E. L., Charlier, A. A., Hoffman, J. I. E. and Guz, A. (1964). Effects of alterations in aortic impedance on the performance of the ventricles. *Circulation Res.* **14,** 283–293.

Yu, P. N. (1969). "Pulmonary Blood Volume in Health and Disease." Lea and Febiger, Philadelphia.

Chapter 19

Synthesis of a Complete Circulation

RICHARD SKALAK

Department of Civil Engineering and Engineering Mechanics,
Columbia University, New York, U.S.A.

1. INTRODUCTION

In many experiments of a hemodynamic nature involving a person, animal or isolated preparation, the system under test consists of an arterial portion, a microvascular bed and a venular portion. The term "complete circulation" in the present chapter is used to designate any system or preparation which contains some part of each category: arterial, capillary and venous networks connected in their usual and natural sequence. The synthesis to be elaborated will cover mathematical models which are feasible and useful to represent such systems depending on the purposes one has in mind. The models and formulae suggested are intended to be suitable for desk computation or programming on a high-speed digital computer. The discussion is directed toward mechanical aspects and wave propagation effects which are observable during a single heart cycle rather than longer term and neural control effects.

Four levels of modeling will be considered: (1) Pure resistance. This is the usual basis of analysis of perfusion experiments such as an isolated organ or single limb when no pulsation is involved. In such tests the effects of blood rheology and vessel distensibility may be explored. It has recently been demonstrated that, surprisingly, there may also be a significant influence of fluid inertia even in steady perfusion experiments. (2) Lumped models. These are "Windkessel" models consisting of networks of discrete resistance, compliance and inertial elements. These may be useful where neither data nor results need to be highly precise. The heart stroke volume can be estimated from the aortic pressure curve by use of such a model. (3) Distributed linear models. These are networks of distributed resistance, compliance and inertia. They are analogous to electrical transmission lines. An approximation to, and an understanding of, many wave propagation effects can be achieved by this kind of model which was first extensively treated by Womersley (1957) and McDonald (1960). (4) Non-linear distributed models. These models are necessary to take account of non-linear terms arising from the change of vessel cross-section with pressure and non-linear terms in the equations of motion of blood. It has been shown that these terms are not negligible and must be included to obtain accurate results. Their inclusion is essential for certain effects like the "pistol shot" sounds (Rockwell, 1969).

In addition to the above models, a general discussion of the energy flow and storage over the period of one heart beat is included. This is a viewpoint which can be utilized in any case and may be useful in evaluating the performance of an actual system or any of the models above.

Historically, conceptual models are usually introduced as a research tool and are as elaborate and precise as possible to facilitate understanding some particular phenomena or measurements. After the validity of a model has been established it may be useful in investigating related phenomena and/or be useful clinically. Commonly models start as research models and may later become utility models. Table 1 gives a brief list of the historical origins and current uses of the four categories of models mentioned above.

The details of each model in Table 1 and references to recent work employing each type will be given in subsequent sections. At this point some comment on the historical entries in Table 1 may be of interest.

An elegant and comprehensive history of the growth of ideas concerning the circulation of the blood is given in a volume edited by Fishman and Richards (1964). The idea that blood circulates in a closed circuit was established by Harvey (1628). Soon thereafter Malpighi (1661) reported the first direct observation of capillaries and Leeuwenhoek (1688) reported observing individual red cells moving single file in capillaries. The first blood pressure measurements were made by Hales (1733) who also gave the first description of the "Windkessel" action of the arteries in storing blood during systole and contracting to maintain flow in diastole.

The first mathematical model of the circulation of blood was developed by Euler in 1775 in a paper which has been largely overlooked and was only published posthumously in 1862. Euler set up the equations for a model consisting of elastic arteries and incompressible, inviscid fluid to represent blood (see Skalak, 1966). Except for the addition of viscous effects, Euler's

TABLE 1

Brief list of the historical origins and current uses of four levels of modeling

Concept	Introduction as a research model	Current utility
1. Pure resistance	Young (1809) Poiseuille (1840)	Slow variations of mean blood pressure. Elasticity of micro-circulation. Rheology of blood.
2. Lumped parameter model (Windkessel)	Otto Frank (1899)	Stroke volume from aortic pressure. Analog models. Analysis of cardiac assist devices.
3. Distributed, linear model (transmission line)	Womersley (1957) McDonald (1960)	Computation of flow from pressure gradient. Space and time distribution of pressure and flow. Input impedance studies.
4. Distributed, non-linear model	Euler (1755) Lambert (1958)	Accurate pressure and flow wave forms. Explanation of pistol shot sounds.

equations are those used in current non-linear models. However, Euler gave no solutions of his equations. They were not solved in the context of blood flow until Lambert (1958) treated them by the method of characteristics.

The first model of the circulation including a quantitative consideration of the pressure drop due to viscosity was discussed by Young (1809). His model started with an aortic segment 9 inches long and $\frac{3}{4}$ inches in diameter followed by 29 generations of bifurcating vessels down to arteriolar size. He estimated that blood must be about four times as viscous as water. His formula for pressure drop in small tubes was not accurate. This was established accurately by the later experiments of Poiseuille (1840).

Young (1809) also extensively discussed the wave propagation in the circulation of blood and derived the equivalent of what is usually known as the Moens–Korteweg formula for the speed of pulse wave propagation (Moens, 1878; Korteweg, 1878). The first comprehensive treatment of wave propagation in blood flow including viscous effects was developed by Womersley (1957) and McDonald (1960). Some of the solutions were derived earlier in other contexts (Witzig, 1914; Iberall, 1950).

The idea of Hales (1733) concerning the elastic action of the arteries was incorporated into a quantitative (Windkessel) theory by Frank (1899) which is the mechanical equivalent of an electrical capacitance and a resistance in parallel. Representation of the circulatory system by lumped parameter networks with more than two elements have been discussed also by Frank and others. Electrical analogs such as those built up by Noordergraaf et al. (1963) are physical analog models of lumped parameter representations of the system. As the number of elements used becomes large, a closer approximation to the behavior of a distributed system is achieved.

2. PURE RESISTANCE MODEL

For any vascular bed, the resistance R (dyn s cm^{-5}) to any steady flow is defined as the pressure drop ΔP (dyn cm^{-2}) divided by the flow Q (cm^3 s^{-1}).

$$R = \Delta P/Q = (P_A - P_V)/Q \qquad (2.1)$$

where the subscripts indicate arterial and venous pressures. This simple concept of resistance is probably the most useful single parameter in evaluating the performance of any vascular bed.

In equation (2.1) the flow Q is assumed to be the same at the arterial and venous ends which implies that there are no losses or inputs between these sections. This is usually the case in a steady perfusion of an intact vascular bed. In the case of pulsatile flow, the instantaneous venous and arterial flows may be different, but the average flow over a period of time will be closely the same (different only by the storage as discussed in Section 6). In this case each of the quantities in (2.1) may be replaced by their time averages to derive a mean resistance. This mean resistance may not be the same as that for a steady flow at the same mean pressures because of non-linearities in the system. This does not usually impede the usefulness of equation (2.1). The question of non-linear effects in pulsatile flows is discussed in Sections 5 and 6. In this section only steady flows will be discussed.

To synthesize a complete circulation one would ideally start with a network in which each vascular segment has a known length, diameter, wall thickness and elasticity. Next, from the known rheology of blood, the discharge through each segment would be established as a function of the inlet, outlet and transmural pressures. The individual segments would then be assembled into a network according to the actual geometry of the system and analyzed by network methods (Koenig and Blackwell, 1961). The key relations in this procedure are obtained by equating the pressures in the three segments joining at any junction and setting the sum of discharges into and out of the junction equal to zero. Solving the system of equations so derived would allow computation of the discharge for given arterial and venous pressures or vice versa so a prediction of resistance would be obtained. Such a model leads also to a prediction of pressures and flows throughout the system. Once such a model is verified by comparison with experiments it can be used to predict the changes of resistance due to altering conditions such as transmural pressure or neurogenic stimuli whose mechanical effects are known.

The ideal procedure suggested above has never been carried out to its full logical extent. In the first place, the geometry of any bed including each and every capillary segment is never known precisely. Difficulties of measurements are discussed by Bergel (Chapter 4). Secondly, even if the geometry were precisely known, the total number of segments would be so large as to make a full network treatment unwarranted if not impossible even using a large digital computer. Thirdly, the rheology of blood under the geometric conditions of a vascular network is not known well enough to make the model described fully reliable. The chief difficulty is that although the rheology of blood in Couette viscometers and in a single, long straight tube is fairly well defined (Charm and Kurland, Chapter 15), the effects of branching and the relatively short segments in most vascular beds are not yet well known. The division of flow at any branch makes it questionable as to what extent the Fåhraeus–Lindqvist (1931) effect is effective. There will always be some "entrance length" phenomena such as discussed by Lew and Fung (1970) and Schultz (Chapter 9). This has bearing on the inertial effects discussed below. Fourthly, the elasticity of walls is difficult to determine (see Chapter 12). Finally, in the capillary blood vessels, the pressure–flow relations are still under discussion (see Chapter 16).

For all these reasons it is generally not feasible to think in terms of a complete, realistic model, but some degree of approximation and restriction of the generality of the model must be adopted to make any progress at all. Two examples of approximate modeling in the literature are given by Burton (1965) and Cumming et al. (1969).

Burton (1965, p. 89) computes the pressure drop in a model of the mesenteric vascular bed of the dog assuming all vessels of a given diameter are identical and in parallel so no network computation is needed. Any vascular bed is not so perfectly regular. Cumming et al. (1969) have made measurements of the arterial portion of a cast of the vasculature of the human lung down to vessels of 800 μm. Below 800 μm three end branches were measured down to vessels of 20 μm. The branching was found to be monopoidal (unequal daughter branches) rather than dichotomous (equal daughter branches). Estimates of the pressure drop down the network were made by assuming (1) that the mean flow is 83 $cm^3 s^{-1}$, and (2) that the flow through each end branch is the same. This assumption again avoids making a full network computation.

The manner of presentation of the data of Cumming et al. (1969) suggests that the next step in modeling a vascular bed could logically be approached in two or more zones. The actual geometry, which is irregular, may be represented exactly down to vessels of a certain size, say 800 μm, on the arterial side. A standard microcirculatory unit from 800 μm arteries to 800 μm veins could be derived from sample measurements on the micro-circulation and finally, the actual irregular venous system above 800 μm vessels could be used. In the case of lungs, information on the geometry of the microcirculation is available (Weibel, 1963) and a theory of flow in the capillaries is also available (Lee and Fung, 1969), but these data have not been assembled in a single model.

The more usual use of the concept of resistance of a complete circulation is not to use a detailed model at all, but to regard the system as a whole as a single entity whose resistance is measured under a variety of controlled con-ditions. Variations in resistance with known changes in external conditions may then be interpreted as reflecting geometric, elastic or rheologic changes. Even this procedure must be used with caution. Experimental curves of flow Q through a vascular bed plotted against the pressure drop ΔP across the bed are generally found to be non-linear and concave toward the flow axis as shown in Fig. 1. There are a variety of possible reasons for the non-linearity of such curves including:

1. Changes in vessel diameters with changes in transmural pressures.
2. Changes in elasticity of the vessel walls due to neuro-humoral agents or neural stimuli.
3. Non-Newtonian behavior of the perfusate.
4. Fåhraeus–Lindqvist effect.
5. Non-linear effects of elastic deformation of erythrocytes in capillaries.
6. Redistribution of flow as the total flow changes.
7. Inertial losses which vary with the Reynolds number and hence are flow dependent.

The distensibility of the vascular bed, item (1) above, is the principal reason the curve shown in Fig. 1 is concave toward the flow axis. As the transmural pressure at any point increases, the diameter of the vessel increases and the flow increases approximately as the fourth power of the diameter in any case. In most test procedures, the action of neuro-humoral agents, item (2), is either the object of the test or is to be eliminated and guarded against. It is, of course, the usual mode of control in the intact animals. Item (3), the non-Newtonian behavior of the perfusing fluid, refers to bulk properties such as might be observed in a Couette viscometer (Chapter 15). Items (4) and (5) are aspects of non-Newtonian behavior which arise when a suspension of particles flows in a tube (Chapters 15, 16). Item (6) is a possible effect due to non-Newtonian behavior of the flow discussed by Benis and Lacoste (1968). Item (7) is an effect due to inertial terms at low but

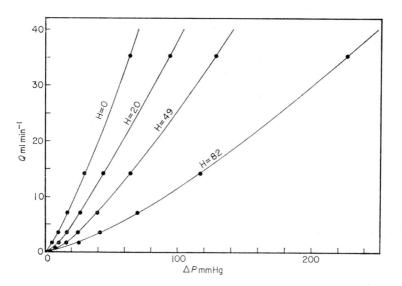

Fig. 1. Pressure–flow curves measured in the isolated hind paw of the dog. Venous pressure was held fixed at 14 mmHg. The abscissa is the pressure drop across the bed, $\Delta P = P_A - P_V$. The perfusing fluid was 5 per cent albumin–Ringer solution with washed red cells in suspension to give the hematocrits shown on each curve. (Data courtesy of Dr. S. Chien. See Benis *et al.* (1970) for methods.)

non-zero Reynolds numbers, which have recently been shown to be of some importance even in the steady perfusion of a vascular bed by Benis *et al.* (1970). The effects are similar to the increased pressure drop in laminar flows at Reynolds numbers of the order of unity which occur in curved tubes (White, 1929) and in tapered tubes (Tanner, 1966). The additional losses vary as the square of the velocity and the total pressure drop is then of the form

$$\Delta P = A\mu Q + BQ^2 \qquad (2.2)$$

where A and B are functions of the vascular geometry and hence vary with transmural pressures.

Benis *et al.* (1970) used the isolated hindpaw of the dog as a test system and held venous pressure constant so A and B in (2.2) depended only on the pressure drop. The coefficient B may be shown to depend on density of the perfusate in general but by using only fluids of equal density, this variation can be eliminated. The parameters A and B for a system may be determined as a function of the pressure drop by performing experiments with two different Newtonian fluids of viscosity μ_1 and μ_2. The term $A\mu Q$ in (2.2) is called the "viscous loss" ΔP_v and the term BQ^2 is called the "inertial loss" ΔP_{In} although both are ultimately dissipated into heat by viscosity. For each test fluid, the ratio r_i of the inertial to the viscous loss at a given pressure drop is

$$r_i = (\Delta P_{In}/\Delta P_v) = \frac{Q_i(\mu_1 Q_1 - \mu_2 Q_2)}{\mu_i(Q_2^2 - Q_1^2)} \qquad (2.3)$$

where $i = 1, 2$ designates the fluids and Q_1, Q_2 are the measured flows. It follows that at each ΔP:

$$A = \frac{\Delta P}{\mu_i Q_i(1+r_i)} \qquad B = \frac{r_i \Delta P}{Q_i^2(1+r_i)}. \qquad (2.4)$$

Benis *et al.* (1970) carried out experiments using a 5 per cent albumin–Ringer solution and a high-viscosity plasma expander as low and high viscosity Newtonian fluids.

After the determination of A and B, (2.2) may be used as an approximate formula when perfusing the same system with blood or a suspension of red cells. An apparent viscosity μ_a may be determined from experimental pressure–flow data by solving for μ_a from the formula

$$\Delta P = A\mu_a Q + BQ^2. \qquad (2.5)$$

The ratio of the observed resistance R_a with a red cell suspension to the resistance R_1 observed at the same pressure drop for a Newtonian fluid with viscosity μ_1 is

$$R_a/R_1 = (A\mu_a + BQ_a)/(A\mu_1 + BQ_1). \qquad (2.6)$$

It follows from (2.6) that ratio of resistances, R_a/R_1, will not in general be equal to the ratio of the viscosities, μ_a/μ_1. The ratio μ_a/μ_1 will be the correct relative viscosity under the conditions of test rather than R_a/R_1.

The relative apparent viscosity μ_a/μ_1 derived by using (2.5) cannot be compared directly to Couette viscometer data because the shear rate is not defined when only ΔP and Q are measured in a test on a vascular bed.

The formula (2.5) results in a pressure–flow curve which is concave to the flow axis as in Fig. 1 in spite of the term Q^2 because the coefficients A and B both decrease as ΔP increases. This is due to the over-riding influence of distensibility.

As the pressure drop approaches zero, the values of A and B appear to approach constants in the data of Benis *et al.* (1970). Then it follows that at sufficiently low values of Q, ΔP is very nearly equal to $A\mu_a Q$. This may seem contradictory to the analyses of Lighthill (1968) and Fitz-Gerald (Chapter 16) in which the pressure drop at low flow rates varies as $Q^{\frac{1}{2}}$ due to the elasticity of red cells in capillary segments. The two approaches may be resolved if μ_a is assumed to vary as $Q^{-\frac{1}{2}}$ at low values of Q as required by the Lighthill (1968) theory. It appears from the experimental observation of red cells by Hochmuth *et al.* (1970) that the $Q^{\frac{1}{2}}$ variation of ΔP should be expected only below some limiting capillary velocity. Above this velocity the red cells are not deformed any further. These effects are also apparent in sieving experiments in which suspensions of red cells are passed through micropore polycarbonate sieves (Gregersen et al., 1967). The $Q^{\frac{1}{2}}$ variation of ΔP produces a curve which is also concave to the flow axis and as yet the influences of red cell elasticity and of vessel distensibility have not been definitively separated.

3. Lumped Parameter Models

The notion of a lumped parameter model was first proposed as a quantitative theory by Frank (1899). The elastic behavior of the arteries is modeled by a single elastic chamber (Windkessel). The rest of the vascular system is represented by a resistance through which any efflux from the elastic chamber must pass. Frank's basic equation is

$$Q_i = \frac{1}{k}\frac{dP}{dt} + \frac{P}{R} \tag{3.1}$$

where Q_i is the inflow from the heart, k is the elastic modulus of the Windkessel, P is the pressure in the Windkessel and R is the exit resistance. As compared to a model consisting only of a resistance, the Windkessel model is an improvement in that it provides for different inflow and outflow curves and a time-dependent pressure. The principal fault of the Windkessel theory is that it assumes the entire arterial system is pressurized at once and thus neglects any possibility of describing a wave propagation. This is particularly in error during the early part of systolic ejection when the inflow, Q_i, rises rapidly from zero. Assuming $Q_i \gg P_D/R$, where P_D is the end diastolic pressure, (3.1) predicts that the rate of pressure rise is proportional to the inflow ($dP/dt \propto Q_i$). But from wave propagation theory and experimental results, the pressure itself is proportional to flow, i.e. $(P-P_D) \propto Q_i$, so that $dP/dt \propto dQ/dt$ as shown in Fig. 2 during the early part of systole.

During diastole, when $Q_i = 0$, and the entire arterial system is more nearly at uniform pressure at each instant, the exponential decay of pressure and flow predicted from (3.1) is closely realized by the vascular system (Aperia, 1940).

The Windkessel model becomes more accurate for the entire cardiac cycle when the pulse wave velocity in the arterial system is high, as under vasoconstrictor drugs which produce high resistance, high pressure and hence high wave velocity (Wetterer, 1954). Taylor (1964) in studying the work done by the heart, notes that the simple Windkessel model is applicable to the arterial system of birds and the branchial arterial system of fish (Mott, 1957).

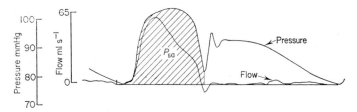

FIG. 2. Tracings of an experimental record taken in the aorta of the dog. The flow curve is scaled so that the peak flow is comparable to peak systolic pressure. Note that the flow and pressure are closely proportional during the early part of systole. The shaded area is the pulse area P_{sa}, used in the pressure–contour method, Eq. (3.2). (Based on Kouchoukos *et al.* (1970), Fig. 6.)

In these cases, as in Frank's original experiments on frogs, (see Cope, 1965, for a translation) the arterial system is relatively stiff and short.

Frank (1926) was well aware of wave propagation effects and suggested (Frank, 1930) that the effective extent of the arterial Windkessel could be taken to equal the wave velocity, c, times the time for systole, while the velocity of flow at the entrance to the aorta be taken proportional to the increment in pressure above end diastolic pressure. These ideas are incorporated in the pulse contour method developed by Hamilton and Remington (1947) based on the Windkessel concept. In a recent study on dogs, Kouchoukos *et al.* (1970) have re-examined the accuracy of stroke volume predicted by the pulse–contour equation given by Warner *et al.* (1953)

$$S_v = KP_{sa}(1 + T_S/I_D) \tag{3.2}$$

where S_v is the stroke volume, K is a constant representing system properties, P_{sa} is the area under the pressure curve measured in the ascending aorta during systole, the pressure at the end of diastole being taken as a base (Fig. 2). T_S and T_D are the lengths of systole and diastole. The term $(1 + T_S/T_D)$ was developed by Remington (1952) to account for the outflow from the arterial system during systole. This is not a rigorous result but is based on the approximation of uniform outflow from the arterial system throughout the cardiac cycle. The results computed using (3.2) and experimental pressure curves are compared to electromagnetic flow meter measurements taken simultaneously in anesthetized open-chested dogs by Kouchoukos *et al.* (1970). A high correlation is demonstrated in a large sampling of cases involving changes of heart rate as well as stroke volume. This is a good example of the utility of a simple model leading to a useful approximation. Kouchoukos *et al.* (1970) also discuss (3.2) from the standpoint of wave propagation.

A practical difficulty in the use of (3.2) is that the coefficient K must be first established for each animal by some other method of measuring stroke volume. Moreover, the constant K appears to vary under the administration of catecholamines and other sympathomimetic drugs.

The simple Windkessel model (3.1) can be represented by an electrical analog which consists of a resistance R and capacitance, $C = 1/k$ in parallel. More elaborate and realistic models using lumped parameters may be developed by adding additional resistive, capacitive and inductive elements. Inductive elements represent the inertia of the fluid. Models with one or two additional elements are discussed by Aperia (1940) and Gomez (1941). With the development of large analog and digital computers it is possible to construct electrical analogs of a vascular bed with a large number of elements (Noordergraaf et al., 1963; Beneken, Chapter 6) or to analyze the theoretical circuit by digital computation. Methods for the analysis of large networks are highly developed (Koenig and Blackwell, 1961) and generalized programs for their solution are often available in libraries of computer programs. As the number of elements becomes large, the approximation to a continuous wave propagation model becomes very close. An analog model of the human systemic arterial tree containing 121 segments has been studied in detail by Westerhof (1968). Even a moderate number of elements can yield realistic results. For example, Rideout and Katra (1969) show a good approximation to the entire pulmonary circulation by a network of twenty-two elements.

Another recent use of lumped parameter models is in the analysis of cardiac pumping assist devices, particularly for intra-arterial counter-pulsation methods (Jones et al., 1968; McMahon et al., 1971a, b). In this application the details of wave propagation are not so important as the gross volumetric and elastic parameters and their variation with time. Jones et al. (1968) find that a simple Windkessel model is adequate to analyze the relative merits and theoretical limits of various types of intra-aortic pumping systems. A more complete analysis of Windkessel theory with a comparison to a linear distributed model is given by Jones (1969). He shows that Windkessel theory is substantially correct except during the early part of systole when wave propagation effects are essential and he develops analytically a first-order correction to the Windkessel result. Extensive reviews and further developments of Windkessel theory are given by Cope (1965) and Wetterer and Kenner (1968).

4. DISTRIBUTED LINEAR MODELS

The greater part of the literature of wave propagation in blood flow deals with linearized distributed parameter models. There are two principal reasons for this. First, such theories contain a large variety of possibilities which can describe and interpret many features of the space and time distribution of pressure and flow wave forms found in actual blood circulations. Second, it is practical to carry out a detailed mathematical analysis for linearized theories far beyond the analysis possible in any non-linear theory. The linear analyses can often suggest the trend of effects to be expected due to changing assumptions such as of wall behavior, blood viscosity, taper and/or bifurcations.

A large number of different linearized models have been considered. Cox (1969) gives a review and comparison of twenty-one contributions by various authors. All of these have certain common features. The analyses are all carried out for a straight, infinite, circular tube filled with a homogenous, isotropic, Newtonian fluid. The fluid representing blood is usually assumed to be incompressible which is a justifiable assumption since the compressibility of blood is so small in comparison to the distensibility of blood vessels. The blood is also assumed to have a constant viscosity which is usually regarded as a reasonable assumption in large blood vessels because the shear rates are high and blood does behave nearly as a Newtonian fluid at high shear rates (see Chapter 15). Furthermore, the dissipation due to the blood viscosity is a minor effect in large blood vessels. In the propagation of pressure and flow pulses into the microcirculation it is probably not accurate to represent blood as a Newtonian fluid.

The most significant differences in the various linearized theories arise from differences in the assumed behavior of the vessel wall. The simplest assumption is that the vessel wall behaves as a series of independent rings so that the transmural pressure at any point is a function of the radial displacement at that point. More elaborate models run the full gamut from an elastic membrane to a thick-walled cylindrical shell treated as visco-elastic continuum (see Cox, 1969). It appears that for many purposes, if a linearized theory is adopted, the simple assumption of independent rings is adequate. There are a variety of other effects which are usually unknown or not evaluated which are more important and hence mitigate against use of more elaborate models. These include effects of non-linearities (discussed below), the complexity of the geometry of any real vascular bed which is important, but rarely known exactly, the lack of precise input data of pressure and/or flow and the lack of knowledge of the physical properties of the wall.

Linearized theories must make certain assumptions in order to linearize the equations of motion of the fluid and tube wall. These are largely justifiable as a first approximation, but are also the main reasons why linearized theory is not adequate for all purposes. First, the non-linear terms in the equations of motion of the fluid are neglected. The terms neglected are the so-called convective terms of the general form $u \cdot \nabla u$. One reason for expecting these to be small is that the mean flow velocity is usually less than 10 per cent of the wave velocity. Secondly, it is assumed that the deflection of the vessel wall is a small percentage of the radius of the vessel. In the systemic arterial system, the change in radius during any one cardiac cycle is usually less than 4 per cent, but the concomitant change in area may not be negligible. Linearization usually implies constant elastic properties of the vessel wall of any one cross-section. But the modulus of elasticity of both arterial and venous vessels varies quite strongly with pressure (Moritz, 1969). The automatic omission of this effect is one of the more serious failings of linearized theory

Both axisymmetric and non-axisymmetric modes of motion can be discussed within the framework of linearized theory. Non-axisymmetric modes are highly dispersive and carry a zero mean pressure over any cross-section so they are not of interest for most purposes (Maxwell and Anliker, 1967). Three types of axisymmetric motion occur which may be referred to as radial, axial and torsional according to the predominant component of the vessel wall displacement at high frequencies. In the axial and torsional modes, the primary motion is that of the tube wall itself with only small accompanying changes in fluid pressure (Moritz, 1969). These modes of motion may be present to some extent *in vivo*, but are of minor importance in the formation and propagation of flow and pressure pulses. The radial mode is responsible for the main wave propagation effects observed. It is also called the pressure mode or Young's mode. It was first discussed by Young (1809) in connection with blood flow. His discussion leads to the well-known formula for the wave velocity, c_0, for an inviscid fluid in an elastic tube:

$$c_0 = (hE/2a\rho)^{\frac{1}{2}} \qquad (4.1)$$

where h and E are the thickness and Young's modulus (named after the same Dr. Young) of the tube wall, a is the tube radius and ρ is the density of the fluid. The velocity c_0 is often referred to as the Moens-Korteweg velocity (Moens, 1878; Korteweg, 1878). The Young's modulus in (4.1) is the effective modulus of the vessel wall in a purely radial distension at an appropriate mean strain.

For the equations, derivations and more detailed discussion of the various modes of motion, the reader is referred to Maxwell and Anliker (1967). The discussion here will be limited to the application of the principal mode (Young's mode) to an entire circulation. The tube wall will be assumed to be linearly elastic and the governing equations reduced to the transmission line equations. This is the theory first used extensively in blood flow by Womersley (1957) and McDonald (1960). The discussions by Gessner (Chapter 10) and Milnor (Chapter 18) in terms of impedances in this volume apply directly also to the case assumed here.

The transmission line equations which result from linearized theory may be written in terms of the pressure, P and the flow, Q:

$$\frac{\partial P}{\partial z} = -RQ - L\frac{\partial Q}{\partial t} \tag{4.2}$$

$$\frac{\partial Q}{\partial z} = -GP - C\frac{\partial P}{\partial t} \tag{4.3}$$

where z is the distance measured axially along the blood vessel, t is the time, R (dyn s cm^{-5}) is the hydraulic resistance, L (dyn s^2 cm^{-5}) is the fluid inertia, analogous to electrical inductance, C (cm^4 dyn^{-1}) is the compliance, analogous to electrical capacitance, and G is the analog of electrical shunt conductance. The term GP may be interpreted in the hydraulic case as a seepage through the vessel walls proportional to the pressure. It is usually assumed to be zero. The pressure and flow are analogous to voltage and current in an electrical transmission line.

Any linearized theory of the Young's mode may be interpreted as giving a prediction of each of the coefficients R, L and C in (4.2) and (4.3). These coefficients will generally be frequency dependent and vary with the model, but the end results often do not depend strongly on the model assumed (Cox, 1969). Typical values are those given by Womersley (1957) and McDonald (1960) for the case of a tube tethered against axial displacement:

$$R = (\rho\omega \sin \theta)/(\pi a^2 M) \tag{4.4}$$

$$L = (\rho \cos \theta)/(\pi a^2 M) \tag{4.5}$$

$$C = 2\pi a^3/Eh \tag{4.6}$$

where M and θ are defined by

$$M\, e^{i\theta} = [1 - 2J_1(i^{\frac{3}{2}}\alpha)/i^{\frac{3}{2}}\alpha J_0(i^{\frac{3}{2}}\alpha)] \tag{4.7}$$

in which α is the dimensionless frequency, often referred to as Womersley's α:

$$\alpha = a(\rho\omega/\mu)^{\frac{1}{2}} \tag{4.8}$$

where ω is the angular frequency in radians/sec ($2\pi f$), f is the frequency in Hz and μ is the viscosity of the fluid. McDonald (1960) tabulates values of M and θ as functions of α. At low frequencies, $\alpha \to 0$, the value of R approaches the Poiseuille resistance, R_0

$$R_0 = 8\mu/\pi a^4. \tag{4.9}$$

In steady flow the term $L\partial Q/\partial t$ is zero and (4.2) becomes Poiseuille's law. The resistance R increases with frequency and may be several times the Poiseuille value, R_0, at high frequencies. The value of the inductance, L, shows less variation with frequency and is never more than $4L_0/3$ where L_0 is the limiting value at high frequency

$$L_0 = \rho/\pi a^2. \tag{4.10}$$

Equation (4.10) corresponds to a uniform distribution of velocity across any cross-section of the vessel.

To apply the results of any linearized theory to a complete vascular bed, each vascular segment between any two branch points is represented by a circular tube of uniform diameter. The appropriate solutions of (4.2) and (4.3) in any segment may be written in the form:

$$P = \text{Re}\{p\,e^{i\omega t}\} \tag{4.11}$$

$$Q = \text{Re}\{q\,e^{i\omega t}\} \tag{4.12}$$

where Re stands for "the real part of" and

$$p = A\,e^{-\gamma z} + B\,e^{\gamma z} \tag{4.13}$$

$$q = \frac{1}{Z_0}(A\,e^{-\gamma z} - B\,e^{\gamma z}) \tag{4.14}$$

in which γ is the complex propagation constant

$$\gamma = [i\omega C(R + i\omega L)]^{\frac{1}{2}} = \delta + i\beta. \tag{4.15}$$

The real part of γ is the attenuation per unit length, δ, and β is the wave number. The phase velocity, c, is

$$c = \omega/\beta \tag{4.16}$$

where ω is the frequency of the wave.

The characteristic impedance of the segment is Z_0

$$Z_0 = [(R + i\omega L)/i\omega C]^{\frac{1}{2}}. \tag{4.17}$$

The impedance Z at any point in the line is defined as the ratio of the complex pressure and flow amplitudes.

$$Z = p/q. \tag{4.18}$$

The constants A and B in (4.13) and (4.14) which determine p and q represent the amplitudes of the pressure waves traveling in the positive and negative z directions. They can be evaluated when any two of the three variables, p, q, Z, are known at one point of the segment. In dealing with a large network representing a vascular bed it is generally convenient to solve for the impedances throughout the network first after which the pressures and flows at all points can be determined from given boundary data of either pressure or flow. Details of impedance formulas are given by Gessner (Chapter 10). Computational procedures are also given by Wiener *et al.* (1966). A method of solution of arbitrary networks of transmission line elements is developed by Dicker (1965).

One of the convenient aspects of computations based on linearized theories is that the component of any wave of one frequency is independent of those at all other frequencies. The mean or steady component of pressure and flow (zero frequency) also adds linearly to those of the oscillating components.

The computation of the mean flow corresponds to assuming a Poiseuille flow in each segment of the vascular network. The use of a branched network of uniform segments allows a spatial variation of elastic constants from segment to segment and the properties may vary with frequency. But there is no way to make the properties dependent on the instantaneous pressure.

The advantage of linearity with respect to addition of various frequency components is offset by the necessity of resolving any input data such as pressure or flow curves into their discrete frequency components and then recombining the results for all frequencies. This is particularly awkward if a record of several cycles is to be analyzed in which there are cardiac cycles of varying length. In this case, a large number of frequencies (terms in the Fourier series expansion) must be retained to reproduce the entire record with reasonable accuracy.

At a bifurcation of a blood vessel, the boundary conditions usually applied in linearized theory are that the pressure in the three vessels at the junction be the same and the inflow equal the outflow at the junction. These assumptions are reasonable in that they must be satisfied exactly in any physical system across any section taken through the junction. But they are crude with respect to the details of flow at and near a bifurcation. It is not possible to have the detailed axisymmetric velocity distributions assumed in the theory at the junction of any three blood vessels. The readjustments which must take place will give rise to additional losses similar to those of an entrance region. Energy is not conserved by the usual assumptions (Martin, 1966). Fortunately, it appears that this is not a large error (Krovetz, 1965).

One way to circumvent the problem of branching is to replace the branching system by a single porous tapered tube (Skalak and Stathis, 1966). The porosity of the tube allows a discharge through the walls which simulates the flow taken off by side branches in the actual system. The efflux through the walls may be taken proportional to pressure which simulates resistive side branches by taking G in (4.3) different from zero. The efflux may also be taken proportional to discharge which simulates branches whose pressure–flow characteristics are similar to those of the main branch.

An artery is simulated by a taper of decreasing diameter in the direction of the mean flow and a venous system is simulated by an expanding section with seepage inward through the walls augmenting the main flow. The porous tapered tube model has been found useful in both linear and non-linear models (Skalak and Stathis, 1967; Rockwell, 1969; Hawley, 1970).

When linearized theories are used assuming a linear, elastic wall behavior and a Newtonian fluid, it is found that the attenuation of waves measured experimentally in large arteries is considerably greater than predicted theoretically (Jones *et al.*, 1968). The increased dissipation is attributed to viscous dissipation in the wall itself. This suggests that a more realistic linear theory could be derived by assuming the wall behaves as a series of separate but viscoelastic rather than elastic rings. With respect to the dissipation in the large arteries, the additional dissipation is a large effect, but with respect to the system as a whole, the energy dissipated in the large arteries is a relatively small amount.

Several linear theories incorporating viscoelasticity of the vessel walls have been explored for single infinite tubes (Cox, 1969), but it does not appear that these have been used to simulate a complete circulation. A difficulty which arises in applying any reasonably complete theory to an entire bed is that if any axial motion of the wall is included, some boundary conditions at each junction must be imposed and some assumption on axial elastic properties of each segment must be made. There does not appear to to be any attempt in the literature to carry out such a modeling of a vascular network. The system of axial waves which would be produced would have little effect on pressure and flow. Hence, linearized models of complete systems can reasonably utilize information from more complete theories only as far as the Young's mode (i.e. radial or pressure mode) is concerned. For such modes, if the results are put in the form of coefficients R, L, C or c, α, Z_0, the system of computation outlined above in (4.2)–(4.18) can be carried out for this model using the Young's mode results.

An example of modeling of a complete circulation is given by Weiner *et al.* (1966) in which the pulmonary circulation is modeled by four lobes, each containing 42 generations of branching vascular segments. Within each lobe, the branching is dichotomous, but each lobe has a somewhat different size and length, measured as a heart to capillary distance. It was found essential to have lobes of different lengths to reproduce the fairly flat input impedance curve of the pulmonary circulation (see Milnor, Chapter 18). The distribution of lengths of different parts of the system is also important in modeling the systemic circulation (Taylor, 1964; McDonald, 1968). Another important feature is the stiffening of the arterial walls with distance from the heart. Taylor (1969) has suggested that this is the kind of distribution favored in optimizing the system with respect to the work done by the heart. Measurements in both the pulmonary circulation (McDonald, 1968) and the systemic circulation (Moritz, 1969) infer this stiffening distally in dogs by the measured increase in wave speeds.

Some of the results of the model of the pulmonary circulation computed by Wiener *et al.* (1966) are shown in Fig. 3. The pressure curves at the right ventricle and left atrium were taken from simultaneous measurements in a dog. The remaining curves shown are computed from the model. The model reproduces, with good accuracy, the flow curves measured simultaneously in the main pulmonary artery and a pulmonary vein in the dog in which the pressure measurements were taken. The flow computed in the capillary bed also resembles closely curves of capillary flow measured by the nitrous oxide method (Linderholm *et al.*, 1962). Recently, erythrocyte flow velocities

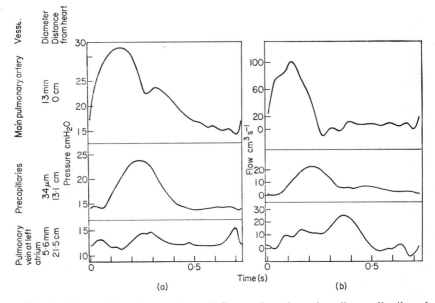

(a)   (b)

FIG. 3. Propagation of pressure and flow pulses through a linear distributed model of the pulmonary circulation of the dog. The top and bottom curves in panel (a) are measured curves of pressure at the arterial and venous ends of the system from which pressures and flows throughout the system were calculated. The diameters listed are the vessel diameters for which the curves shown were computed. Based on Wiener *et al.* (1966).

have been measured in the mesenteric microvessels of the cat down to vessel diameters of 12 μm (Gaehtgens *et al.*, 1970). Their results show flow pulsations exist in the microcirculation of the mesentery of a somewhat similar form to that shown in Fig. 3, but with a much larger mean flow component.

In any realistic model of either the pulmonary or systemic circulation the microcirculation will always be the site of the principal resistance to mean flow. Hence, it is often assumed, when modeling the arterial system only, that the microcirculation may be replaced by a single constant resistance. This may be quite satisfactory for a study of wave forms in the larger arteries, but cannot give accurate results for pressure and flow in the microcirculation itself. The model of the pulmonary circulation (Wiener *et al.*,

1966) and the measurements of Gaehtgens *et al.* (1970) mentioned above, show that the wave forms of pressure and flow continue to change throughout the microcirculation. The microcirculation is generally short compared to any wave propagation speed, but this does not mean that it may be accurately replaced by a pure resistance. It does mean that it can be accurately replaced by a lumped parameter system and since the inertia will generally be a relatively small term, only resistance and capacitance are effective. The presence of capacitance is essential if any differences in wave forms is to be reproduced within the microcirculation. The use of a reasonable distributed parameter model automatically includes such an effect.

A complete model also includes a description of pressure and flow in the venous portion of the system. Linearized theory is probably least accurate for any venous system because the non-linearities in the veins are more severe than in the arterial system (Yates, 1969). Nevertheless, an approximation to observed wave forms has been achieved in the case of the pulmonary circulation (Wiener *et al.*, 1966) using linear theory. In the systemic circulation no examples of a complete circulation model of the distributed linear type appear to have been published but it may be expected that linear theory will be at least accurate in the systemic venous system.

5. Non-linear Distributed Models

As methods of measurement and of analysis have improved, it has become more and more clear that although linear distributed models can give much insight into the mechanics of blood flow, accurate description of the progressive changes in wave forms observed in the major arteries and veins requires taking certain non-linear effects into account. Although no closed form analytic solutions for any non-linear case of a blood flow model have been derived, it is now entirely feasible to carry out extensive, accurate numerical computations by the use of high-speed digital computers. Such computations can readily include changes of wall properties with distance along a vessel, with pressure, and even with time. Besides the non-linear wall properties, the most important non-linear effects to be included are the convective acceleration and the change in area of the lumen of each vessel with pressure.

The various steps discussed herein, from a pure resistance, to a Windkessel model, to a linear distributed and finally to a non-linear model are about equal in their degree of improvement in the respective possibilities for accurate representation of a complete circulation, but each is useful for various purposes.

Equations describing a non-linear distributed model of blood flow were first written by Euler in a remarkable paper dated 1775. He even suggested a pressure radius relation which gives an increasing wave velocity with increasing pressure (see Skalak, 1966). However, he was not able to solve his equations at all, nor has anyone else since, but we have since learned to integrate numerically using the method of characteristics or finite differences. Euler's equations were derived independently by Lambert in 1958 who first suggested using the method of characteristics for non-linear blood flow computations.

The non-linear theories that have been developed for blood flow are all one-dimensional as far as the treatment of the blood itself is concerned. This means that the pressure and velocity of flow are considered to be functions of axial distance z along the vessel and of time, but no detailed description of the variation of pressure or velocity across a cross-section is attempted. In this sense the non-linear theories are cruder than linearized theories which can predict detailed velocity distributions which have been verified closely in properly conducted experiments. As will be explained below, it is possible to some extent to incorporate some of the coefficients derived from linear theory into non-linear equations.

The basic equations of the usual one-dimensional non-linear approach are (Rudinger, 1966; Skalak, 1966):

the equation of continuity

$$\frac{\partial A}{\partial t} + \frac{\partial(AV)}{\partial z} + \psi = 0 \qquad (5.1)$$

the equation of motion

$$\frac{\partial V}{\partial t} + V\frac{\partial V}{\partial z} = -\frac{1}{\rho}\frac{\partial P}{\partial z} + f \qquad (5.2)$$

and an equation describing the vessel wall behavior

$$A = A(P, z, t) \qquad (5.3)$$

where A is the cross-sectional area, assumed to be a known function of pressure, P, distance, z, along the tube and time, t, in (5.3). The term ψ in (5.1) represents the efflux through the walls per unit length. This is a convenient way to treat branches, as explained above for the linear model. The term f represents the net effect of shear stresses due to viscosity at the boundary of the vessel. Its dependence on the mean velocity, V, and other parameters of the problem must be supplied from some other theory or experiments. Some typical cases are discussed below.

The theory of characteristics of hyperbolic equations such as (5.1) and (5.2) shows that for certain paths in the (z, t) plane, the partial differential equations become ordinary differential equations. Using (5.3), the slopes of the characteristics of (5.1) and (5.2) are found to be

$$\frac{dz}{dt} = V \pm c \tag{5.4}$$

where c is the local value of wave velocity of the radial or Young's mode:

$$c = \left[A \Big/ \left(\rho \frac{\partial A}{\partial P} \right) \right]^{\frac{1}{2}}. \tag{5.5}$$

For a linearly elastic wall of effective Young's modulus E, (5.4) reduces to the Korteweg-Moens velocity (4.1).

In general (5.1) and (5.2) reduce along the characteristic directions to

$$\frac{dV}{dt} \pm \frac{1}{\rho c} \frac{dP}{dt} = f \mp \frac{Vc}{A} \left(\frac{\partial A}{\partial z} \right) \mp \frac{c}{A} \left(\frac{\partial A}{\partial t} \right) \mp \frac{\psi c}{A} \tag{5.6}$$

where the alternate signs apply to the positive and negative characteristics indicated in (5.4).

The velocity V in (5.1) and (5.2) is the average velocity (Q/A) where Q is the discharge or flow. The form of the convective acceleration term $[V(\partial V/\partial z)]$ in (5.2) implies that the velocity distribution is uniform over the cross-section which is in reality never realized. Various suggestions have been proposed based on linearized theories which predict a detailed velocity distribution.

The results of any linearized theory are most conveniently incorporated if basic equations are written in terms of the discharge, $Q = AV$, and the area, A, instead of in terms of A, V. The resulting equations are (Fox and Saibel, 1965; Stathis, 1967; Hawley, 1970):

the equation of continuity

$$\frac{\partial A}{\partial t} + \frac{\partial Q}{\partial z} + \psi = 0 \tag{5.7}$$

and the equation of motion

$$\frac{\partial Q}{\partial t} + \frac{\partial}{\partial z} \int_A v^2 \, dA = -\frac{A}{\rho} \frac{\partial P}{\partial z} + Af. \tag{5.8}$$

In (5.8) v is the velocity at any point of the cross-section A. If the velocity distribution is uniform, then $v = V$ and (5.6) and (5.7) can be reduced to (5.1) and (5.2). The term Af in (5.8) is related to the force exerted by the shear stress τ_0 at the vessel wall:

$$Af\rho = 2\pi a \tau_0 \tag{5.9}$$

where a is the radius of the vessel. Eq. (5.9) defines f in (5.2) also.

If a non-uniform velocity profile is used to approximate the integral in

(5.8), the integral at any instant can be written in the form

$$\int_A v^2 \, dA = \lambda \frac{Q^2}{A} \tag{5.10}$$

where λ is a coefficient which would be a function of both z and t to have an exact result in general. Hawley (1970) shows that for typical velocity profiles measured experimentally (Ruterbories, 1966) that the value for λ of 4/3 which holds for Poiseuille flow is a good approximation. This is also in agreement with the fact that in the Womersley theory the ratio (L/L_0) ranges from 1 to 4/3. A more detailed approximation based on Womersley's solution is given by Stathis (1967).

Some approximation of the frictional term Af in (5.9) is also required before computations can proceed. A reasonable approximation can be developed from the Womersley solution. The shear stress at the wall in that case can be expressed in the form (Lambossy, 1952, Stathis, 1967)

$$\tau_0 = \frac{\rho}{2\pi a} \left[-\tau_1 \omega Q + (1+\tau_2) \frac{\partial Q}{\partial t} \right] \tag{5.11}$$

where τ_1 and τ_2 are constants which are frequency dependent. They are given by

$$\tau_2 + i\tau_1 = J_0(i^{\frac{3}{2}}\alpha)/J_2(i^{\frac{3}{2}}\alpha) \tag{5.12}$$

where α is the Womersley α, Eq. (4.8), and J_0 and J_2 are Bessel functions. Since τ_0 is frequency dependent, a typical frequency, such as the first or second harmonic of the heart rate must be used in evaluating (5.11) and (5.12).

Another approximation used by Rockwell (1969) and Hawley (1970) is the Blasius formula which holds for turbulent flow at moderate Reynolds number. In this case

$$\tau_0 = \mp 0.0396 \frac{Q^2}{Re^{\frac{1}{4}} \rho A^2} \tag{5.13}$$

where Q is the instantaneous flow and the $-$ or $+$ sign is chosen for Q positive or negative respectively, and

$$Re = \frac{VD\rho}{\mu} = \text{Reynolds number} \tag{5.14}$$

in which D is the diameter of the tube.

In the large arteries, the influence of fluid friction is small and it does not greatly matter what frictional value is used although the laminar formula (5.11) appears to give the best results (Hawley, 1970). In the microcirculation, where Reynolds numbers become very small, the laminar flow approximation should be preferred. In this range, $(\alpha \to 0)$, Eq. (5.11) approaches the result of Poiseuille's law:

$$\tau_0 = -8\mu Q/DA. \tag{5.15}$$

In any case, whether (5.1) and (5.2) or (5.7) and (5.8) are utilized it is necessary to assume also a relation of the form of (5.3) giving the area as a function of location and pressure. This is an important assumption because it controls the small amplitude wave speed, c, defined by (5.5). If the wall is treated as a series of separate rings with a constant effective Young's modulus, it will be found that the wave speed c given by (5.5) decreases with pressure increasing. This is contrary to measurements made by Anliker *et al.* (1968) in the canine aorta. They find that the wave speed increases linearly with pressure. Rockwell (1969) has incorporated this experimental result directly by integrating (5.5) to find a relation of the form (5.3). Starting with the assumption of a wave speed linear in p and linear in z:

$$c = (c_1 + c_2 P)(1 + nz) \qquad (5.16)$$

where c_1, c_2 and n are constants, the end result is

$$A(P, z) = A_0(P_0) \exp\left(-\kappa z + \frac{P - P_0}{\rho c c_0}\right) \qquad (5.17)$$

where $A_0(P_0) \exp(-\kappa z)$ represents the area at the reference pressure P_0 as a function of z and κ is a constant which describes the tapering of the artery; c_0 is the value of c (5.16) at $P = P_0$.

Two other models of the vessel wall behavior are developed by Hawley (1970). One is a series of linearly visco-elastic rings and the other is a membrane under axial tension. In this last model, the axial displacement of the membrane wall is neglected. Since the one-dimensional non-linear theory simulates the Young's mode only, no theory of the wall behavior involving both radial and axial displacement of the wall can be incorporated in this type of theory. If axial displacements were included, axial modes could also be reproduced within the non-linear theory. There would then be four characteristic curves through each point instead of the usual two and the numerical procedures would be accordingly more complicated.

The seepage, ψ, through the vessel wall in (5.1) or (5.7) must also be related to P or Q at each point if seepage through the wall is used to simulate side branches. If the branching being simulated is a regular dichotomous branching, then it is appropriate to assume the seepage, ψ, is proportional to Q at any time and location (Stathis, 1967). Another alternative is to assume the efflux ψ is proportional to the pressure, P, at any point. This assumption has been used to model the canine aorta by Rockwell (1969) and Hawley (1970).

The assumption of seepage, ψ, proportional to the pressure is equivalent to assuming each side branch may be represented by a single, constant resistance. This is the most elementary model (Table 1) that seems at all reasonable. The representation of side branches can undergo the same evolution indicated in Table 1. The next level of complexity would be to replace the distributed seepage by discrete Windkessel models at the points at which the side branches leave as suggested by Jones (1969). This would be feasible computationally since a fixed space grid can be chosen so that the branch point is the boundary between two segments of the finite difference scheme. The information from the characteristics entering such a point would be coupled to the properties of the Windkessel representing the side branch.

It would also be possible to use a tapered porous tube analyzed by linearized theory to represent each side branch (Stathis, 1967). A more sophisticated model would be to treat all arteries and veins above a certain diameter as a distributed non-linear model and to interconnect arteries and veins by standardized "microvascular beds." Such beds would in turn be modeled by a network of distributed elements depending on the organ or tissue being represented.

No models of any complete circulation have been analyzed by non-linear methods as yet, but two similar treatments of the arterial system of the dog have demonstrated realistic results (Rockwell, 1969; Hawley, 1970). Each of these authors has represented the canine aorta plus some portion of the external iliac artery by a single porous tapered tube. All side branches are replaced by appropriate seepage through the tube walls. The seepage is adjusted in each case so that its distribution along the length of the aorta is similar to the known distribution of mean flow from the aorta and its continuation.

In the model of Rockwell (1969) the proximal input data was an inflow curve of the rate of cardiac ejection vs time for one cardiac cycle taken from experimental data. This was found to be more satisfactory than assuming the pressure to be given and computing the flow. This appears to be a general characteristic of any kind of model of a complete circulation, i.e. it is more difficult to arrive at a model which will yield realistic results for the flow using experimental pressure curves as input data than it is to obtain realistic pressure curves using experimental inflow curves as input data.

The results of Rockwell (1969) reproduce many features of the natural pulse such as the incisura, growth and decay of the pulse pressure with distance from the heart and the development of the dicrotic wave as shown in Fig. 4. There is also a steepening of the wave front with distance from the heart. This is a feature which appears to depend on the presence of the non-linear terms.

Rockwell's model also predicts the development of very steep fronted waves when cardiac ejection is assumed to be followed by marked regurgitation as in aortic insufficiency. The development of a very sharp and large rise in pressure is similar to the development of shock waves in air or other

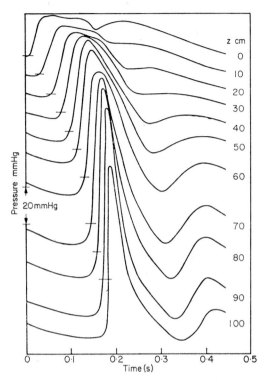

FIG. 4. Pressure curves computed in a non-linear distributed model of the canine aorta and its continuation. The distances shown are measured from the heart. All curves shown were computed from an assumed curve of inflow from the heart. The pressure corresponding to 80 mmHg is marked on each curve. From Rockwell (1969).

compressible media and is a logical explanation of the so-called pistol shot sounds heard in patients with incompetent aortic valves.

Another interesting result is that if the tapered tube model is continued to a point where the arterial diameter is less than 10 per cent of that at the entrance of the aorta, then a termination of a pure resistance appears to give realistic results for a variety of conditions such as changing heart rate and simulating exercise conditions. This judgment is made on the basis of the wave forms in the aorta and does not necessarily imply that the same conclusion holds if a complete system of wave forms in the microcirculation and the venous system are to be reproduced also. This remains to be explored.

In the model developed by Hawley (1970), using isolated linearly elastic rings to represent the arteries, the results show less steepening of the wave fronts distally than in Rockwell's (1969) model, particularly in the flow pulse. This is probably due to the fact that the elementary wave speed (5.5) does not increase with pressure for linear elasticity of the walls. The results computed by Hawley (1970) assuming a membrane under longitudinal tension to represent the arterial wall are more realistic.

The numerical method usually used in computing pressure and flow in non-linear models is the method of characteristics in which computations are generally advanced in time by using (5.6) along the two characteristics through a given point (Streeter *et al.*, 1963; Barnard *et al.*, 1966). This method works if the wall is non-linear, but elastic, because (5.1) and (5.2) then have two real characteristics. However, Hawley has pointed out that the method fails if not all the characteristics are real. Hawley shows this occurs if the wall is assumed to be visco-elastic. In this case, and in the usual elastic case, a finite difference scheme can be used instead. The details of the differencing scheme and numerical handling of boundary conditions are important to achieving accurate, stable results (see Hawley, 1970).

The one-dimensional non-linear models of the circulation are the best representation of the wave propagation in the vascular system that has been achieved to date. It is deficient, however, in that being one-dimensional, it cannot describe the stress state in the vessels' walls completely, particularly at bifurcations and bends. Likewise it cannot yield descriptions of the detailed fluid motions and pressure fields generated at bifurcations and bends. These local considerations of fluid flow and stress distributions may be of considerable importance to the development of atherosclerosis, aneurisms and stenosis. The present wave propagation theories can provide gross pressure and flow curves as inputs to models of such local situations which must then be analyzed by more detailed models if more detailed information is to be derived.

6. Energy and Power

An accounting of the forms and distribution of energy within any circulation is of interest because any energy dissipated from mechanical forms into heat must come from the work done by the heart. It also provides an alternate viewpoint from which to evaluate the performance of the cardiovascular system which may give a better insight than considering only pressure and flow waves. Questions of efficiency and optimization usually imply measures related to energy and power. Taylor (1964) has given a discussion of the systemic circulation from the stand-point of optimization both for Windkessel and distributed models.

The law of conservation of energy applies with equal stringency to any of the models discussed above (Sections 2–5) but the forms of energy recognized within each model vary, so the appropriate statement of conservation of energy varies also. In what follows, the most general statement of conservation of energy as it applies to the blood in any circulation will be given first and the appropriate reductions in special cases will be indicated subsequently. Only mechanical forms of energy and their dissipation into heat will be considered. This specifically omits energies associated with electrical, chemical and heat conduction effects.

Consider all the blood within any complete circulation as a certain multiply-connected volume, $\mathcal{R}$. An appropriate statement of the conservation of energy for any viscous, incompressible fluid is (Aris, 1962)

$$\frac{\partial}{\partial t} \int \int_{\mathcal{R}} \int (\tfrac{1}{2}\rho v^2 + \rho g h) \, \mathrm{d}v = - \int \int_{S} (\tfrac{1}{2}\rho v^2 + \rho g h) V_n \, \mathrm{d}s + W_s - \Phi \qquad (6.1)$$

where v is the vector velocity at any point of $\mathcal{R}$, g is the gravitational constant, h is the distance above a fixed horizontal datum plane, $\mathrm{d}v$ is a volume element of $\mathcal{R}$, S is the surface of $\mathcal{R}$, V_n is the velocity component normal to S taken positive outwards, $\mathrm{d}s$ is a surface element of S, W_s is the rate of work done on the boundary S by pressures and viscous stresses on S and Φ is the rate at which energy is dissipated into heat within $\mathcal{R}$ by the action of viscosity. This equation applies equally whether the flow is laminar or turbulent, steady or pulsatile, viscous or non-viscous, and whether the fluid is Newtonian or non-Newtonian. The left-hand side of (6.1) is the rate at which energy in $\mathcal{R}$ is increasing. The right-hand side is the influx of energy across S, plus the rate at which work is done on S, (W_s), minus the rate of dissipation, Φ.

Note that for an incompressible fluid the only forms of energy which are properly recognized as being contained in the fluid itself are the kinetic energy, $\tfrac{1}{2}\rho v^2$, per unit volume, and the potential (gravitational) energy, $\rho g h$, per unit volume. Pressure is not a form of energy of the fluid although it is often so regarded. To see that it is not, consider 1000 cm^3 of an incompressible fluid in a container of compliance $0\cdot1 \text{ cm}^3$ per 100 mmHg, which can easily be achieved by a thin metal bottle. Let the opening of the bottle be closed by a rigid piston which is then pushed in to raise the pressure from zero to 100 mmHg ($133\,000 \text{ dyn cm}^{-2}$). The work done by the piston is the average pressure times the volume displaced or 6650 dyn cm (ergs). This energy is stored in the walls of the bottle as strain (elastic) energy. None is stored in the fluid. If pressure were an energy per unit volume of the fluid, the pressurized fluid would contain 133×10^6 dyn cm. No such energy exists by the law of conservation of energy. If the piston is slowly released, there is a work of 6650 dyn cm done on it by the fluid, but this energy comes from the container walls, not the fluid. In this situation, as in blood flow, pressure is a means of transmitting energy but does not endow the fluid itself with energy by virtue of being pressurized. The work done by boundary pressures is contained in the term W_s in (6.1).

The appropriate reduction of the energy equation (6.1) for a complete circulation with one arterial inlet section (subscript A) and a venous outlet section (subscript V) is (Skalak *et al.*, 1966)

$$Q_A(P_A + \tfrac{1}{2}\rho V_A^2) - Q_V(P_V + \tfrac{1}{2}\rho V_V^2) = \frac{\partial}{\partial t} \int_\mathscr{R} \tfrac{1}{2}\rho v^2 \, dv + \int_{S_w} PV_n \, ds + \Phi \qquad (6.2)$$

where Q, P, V are the instantaneous flow, pressure and velocity averaged over the cross-section of a blood vessel, and S_w is the part of S which is the surface of the blood vessels' walls. The terms $Q_A P_A$, $Q_V P_V$ and $\int_{S_w} PV_n \, ds$ all derive from the term W_s in (6.1). The terms $(Q_A P_A - Q_V P_V)$ represent the net rate at which work is done by pressures at the inlet and outlet sections and are better called flow work rather than pressure energy. The term $\int_{S_w} PV_n \, ds$ is the rate at which the fluid does work on the vessel walls. If the walls are elastic, the net contribution of this term over a cycle is zero. It is the mechanism by which strain energy is developed in the walls and subsequently returned.

The rate of dissipation Φ may be expressed, in general, as a volume integral (Aris, 1962)

$$\Phi = \int \int_\mathscr{R} \int \tau_{ij} e_{ij} \, dv \qquad (6.3)$$

where τ_{ij} represents the viscous stress tensor and e_{ij} is the strain rate tensor. Usually there is no hope of evaluating Φ from (6.3) in any experimental blood flow, but it may be evaluated from (6.2) if all the other terms are approximated (see Skalak *et al.*, 1966). Figure 5 shows some numerical results computed in this way for the pulmonary circulation of the dog. Each of the terms in (6.2) and Fig. 5 has the units of dyn cm s^{-1} or ergs s^{-1}. These are units of work per unit time or power (10^4 ergs s$^{-1} = 1$ mW). In Fig. 5 and (6.2) the terms of the general equation (6.1) involving gravitational energy are omitted because the arterial and venous sections are assumed to be close to each other so that the net effect of gravity is negligible.

One item of interest that can be discussed more fully from the standpoint of energy is the concept of resistance and the losses associated with pulsatile as opposed to steady flow. Milnor (Chapter 18) discusses the relative size of various terms in the pulmonary circulation where pulsatility is more important from the standpoint of energetics than in the systemic circulation. The present discussion will be limited to theoretical aspects to form a bridge to the data and computations presented by Milnor in Chapter 18.

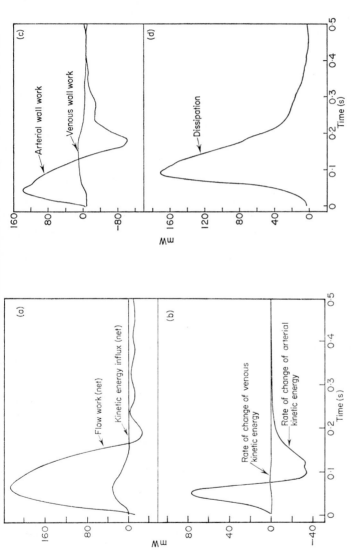

FIG. 5. The rates of input energy (power) and its distribution in the pulmonary circulation of the dog at rest. (a) Net rates of power input from flow work and kinetic energy influx. These net rates are arterial inputs minus venous efflux given by the left-hand side of Eq. (6.2). (b) The rate of change of kinetic energy within the system, given by the first term on the right in Eq. (6.2). (c) The rate of work done on the vessels' walls, given by the second term on the right of Eq. (6.2). This term represents strain energy of the arterial walls primarily. (d) The rate of dissipation of energy into heat by viscosity, given by the last term in Eq. (6.2). Note that the shape of the dissipation curve is similar to the contour of the flow pulse through the microvascular bed shown in Fig. 3. Based on Skalak et al. (1966).

In a single rigid tube in which there is a steady viscous flow, the rate of energy dissipation is

$$\Phi = Q^2 R_0 \mathscr{L} \tag{6.4}$$

where $\mathscr{L}$ is the length of the tube and R_0 is the Poiseuille resistance (4.9). By virtue of Poiseuille's law, (6.4) is also equal to

$$\Phi = \Delta P Q \tag{6.5}$$

where ΔP is the pressure across the tube. Now if the discharge varies slowly (so Poiseuille's law holds at any instant), the average rate of dissipation will be equal to

$$\bar{\Phi} = R_0 \mathscr{L} \frac{1}{T} \int_0^T Q^2 \, dt \tag{6.6}$$

where T is the time interval (cardiac cycle) under consideration. But the dissipation will not be equal to $\bar{\Delta P} \bar{Q}$ where $\bar{\Delta P}$ and $\bar{Q}$ are the mean pressure drop and mean flow rate. Moreover, if the system were such that the kinetic energy were less at the exit than at the entrance, the estimate $\bar{\Delta P} \bar{Q}$ would be further in error (Milnor, Chapter 18; Fishman, 1963). These discrepancies suggest an alternative definition of resistance, called the "effective resistance", may be useful in addition to the usual definition $R = (\bar{\Delta P}/\bar{Q})$, (Eq. (2.1). The effective resistance R_e is defined as that constant resistance which will result in the actual dissipation under a uniform flow equal to the mean flow:

$$R_e = \bar{\Phi}/(\bar{Q})^2. \tag{6.7}$$

It will be found that in a typical complete circulation R_e is greater than R, (Skalak et al., 1966). The use of R_e is not recommended for routine use because it entails much more data and computations to estimate than the usual resistance R. Moreover, changes in R are generally indicative of changes in R_e. But R_e may be useful if questions of the effect of pulsatility and kinetic energy are raised because these are taken into account in computing R_e.

A related issue is the use of a uniform velocity distribution across the inlet and outlet cross-sections assumed in deriving (6.2) from (6.1). The terms involving V^2 on the left-hand side of (6.2) should be multiplied by a factor σ given by

$$\sigma = \frac{1}{AV^3} \int_A v^3 \, ds \tag{6.8}$$

where A is the cross-section of the blood vessel and V is the mean velocity. The value of σ could be several times unity, but for arterial inflow where the velocity profile is fairly flat (Schultz, Chapter 9), σ may be only a little greater than unity.

In the simple Windkessel theory, Eq. (3.1), an energy equation can be formed by multiplying (3.1) by P and rewriting the resultant equation in the form

$$P_A Q_A = P_A \frac{d\mathscr{R}}{dt} + \Phi \tag{6.9}$$

where the P and Q_i of (3.1) are replaced by P_A and Q_A in the present terminology. The term

$$\frac{d\mathscr{R}}{dt} = \frac{1}{k}\frac{dP}{dt}$$

is the rate of change of the volume of the Windkessel and is an approximation of the term $\int_{S_w} PV_n \, ds$ of (6.2). The dissipation Φ in (6.9) is the approximation

$$\Phi = RQ_V^2 \tag{6.10}$$

where $Q_V = P_A/R$ is the venous flow which is also the flow through the resistive component of the Windkessel model. Comparing (6.9) to (6.2) shows that the Windkessel model neglects all kinetic energy terms and assumes venous pressure to be zero. Any attempt to use an improved energy equation in connection with a Windkessel model will lead to some inconsistency since (6.9) follows from (3.1).

The situation is similar for the linearized model described by (4.2) and (4.3). Multiplying (4.2) by Q, (4.3) by P, and adding one arrives, after some manipulation and integration over the length of the line, $\mathscr{L}$, at the equation:

$$Q_A P_A - Q_V P_V = \frac{\partial}{\partial t} \int_{\mathscr{L}} \tfrac{1}{2}\rho V^2 A \, dz + \int_{\mathscr{L}} P \frac{\partial A}{\partial t} \, dz + \Phi. \tag{6.11}$$

In the derivation of (6.11) the seepage GP in (4.3) was set equal to zero and R, L, and C were assumed to be constant within each segment of the vascular network. The values Q_A, P_A, Q_V, P_V enter (6.11) through limits of the integration over z. The term containing $\tfrac{1}{2}\rho V^2$ is derived using (4.10) for L in (4.2). The term $P(\partial A/\partial t)$ is derived from $PC(\partial P/\partial t)$ by using (4.3) and the equation of continuity (5.7) with $\psi = 0$. In the present case, the dissipation Φ is given by

$$\Phi = \int_{\mathscr{L}} RQ^2 \, dz. \tag{6.12}$$

Comparing (6.11) with (6.2) shows that the linearized distributed parameter model contains all the appropriate terms of the general energy equation with the exception of the influx of kinetic energy terms on the left-hand side of (6.2). Any attempt to add on such terms after using a linearized model must lead to an inconsistency if the several terms of the energy equation are computed separately because (6.11) follows from (4.2) and (4.3).

A similar manipulation can be carried out for the non-linear distributed model equations starting with (5.7) and (5.8) with seepage ψ set equal to zero. Multiplying (5.8) by ρQ and integrating over the length, $\mathscr{L}$, of the system, yields after some manipulation

$$Q_A(P_A + \tfrac{1}{2}\rho V_A^2) - Q_V(P_V + \tfrac{1}{2}\rho V_V^2) = \frac{\partial}{\partial t} \int_{\mathscr{L}} \tfrac{1}{2}\rho V^2 A\, dz + \int_{\mathscr{L}} P \frac{\partial A}{\partial t} + \Phi. \quad (6.13)$$

In (6.13) the dissipation takes on the form

$$\Phi = \int_{\mathscr{L}} \rho Q f\, dz = \int_{\mathscr{L}} V(2\pi a\tau_0)\, dz \quad (6.14)$$

in which $(2\pi a\tau_0)$ may be identified as the force per unit length due to viscous stresses. In deriving (6.13), the factor λ in (5.10) was taken equal to unity for simplicity. In both (6.13) and (6.11) the term $(\partial A/\partial t)dz$ plays the role of $V_n ds$ in (6.2). Comparing (6.13) with (6.2), it may be seen that there is a complete accounting for all terms of the general energy equation (6.2) by the non-linear result (6.13). Hence only the distributed parameter non-linear theory accounts properly for all forms of mechanical energy.

The omission of the influx of kinetic energy terms in the distributed linearized theory is not a serious discrepancy in the systemic circulation because the kinetic energy is at most about 3 per cent of the energy supplied. The great bulk of the input energy is flow work. In the pulmonary circulation the kinetic energy is a somewhat greater percentage (Milnor, Chapter 18). Nevertheless, the discussion of energetics in terms of linearized theory impedance curves leads to the significant conclusion that increasing heart rate is a more efficient means of increasing cardiac output than increasing stroke volume (Milnor, Chapter 18). Similar conclusions may be drawn from the study of energetics and design of the cardiovascular system by Taylor (1964) using only a simple Windkessel theory. These studies show that even relatively crude models can be adequate to discover trends and to lead to useful results.

REFERENCES

Anliker, M., Histand, M. B. and Ogden, E. (1968). Dispersion and attenuation of small artificial pressure waves in canine aorta. *Circulation Res.* **23**, 539–551.

Aperia, A. (1940). Hemodynamical studies. *Skand. Arch. Physiol.* **83**, Suppl. 16.

Aris, R. (1962). "Vectors, Tensors, and the Basic Equations of Fluid Mechanics." Prentice-Hall, Englewood Cliffs.

Barnard, A. C. L., Hunt, W. A., Timlake, W. P. and Varley, E. (1966). A theory of fluid flow in compliant tubes. *Biophys. J.* **6**, 717–746.

Benis, A. M. and Lacoste, J. (1968). Study of erythrocyte aggregation by blood viscometry at low shear rates using a balance method. *Circulation Res.* **22**, 29–41.

Benis, A. M., Usami, S. and Chien, S. (1970). Effect of hematocrit and inertial losses on pressure-flow relations in the isolated hind paw of the dog. *Circulation Res.* **27**, 1047–1068.

Burton, A. C. (1965). "Physiology and Biophysics of the Circulation." Year Book Medical Publishers, Chicago.

Cope, F. W. (1965). Elastic reservoir theories of the human circulation with applications to clinical medicine and to computer analysis of the circulation. *Adv. Biol. Med. Phys.* **10**, 277–356.

Cox, R. H. (1969). Comparison of linearized wave propagation models for arterial blood flow analysis. *J. Biomechanics* **2**, 251–265.

Cumming, G., Henderson, R., Horsfield, K. and Singhal, S. S. (1969). The functional morphology of the pulmonary circulation. *In* "The Pulmonary Circulation and Insterstitial Space" (A. P. Fishman and H. H. Hecht, eds.), University of Chicago Press, Chicago.

Dicker, D. (1965). Analysis of distributed parameter networks—a general method. *Proceedings 3rd Annual Allerton Conference on Circuit and System Theory*, University of Illinois, Urbana.

Euler, L. (1862). Principia pro motu sanguinis per arterias determinado. *Opera posthuma mathematica et physica anno 1844 detecta*, ediderunt P. H. Fuss et N. Fuss. Petropoli: Apud Eggers et socios, **2**, 814–823.

Fishman, A. P. (1963). Dynamics of the pulmonary circulation. *In* "Handbook of Physiology", Section 2, Volume 2, (W. H. Hamilton and P. Dow, eds.), pp. 1667–1743, American Physiological Society, Washington, D.C.

Fishman, A. P. and Richards, D. W. (1964). "Circulation of the Blood: Men and Ideas." Oxford University Press, London.

Fox, E. A. and Saibel, E. (1965). A formulation of the problem of flow through tubes. *Proceedings 4th International Congress on Rheology*, Volume 4, pp. 125–133, Wiley, New York.

Frank, O. (1899). Die Grundform des arteriellen Pulses. *Z. Biol.* **37**, 483–526.

Frank, O. (1926). Die Theorie der Pulswellen. *Z. Biol.* **85**, 91–130.

Frank, O. (1930). Schatzung des Schlagvolumens des menschlichen Herzens auf Grund der Wellen- und Windkesseltheorie. *Z. Biol.* **90**, 405–409.

Gaehtgens, P., Meiselman, H. J. and Wayland, H. (1970). Erythrocyte flow velocities in mesenteric microvessels of the cat. *Microvasc. Res.* **2**, 151–162.

Gomez, D. M. (1941). "Hemodynamique et Angiocinetique Etude Rationnelle des Lois Regissant les Phenomenes Cardio-vascularies." Hermann, Paris.

Gregersen, M. I., Bryant, C. A., Hammerle, W. E., Usami, S. and Chien, S. (1967). Flow characteristics of human erythrocytes through polycarbonate sieves. *Science, N.Y.* **157**, 825–827.

Hales, S. (1733). "Statical essays. Haemastaticks II." Innays and Manby, London. Reprinted 1964 by Hafner Publishing Co., New York.

Hamilton, W. F. and Remington, J. W. (1947). The measurement of the stroke volume from the pressure pulse. *Amer. J. Physiol.* **148**, 14–24.

Harvey, W. (1628). "Exercitatio Anatomica de Motu Cordis et Sanguinis in Animalibus." An English translation with annotations by C. D. Leake, 4th Ed. (1958). Thomas, Springfield.

Hawley, J. K. (1970). Studies of mathematical models of aortic blood flow. Ph.D. Dissertation: Rensselaer Polytechnic Institute, Troy, New York.

Hochmuth, R. M., Marple, R. N. and Sutera, S. P. (1970). Capillary blood flow. I. Erythrocyte deformation in glass capillaries. *Microvasc. Res.* **2**, 409–419.

374   R. SKALAK

Iberall, A. S. (1950). Attenuation of oscillatory pressures in instrument lines. *J. Res. Nat. Bur. Standards* **45**, 85–108.

Jones, E., Chang, I. D. and Anliker, M. (1968). Effects of viscosity and external constraints on wave transmission in blood vessels. SUDAAR No. 334, Stanford University, Stanford, California.

Jones, R. T., Petschek, H. E. and Kantrowitz, A. R. (1968). Elementary theory of synchronous arterio-arterial blood pumps. *Med. Biol. Eng.* **6**, 303–312.

Jones, R. T. (1969). Blood flow. *Annu. Rev. Fluid Mech.* **1**, 223–244.

Koenig, H. E. and Blackwell, W. A. (1961). "Electromechanical System Theory". McGraw-Hill, New York.

Korteweg, D. J. (1878). Über die Fortpflanzungesgeschwindigkeit des Schalles in elastischen Röhren. *Ann. Phys. und Chem. Ser.* 3 **5**, 525–542.

Kouchoukos, N. T., Sheppard, L. C. and McDonald, D. A. (1970). Estimation of stroke volume in the dog by a pulse contour method. *Circulation Res.* **26**, 611–623.

Krovetz, L. J. (1965). The effect of vessel branching on haemodynamic stability. *Phys. Med. Biol.* **10**, 417–427.

Lambert, J. W. (1958). On the non-linearities of fluid flow in non-rigid tubes. *J. Franklin Inst.* **266**, 83–102.

Lambossy, P. (1952). Oscillations forcées d'un liquid incompressible et visqueux dans un tube rigid et horizontal. Calcul de la force de frottement. *Helv. Phys. Acta* **25**, 371–386.

Lee, J. S. and Fung, Y. C. (1969). Stokes flow around a circular cylindrical post confined between two parallel plates. *J. Fluid Mech.* **37**, 657–670.

Leeuwenhoek, A. V. (1688). On the circulation of the blood. Latin texts of his 65th letter to the Royal Society. Facsimile with introduction by A. Schierbeek, N. B. deGraaf, 1962.

Lew, H. S. and Fung, Y. C. (1970). Entry flow into blood vessels at arbitrary Reynolds number. *J. Biomechanics* **3**, 23–38.

Lighthill, M. J. (1968). Pressure-forcing of tightly fitting pellets along fluid-filled elastic tubes. *J. Fluid Mech.* **34**, 113–143.

Linderholm, H., Kimbel, P., Lewis, D. and DuBois, A. B. (1962). Pulmonary capillary blood flow during cardiac catheterization. *J. Appl. Physiol.* **17**, 135–141.

McDonald, D. A. (1960). "Blood Flow in Arteries." Williams and Wilkins, Baltimore.

McDonald, D. A. (1968). Hemodynamics. *Annu. Rev. Physiol.* **30**, 525–556.

McMahon, T. A., Clark, C., Murthy, V. S. and Shapiro, A. H. (1971a). Intra-aortic balloon experiment in a lumped element hydraulic model of the circulation. *J. Biomechanics*, **4**, 335–350.

McMahon, T. A., Jaffrin, M. Y., Murthy, V. S. and Shapiro, A. H. (1971b). Intra-aortic balloon for left heart assistance: an analytic model. *J. Biomechanics*, **4**, 351–367.

Malpighi, M. (1661). De pulmonibus. *In* "Observationes Anatomicae", Bologna.

Martin, J. D. (1966). An extension to the theory of wave reflections. *In* "Biomedical Fluid Mechanics Symposium", pp. 70–77, A.S.M.E., New York.

Maxwell, J. A. and Anliker, M. (1967). Dispersion and dissipation of waves in blood vessels. SUDAAR No. 312, Stanford University, Stanford, California.

Moens, A. I. (1878). "Die Pulskurve." Brill, Leiden.

Moritz, W. E. (1969). Transmission characteristics of distension, torsion and axial waves in arteries. SUDAAR No. 373, Stanford University, Stanford, California.

Mott, J. C. (1957). The cardiovascular system. *In* "The Physiology of Fishes", (M. E. Brown ed.), Vol. 2, Academic Press, New York and London.

Noordergraaf, A., Jager, G. N. and Westerhof, N. (1963). "Circulatory Analog Computers." North-Holland, Amsterdam.

Poiseuille, J. L. M. (1840). Recherches expérimentales sur le mouvement des liquides dans les tubes de très petits diamètres. *C.R. Acad. Sci., Paris* **11**, 961–967; **11**, 1041–1048; **12**, 112–115 (1841); **15**, 1167–1186 (1842).

Remington, J. W. (1952). Volume quantitation of the aortic pressure pulse. *Fed. Proc.* **11**, 750–761.

Rideout, V. C. and Katra, J. A. (1969). Computer simulation study of the pulmonary circulation. *Simulation* **12**, 239–245.

Rockwell, R. L. (1969). Non-linear analysis of pressure and shock waves in blood vessels. Ph.D. Dissertation: Stanford University, Stanford, California.

Rudinger, G. (1966). Review of current mathematical methods for the analysis of blood flow. *In* "Biomedical Fluid Mechanics Symposium". A.S.M.E., New York.

Ruterbories, B. H. (1966). Velocity and pressure measurements of pulsating flow in a flexible tube. Ph.D. Thesis: Case Institute of Technology, Cleveland, Ohio.

Skalak, R. (1966). Wave propagation in blood flow. *In* "Biomechanics" (Y. C. Fung, ed.), pp. 20–46, A.S.M.E., New York.

Skalak, R., Wiener, F., Morkin, E. and Fishman, A. P. (1966). The energy distribution in the pulmonary circulation. I. Theory. *Phys. Med. Biol.* **11**, 287–294. II. Experiments. *Phys. Med. Biol.* **11**, 437–449.

Skalak, R. and Stathis, T. C. (1966). A porous tapered elastic tube model of a vascular bed. *In* "Biomechanics" (Y. C. Fung, ed.), pp. 68–81, A.S.M.E., New York.

Skalak, R. and Stathis, T. C. (1967). A comparison of linear and non-linear theories of blood flow. *In* "Digest of the 7th International Conference on Medical and Biological Engineering", p. 56, Stockholm, Sweden.

Stathis, T. C. (1967). Pulsatile flow in a tapered porous, elastic tube. Doctoral Dissertation: Columbia University, New York.

Streeter, V. L., Keitzer, W. F. and Bohr, D. F. (1963). Pulsatile pressure and flow through distensible vessels. *Circulation Res.* **13**, 3–20.

Tanner, R. I. (1966). Pressure losses in viscometric capillary tubes of slowly varying diameter. *Brit. J. Appl. Phys.* **17**, 663–669.

Taylor, M. G. (1964). Wave travel in arteries and the design of the cardiovascular system. *In* "Pulsatile Blood Flow" (E. O. Attinger, ed.), pp. 343–372, McGraw-Hill, New York.

Taylor, M. G. (1969). Arterial impedance and distensibility. *In* "The Pulmonary Circulation and Interstitial Space" (A. P. Fishman and H. H. Hecht, eds.), pp. 343–354, University of Chicago Press, Chicago.

Warner, H. R., Swan, H. J. C., Connolly, D. C., Tompkins, R. G. and Wood, E. H. (1953). Quantitation of beat-to-beat changes in stroke volume from aortic pulse contour in man. *J. Appl. Physiol.* **5**, 495–507.

Weibel, E. R. (1963). "Morphometry of the Human Lung." Academic Press, New York and London.

Westerhof, N. (1968). Wave reflection in the human systemic arterial tree. Ph.D. Thesis: University of Pennsylvania, Philadelphia, Pa.

Wetterer, E. (1954). Flow and pressure in the arterial system, their hemodynamic relationship, and the principles of their measurement. *Minn. Med.* **37**, 77–86.

16*

R. SKALAK

Wetterer, E. and Kenner, Th. (1968). "Grundlagen der Dynamik des Arterien-pulses." Springer-Verlag, Berlin.

White, C. M. (1929). Streamline flow through curved pipes. *Proc. Roy. Soc.* A, **123**, 645–663.

Wiener, F., Morkin, E., Skalak, R. and Fishman, A. P. (1966). Wave propagation in pulmonary circulation. *Circulation Res.* **19**, 834–850.

Witzig, K. (1914). Uber erzwungene Wellenbewegungen zäher, inkompressibler Flussigkeitan in elastischen Röhren. Inaugural Dissertation: Universitat Bern. Wyss Erben, Bern.

Womersley, J. R. (1957). An elastic tube theory of pulse transmission and oscillatory flow in mammalian arteries. Wright Air Development Center, WADC Rpt. TR 56–614.

Womersley, J. R. (1958). Oscillatory flow in arteries. The constrained elastic tube as a model of arterial flow in pulse transmission. *Phys. Med. Biol.* **2**, 178–187.

Yates, W. G. (1969). Experimental studies of the variations in the mechanical properties of the canine abdominal vena cava. Ph.D. Dissertation: Stanford University, Stanford, California.

Young, T. (1809). On the functions of the heart and arteries. *Philos. Trans.* **99**, 1–31.

Author Index (Volume 2)

Numbers in *italics* refer to pages where references are listed at the end of chapters.

Subject Index, Vols. 1 and 2

G *refers to the Glossary and those page numbers in bold refer to Vol. 2*

A

Acceleration, convective, **359, 361**
  of blood flow, 262, 265, 268, 273
Action potential, 229
Active state (see Myocardium)
Active tension, 80, **88**
Adventitia, G (see Histology of Blood Vessels)
Afterload (see Myocardium)
Age changes in arteries (see Elasticity)
Aliasing error, 333
Alveolar pressure, **225, 323, 326**
Amplitude distortion (see Frequency response)
Anaesthetics, transport by blood stream, 208
Analogue computer (see Computers)
Aneurysm, G., **112, 126, 141, 154, 366**
Angiogram, G (see X-rays)
Angiometer (see Transducers)
Anisotropy (see Elasticity)
Anticoagulants and blood rheology (see Rheology)
Aorta
  elasticity (see Elasticity)
  flow in, 52, 59, 268, 289, 294, 297, 308, **309, 311, 327, 350**
  pressure in, 4, 227, **350, 365**
  (see Heart in Glossary)
Aortic stenosis, 269, 307, **112, 130**
Aortic valve (see Valves)
Aortic wall
  histology, **13, 68, 126**
  smooth muscle, **87**
Artery, G (see individual vessels, and below)
Arterial stenosis, **111**
Arterial wall
  age changes in elasticity (see Elasticity)
  histology, **42, 68, 71, 126, 244**
  thickness, 55, **5, 68**

Arteries
  conduit, **97, 100**
  elastic, 2, **68**
  muscular, 2, **68**
  (see Femoral, Carotid, Renal arteries)
Arteriole, G, 4, **68, 82, 94, 188, 190, 319**
  flow velocity in, **189**
Arteriosclerosis, Atherosclerosis, G, **126, 142, 152, 366**
Atrium, 282, **328**
Attenuation, G, 132, 321 (see Frequency response)
  of waves in vessels, **226, 318, 355**
Autocorrelation, 333
Autonomic nervous system, **93, 321**
Autoregulation, 143, 164, 189, **95, 322**
Axial stream (see Marginal layer)
Axial train, **208, 227**

B

Bandwidth (see Frequency response)
Baroreceptor, G, **189**
Baroreceptor reflexes, 121, 142, 144, 149, 152, 343, **97, 322**
Basement membrane (see Capillaries)
Bifurcations in blood vessels, 325, **141, 145, 153, 186, 301, 317, 356, 366**
Blasius formula, **362**
Blood, G, **158, 212, 346, 349**
Blood cells, G, 4 (see Rheology)
Blood volume, 4, 122, 126, 150, **188**
Bode plot, G, 147, 153, 161
Bolus flow, **209, 216, 218, 227, 230**
Boundary conditions, **298**
Boundary layer, G, **142, 146**
Branching coefficient, **326, 301**
Bronchial arteries, **302**
Bulk modulus (see Elasticity)

C

Calcium, 229

389